MRCS Core Modules:

The Complete Test

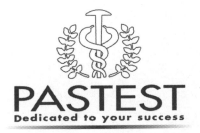

PASTEST

Dedicated to your success

MRCS Core Modules:

The Complete Test

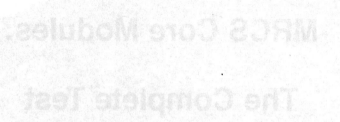

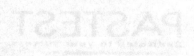

PASTEST

MRCS Core Modules:

The Complete Test

Christopher L H Chan
BSc (Hons) MBBS FRCS
Overseas Colorectal Surgical Fellow
Concord General Hospital
University of Sydney

SpR (General Surgery)
S E Thames

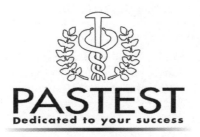

PASTEST
Dedicated to your success

© 2003 PasTest Ltd
Egerton Court
Parkgate Estate
Knutsford
Cheshire WA16 8DX

Telephone: 01565 752000

First published 2003

ISBN 1 901198 14 6

A catalogue record for this book is available from the British Library.

The information contained within this book was obtained by the author from reliable sources. However, while every effort has been made to ensure its accuracy, no responsibility for loss, damage or injury occasioned to any person acting or refraining from action as a result of information contained herein can be accepted by the publishers or author.

PasTest Revision Books and Intensive Courses
PasTest has been established in the field of postgraduate medical education since 1972, providing revision books and intensive study courses for doctors preparing for their professional examinations.
Books and courses are available for the following specialties:
MRCP Part 1 and Part 2, MRCPCH Part 1 and Part 2, MRCS, MRCOG, MRCGP, DRCOG, MRCPsych, DCH, FRCA and PLAB.
For further details contact:
PasTest, Freepost, Knutsford, Cheshire WA16 7BR
Tel: 01565 752000   Fax: 01565 650264
E-mail: enquiries@pastest.co.uk
Web site: www.pastest.co.uk

Typeset by Breeze Limited, Manchester.
Printed by MPG Books Ltd, Bodmin, Cornwall.

CONTENTS

PREFACE

This book is primarily intended for candidates sitting the Core MCQ section of the MRCS/AFRCS examinations. The multiple true false and extended matching questions and practice papers have been specifically structured to reflect the syllabus of all the Surgical Royal Colleges of GB and Ireland.

The goal of such a book is to help assess knowledge and provide an adjunct to reading, in addition to alerting one to areas that require further study. This book covers many of the 'most popular' topics that appear in the MRCS/AFRCS examinations. MCQ practice will increase overall knowledge and detailed explanations have been written to aid revision. The explanations should also be useful to candidates in other parts of the examination.

I hope that this book will not be restricted only to candidates sitting the MRCS/AFRCS examination but will be of use to Final Year medical students.

Christopher L H Chan
April 2003

CONTRIBUTORS

Contributor Coordinator:

Victoria Chamberlain MB ChB, MRCS, Wellington Hospital, Wellington, New Zealand

Contributors:

Steven J Arnold MSc (Hons), MRCS (Eng), East Surrey Hospital, Redhill, Surrey

Robert Attaran BSc (Hons), MBChB (Hons), University College London Hospital, London

Sunil Auplish MBBS, BSc (Hons), MRCS, Orthopaedic SpR, Oxford rotation

Philip J Blackie BSc (Hons), MBBS (London), Senior House Officer in Anaesthetics, King's College Hopital, London

Victoria Chamberlain MB ChB, MRCS, Wellington Hospital, Wellington, New Zealand

Joseph A Dawson MBBS MRCS (Eng), Basic Surgical Trainee, The Warwickshire & Worcestershire Basic Surgical Training Scheme

Richard J D Hewitt BSc MBBS, Senior House Officer in Neurosurgery, St Bartholomew's and the London Hospitals, London

Kismet Hossain-Ibrahim MBBS, BSc (Hons), MRCS (Eng), MRCS (Ed), Research Assistant, Department of Anatomy, University College London

Stephen J Washington MB ChB, Senior House Officer in Plastic Surgery, Christie Hospital, Manchester

MCQ EXAMINATION TECHNIQUE

The MCQ section of the MRCS comprises two written papers, one for the Core modules and another for the System modules. Each paper consists of 65 multiple choice stems and 60 extended matching items. Candidates are allowed 2 ½ hours per paper.

Pacing yourself accurately during the examination to finish on time, or with time to spare, is essential. There are two common mistakes which cause good candidates to fail the MRCS written examinations. These are neglecting to read the directions and questions carefully enough, and failing to fill in the computer answer card properly. You must read the instructions given to candidates at the beginning of each section of the paper to ensure that you complete the answer sheet correctly.

You must decide on a strategy to follow with regard to marking your answers. The answer sheet is read by an automatic document reader that transfers the information to a computer. It is critical that the answer sheet is filled in clearly and accurately using the pencils provided. Failure to fill in your name and your examination correctly could result in the rejection of your paper.

Some candidates mark their answers directly on to the computer sheet as they go through the questions, others prefer to make a note of their answers on the question paper and reserve time at the end to transfer their answers on to the computer sheet. If you choose the first method, there is a chance that you may decide to change your answer after a second reading. If you do change your answer on the computer sheet, you must ensure that your original is thoroughly erased. If you choose the second method, make sure that you allow enough time to transfer your answers methodically onto the computer sheet, as rushing at this stage could introduce some costly mistakes. You will find it less confusing if you transfer your marks after you have completed each section of the examination. You must ensure that you have left sufficient time to transfer your marks from the question paper to the answer sheet. You should also be aware that no additional time will be given at the end of the examination to allow you to transfer your marks.

If you find that you have time left at the end of the examination, there can be a temptation to re-read your answers time and time again, so that even those that seemed straightforward will start to look less convincing. In this situation, first thoughts are usually the best; don't alter your initial answers unless you are sure.

MCQ Examination Technique

You must ensure that you read the question (both stem and items) carefully. Regard each item as being independent of every other item, each referring to a specific quantum of knowledge. The item (or the stem and the item taken together) make up a statement as 'True' or 'False'. The number of stems will vary for each question. For this reason, a mark will not necessarily be required for each column of the answer sheet. For every correct answer you will gain a mark (+1). For the MRCS (London) examination, marks will not be deducted for a wrong answer. Equally, you will not gain a mark if you mark both true and false.

The MRCS exams in England are not negatively marked . For this reason you should answer every question as you have nothing to lose. If you do not know the answer to a question, you should make an educated guess – you may well get the answer right and gain a mark.

If you feel that you need to spend more time puzzling over a question, leave it and, if you have time, return to it. Make sure you have collected all the marks you can before you come back to any difficult questions.

Multiple choice questions are not designed to trick or confuse you, they are designed to test your knowledge of medicine. Accept each question at face value, do not look for hidden meanings.

The aim of this book is to give you two different methods of revising for the Core modules paper containing a mixture of MCQs and EMQs. Firstly, there are five chapters covering each of the five Core modules containing a mixture of MCQs and EMQs. This gives you a range of questions to test your knowledge on specific subjects. These are then followed by two practice papers to give you the chance to experience answering questions in exam format. You could also time yourself to see how well you manage to answer your questions in the 2 $\frac{1}{2}$ hours allowed.

Working through the questions in this book will help you to identify your weak subject areas. In the last few weeks before the exam it will be important for you to avoid minor unimportant areas and concentrate on the most important subject areas covered in the exam.

ABBREVIATIONS

α-FP	alpha-fetoprotein
AAA	abdominal aortic aneurysm
ABC	airway, breathing, circulation
ACE	angiotensin-converting enzyme
ACTH	adrenocorticotrophic hormone
ADH	antidiuretic hormone
ADRS	adult respiratory distress syndrome
AF	atrial fibrillation
Ag	antigen
AIDS	acquired immune deficiency syndrome
ANOVA	analysis of variance
AP	anteroposterior
APC	activated protein C/acetylsalicylic acid/adenomatous polyposis coli
APTT	activated partial thromboplastin time
APUD	amine precursor uptake and decarboxylation
ARDS	adult respiratory distress syndrome
ARF	acute renal failure
ASA	American Society of Anesthesiologists
ASD	atrial septal defect
ATLS	Advanced Trauma Life Support (guidelines)
ATP	adenosine triphosphate
AXR	abdominal X-ray
β-hCG	beta-human chorionic gonadotrophin
bd	*bis die* (twice a day)
BMI	body mass index
BP	blood pressure
bpm	beats per minute
BRCA1	breast cancer gene type 1
BXP	balanitis xerotica obliterans
CABG	coronary artery bypass graft(ing)
CCF	congestive cardiac failure
CD	cluster of differentiation
CEA	carcinoembryonic antigen
CIN	cervical intraepithelial neoplasia
CMF	cyclophosphamide, methotrexate and 5-FU
CN	cranial nerve
CO	cardiac output
COPD	chronic obstructive pulmonary disease
CPAP	continuous positive airway pressure
CSF	cerebrospinal fluid/colony-stimulating factor
CSH	chronic subdural haematoma
CT	computed tomography
CVA	cardiovascular accident
CVP	central venous pressure
CXR	chest X-ray

Abbreviations

Da	dalton
DAI	diffuse axonal injury
DCIS	ductal carcinoma *in situ*
DIC	disseminated intravascular coagulopathy
2,3-DPG	2,3-diphosphoglycerate
DPL	diagnostic peritoneal lavage
DVT	deep vein thrombosis
EACA	epsilon-aminocaproic acid
ECG	electrocardiogram/graphy
ECHO	echocardiogram
EMD	electromechanical dissociation
erbB2	after avian *erythroblastosis virus*, type *B2* (an oncogene)
ERCP	endoscopic retrograde cholangiopancreatography
ERDF	endothelium-derived relaxing factor (now known to be nitric oxide)
ESR	erythrocyte sedimentation rate
FBC	full blood count
FDP	fibrin degradation products
FEV_1	forced expiratory volume in 1 second
FFP	fresh-frozen plasma
FiO_2	fractionated concentration of oxygen in inspired gas
FNAC	fine-needle aspiration cytology
FOBT	faecal occult blood testing
FRC	functional residual capacity
FVC	forced vital capacity
G	growth (stage of the cell cycle)
GABA	gamma-aminobutyric acid
GCS	Glasgow Coma Score
GFR	glomerular filtration rate
GI	gastrointestinal
GTN	glyceryl trinitrate
GVHD	graft-versus-host disease
$[H^+]$	hydrogen ion concentration
H-*ras*	Harvey *rat* sarcoma virus
Hb A1c	Hb A_{1c}
HBe	hepatitis B early (antigen)
HBs	hepatitis B surface (antigen)
HBV	hepatitis B virus
HDU	high-dependency unit
5-HIAA	5-hydroxyindoleacetic acid
HiB	*Haemophilus influenzae* B
HIV	human immunodeficiency virus
hMLH1	human MutL homologue type 1 (associated with HNPCC)
hMSH2	human MutS homologue type 2 (associated with HNPCC)
HNPCC	hereditary non-polyposis colon cancer
HPV	human papillomavirus
HR	heart rate
HRT	hormone replacement therapy

Abbreviations

5-HT	5-hydroxytryptamine (serotonin)
HTLV-I	human T-cell leukaemia virus
Hz	hertz
I:E	inspiration:expiration
IL-1	interleukin-1
INR	international normalised ratio
IPPV	intermittent positive-pressure ventilation
ITU	intensive therapy unit
IU	international units
IVC	inferior vena cava
IVU	intravenous urography
J	joule (1 kcal = ~4.186 J)
JVP	jugular venous pressure
K-*ras*	after Kirsten *rat sarcoma* virus (an oncogene)
kcal	kilocalorie (dietary; 1 kcal = ~4.186 J)
kph	kilometres per hour
LCIS	lobular carcinoma *in situ*
LDH	lactate dehydrogenase
LFT	liver function test
LMWH	low-molecular-weight heparin
M	mitosis (stage of the cell cycle)
MCV	mean corpuscular/cell volume
MEN	multiple endocrine neoplasia
MODS	multiple organ dysfunction syndrome
mph	miles per hour
MRI	magnetic resonance imaging
MRSA	methicillin-resistant *Staphylococcus aureus*
myc	after avian *myelocytomatosis* virus (an oncogene)
Nd–YAG	neodymium–yttrium aluminium garnet (laser)
NPI	Nottingham Prognostic Index
NSAID	non-steroidal anti-inflammatory drug
NSCLC	non-small-cell lung carcinoma
o.d.	*omni die* (daily)
OPCS	Office of Population Censuses and Surveys
p	probability
p53	gene (produces the 53-kDa phosphoprotein)
PA	posteroanterior
$PaCO_2$	partial pressure of carbon dioxide in arterial blood
PaO_2	partial pressure of oxygen in arterial blood
PAOP	pulmonary artery occlusion pressure
Pap	Papanicolaou (cervical smear)
PASG	pneumatic antishock garment
PCA	patient-controlled analgesia
PCO_2	partial pressure of carbon dioxide
PCR	polymerase chain reaction
PDS	Polydioxanone sutures
PE	pulmonary embolism

Abbreviations

PEA	pulseless electrical activity
PEEP	positive end-expiratory pressure
PMC	pseudomembranous colitis
PMN	polymorphonuclear neutrophils
PO_2	partial pressure of oxygen
PSA	prostate specific antigen
PT	prothrombin time
RB1	retinoblastoma type 1 gene
RBC	red blood cell
s	seconds
S	synthesis (stage of the cell cycle)
SA	sinoatrial
SCC	squamous-cell carcinoma
SCLC	small-cell lung carcinoma
SD	standard deviation
SIADH	syndrome of inappropriate secretion of antidiuretic hormone
SV	stroke volume
SVC	superior vena cava
SVR	systemic vascular resistance
$t_{1/2}$	half-life
tds	ter die sumendum (i.e. three times per day)
TED	thromboembolic disease
TEDS	thromboembolic deterrent stockings
TENS	transcutaneous electrical nerve stimulation/transepidermal neurostimulation
TF	tissue factor
TIBC	total iron-binding capacity
TNM	tumour, node, metastasis (staging)
tPA	tissue plasminogen activator
TPN	total parenteral nutrition
TSH	thyroid stimulating hormone
TT	thrombin time
TURP	transurethral resection of the prostate
U	unit
U&E	urea and electrolytes
UICC	International Union against Cancer (translation)
URTI	upper respiratory tract infection
USS	ultrasound scan
UTI	urinary tract infection
V/Q	ventilation–perfusion
VSD	ventricular septal defect
vWF	von Willebrand factor
WCC	white cell count
WHO	World Health Organization

CHAPTER 1: PERIOPERATIVE MANAGEMENT 1

1.1   Metastatic calcification is associated with

❑ A   hyperparathyroidism
❑ B   carcinoma of the lung
❑ C   rheumatoid arthritis
❑ D   healing tuberculous lesions
❑ E   atherosclerosis
❑ F   aortic stenosis

1.2   Perioperative complications due to poorly controlled diabetes include

❑ A   increased susceptibility to fluid and electrolyte derangement
❑ B   ketoacidosis
❑ C   non-clostridial, gas-forming wound infections
❑ D   fungal mouth infections
❑ E   haematoma formation

1.3   Theme: Viral hepatitis

A   Hepatitis A
B   Hepatitis B
C   Hepatitis C
D   Hepatitis D
E   Hepatitis E

For each of the statements below select the most likely answer from the list above. Each option may be used once, more than once, or not at all.

❑   1.   Immunisation against hepatitis B infection will also protect against infection with this virus.

❑   2.   Is an aetiological agent in hepatocellular carcinoma, and has a vaccine.

❑   3.   Infection with this virus carries a high mortality rate in pregnant women.

❑   4.   This is a DNA virus.

1.4   Arterial emboli can be caused by

❑   A   atrial myxoma
❑   B   mitral stenosis
❑   C   pulmonary stenosis
❑   D   atrial fibrillation

1.5   During exercise

❑   A   cardiac output can increase sixfold
❑   B   there is a decrease in PaO_2 and $PaCO_2$
❑   C   anticipation of exercise can cause an increase in respiratory rate
❑   D   an increase in systolic and diastolic blood pressure is seen
❑   E   renal blood flow is increased
❑   F   there is a decrease in negative intrathoracic pressure

1.6   Theme: Classes of antibiotic

A   Macrolide
B   Quinolone
C   Glycopeptide
D   Monobactam

For each of the antibiotics listed below, select its correct antibiotic class from the list above. Each option may be used once, more than once, or not at all.

❑   1. Aztreonam

❑   2. Norfloxacin

❑   3. Erythromycin

❑   4. Vancomycin

1.7   The following may reduce intraoperative heat loss:

❑   A   condenser–humidifier in the breathing circuit
❑   B   low-flow anaesthesia
❑   C   laminar flow in an orthopaedic theatre
❑   D   use of a 'bowel bag' during laparotomy
❑   E   use of volatile surgical-preparation sterilising agents

1.8   In metabolic acidosis

❏   A   there is a negative base excess
❏   B HCO_3^- is the main intracellular buffer
❏   C   proteins and phosphates are the main extracellular buffer
❏   D   compensation occurs by an increase in alveolar ventilation
❏   E   bicarbonate infusion is the mainstay of treatment

1.9   Theme: Hospital infections

A   *Staphylococcus aureus* (MRSA)
B   *Streptococcus pyogenes*
C   *Legionella pneumonia*
D   *Pseudomonas aeruginosa*
E   *Escherichia coli*
F   *Yersinia enterolitica*
G   *Candida albicans*

From the list above choose the most common causative organism for the following infections. Each option may be used once, more than once, or not at all.

❏   1.   A 25-year-old man on prednisolone for asthma and antibiotics develops acute dysphagia.

❏   2.   A sudden outbreak of urinary catheter infections in an all-male geriatric ward.

❏   3.   Infection in a ward traced back to a member of staff.

❏   4.   A 35-year-old patient on immunosuppressive therapy and ventilated, develops a hyperaemic and ulcerated oesophagus seen on endoscopy.

1.10   In diabetic emergencies

❏   A   hypoglycaemia most commonly occurs in type II diabetes
❏   B   diabetic ketoacidosis is a typical feature of type II diabetes
❏   C   hyperosmolar coma is usually caused by ketoacidosis
❏   D   if the cause of coma is not known, insulin should be given until the diagnosis is confirmed
❏   E   glucose is useful in the initial treatment of diabetic ketoacidosis

1.11 Inflammation is characterised by

- ❏ A increased blood flow
- ❏ B decreased vascular permeability
- ❏ C recruitment of cells that phagocytose microbes and damaged tissue
- ❏ D secretion of preformed mediators
- ❏ E an inflammatory response that is independent of the burden of tissue injury

1.12 Conditions appropriate for day surgery include

- ❏ A inguinal hernia repair in a man with a BMI >30
- ❏ B recurrent inguinoscrotal hernia
- ❏ C hernia repair in a man who would have to drive home alone after the operation
- ❏ D emergency hernia repair in a 32-year-old man
- ❏ E hernia repair in a man with well-controlled angina
- ❏ F American Society of Anesthesiologists (ASA) grade 3 disease

1.13 Theme: Suture material

- A Absorbable, braided, synthetic
- B Absorbable, monofilament, synthetic
- C Non-absorbable, braided, natural material
- D Non-absorbable, monofilament, synthetic

For each of the suture materials listed below, select the most appropriate description from the list above. Each option may be used once, more than once, or not at all.

- ❏ 1. Polyglactic acid (Vicryl)

- ❏ 2. Nylon

- ❏ 3. Polyglyconate (Maxon)

- ❏ 4. Polypropylene (Prolene)

- ❏ 5. Polydioxanone sutures (PDS)

- ❏ 6. Polyglycolic acid (Dexon)

- ❏ 7. Silk

1.14 Phagocytic cells include

- ❏ A mast cells
- ❏ B neutrophil polymorphs
- ❏ C B lymphocytes
- ❏ D T lymphocytes
- ❏ E Kupffer's cells

1.15 Theme: Bacterial infections

A *Staphylococcus aureus*
B *Staphylococcus epidermidis*
C *Cryptococcus* spp.
D *Actinomyces* spp.
E *Bacteroides* spp.
F *Streptococcus pneumoniae*

From the list above choose the most common causative organism for the following infections. Each may be used once, more than once, or not at all.

- ❏ 1. This pathogen is the commonest cause of primary peritonitis.

- ❏ 2. A 3-month-old baby presents to A&E crying with a painful, red, swollen fingernail.

1.16 Preoperative work-up for general anaesthesia

- ❏ A all patients over 40 years of age should have an ECG
- ❏ B all smokers should have a CXR
- ❏ C premedication is not given until a consent form is signed
- ❏ D an FEV_1/FVC of 70% is insignificant

1.17 In strenuous exercise the following may occur:

- ❏ A increased stroke volume
- ❏ B rise in $PaCO_2$
- ❏ C rise in blood pressure
- ❏ D tachycardia
- ❏ E rise in mixed venous blood O_2 saturation

1.18   Recognised causes of hypokalaemia include

❏   A   villous adenoma of the rectum
❏   B   captopril therapy
❏   C   Conn's syndrome
❏   D   pyloric stenosis
❏   E   pseudo-obstruction

1.19   Theme: Bacterial infections

A   *Staphylococcus aureus*
B   *Streptococcus pneumoniae*
C   *Cryptococcus neoformans*
D   *Actinomyces israelii*
E   *Bacteroides* spp.
F   *Streptococcus viridans*

From the list above choose the most common causative organism of the following infections. Each may be used once, more than once, or not at all.

❏   1.   A young woman presents with a breast abscess. She has a 2-month-old baby and has been breast-feeding.

❏   2.   An immunocompromised man presents with a lung abscess.

❏   3.   A young woman presents a few weeks after an appendicectomy. A discharging fistula is noted in the right iliac fossa.

1.20   The following are causes of hyperkalaemia:

❏   A   dopamine infusion
❏   B   metabolic alkalosis
❏   C   suxamethonium chloride
❏   D   burns
❏   E   diabetic ketoacidosis

1.21   Diathermy

❏   A   involves a high-radiofrequency current
❏   B   is dangerous with earthed metal
❏   C   is dangerous in the presence of volatile anaesthetic gases
❏   D   is contraindicated in patients with a pacemaker

1.22 Metabolic alkalosis is commonly seen in patients with

❑ A pancreatic fistula
❑ B aspirin poisoning
❑ C protracted vomiting
❑ D hypoglycaemia
❑ E hyperventilation
❑ F acute renal failure

1.23 Theme: Local anaesthetics

A 1% lidocaine (lignocaine) + 1:200,000 adrenaline (epinephrine)
B 0.5% bupivacaine + 1:200,000 adrenaline
C 1% lidocaine
D Prilocaine
E Tetracaine (amethocaine)
F Lidocaine gel

Select the appropriate anaesthetic from the list above for each procedure listed below. Each option may be used once, more than once, or not at all.

❑ 1. Digital nerve block

❑ 2. After open inguinal hernia repair

❑ 3. Bier's block

❑ 4. Suturing of scalp lesion

1.24 Factors predisposing to DVT include

❑ A prolonged anaesthesia
❑ B disseminated malignancy
❑ C oral contraceptive pill
❑ D preoperative dehydration
❑ E pneumatic calf compression

1.25   Hypertension

❑   A   needs to be corrected preoperatively in a patient over 50 years of age
❑   B   is defined as a diastolic BP of 85 mmHg
❑   C   caused by phaeochromocytoma has a surgical mortality rate of 30%
❑   D   needs correction prior to emergency surgery

1.26   For suitability for day surgery under general anaesthesia, the patient

❑   A   should have a friend or relative to stay with them on the first night
❑   B   could be undergoing haemorrhoidectomy
❑   C   may have a body mass index (BMI) of 34
❑   D   could be undergoing a laparoscopic cholecystectomy
❑   E   could be ASA grade 3
❑   F   could have insulin-controlled diabetes mellitus
❑   G   could be undergoing an axillary clearance for breast cancer

1.27   Theme: Nosocomial infections

A   *Staphylococcus aureus*
B   *Streptococcus pyogenes*
C   *Escherichia coli*
D   *Legionella pneumophilia*
E   *Clostridium difficile*
F   *Pseudomonas aeruginosa*
G   *Streptococcus viridans*

From the list above choose the most common causative organism of the following infections. Each may be used once, more than once, or not at all.

❑   1.   A group of elderly patients on a ward all develop chest infections and the microbiologist informs you that it is the same organism causing the infections.

❑   2.   An inpatient develops infective endocarditis after his prosthetic aortic valve replacement.

1.28   The following are associated with the acute response to injury:

❏   A   increased plasma catecholamines
❏   B   increased liver glycogen levels
❏   C   reduced insulin levels
❏   D   relative hypoglycaemia
❏   E   raised plasma fatty acids

1.29   Incidence of postoperative wound infection in abdominal surgery is increased with

❏   A   extensive diathermy use
❏   B   not wearing masks
❏   C   inadequate haemostasis
❏   D   well-controlled diabetes mellitus
❏   E   steroid therapy
❏   F   ciclosporin treatment

1.30   Human immunodeficiency virus (HIV)

❏   A   has been contracted by droplet aerosol created by orthopaedic power tools
❏   B   leads to a persistently elevated antigen titre
❏   C   most frequently leads to a reversal of the CD4/CD8 lymphocyte ratio
❏   D   has a transmission rate of about 1% following percutaneous exposure
❏   E   is less infectious than hepatitis B

1.31   Osteomyelitis

❏   A   most commonly arises in adults as a result of a haematogenous infection from a primary focus elsewhere in the body
❏   B   is most commonly caused by *E. coli* in neonates
❏   C   in adults is most commonly due to *Staphylococcus* spp.
❏   D   may not be apparent on X-ray for up to 14 days after the onset of symptoms
❏   E   early high-dose intravenous antibiotics are part of the treatment regimen

1.32   Theme: Bone and joint sepsis

A   *Mycobacterium tuberculosis*
B   *Staphylococcus aureus*
C   *Haemophilus influenzae*
D   *Gonococcus* spp.
E   *Salmonella typhi*
F   Haemolytic *Streptococcus* spp.
G   *Clostridium perfringens*
H   *Clostridium difficile*

For each clinical situation below, select the organism that is the most likely cause of the pathology from the list above. Each option may be used once, more than once, or not at all.

❑   1.   A 20-year-old man, with a history of drug abuse, presents with soft tissue swelling, tenderness and erythema of the left forearm. There are multiple tender lymph nodes in his axillas.

❑   2.   A child with known sickle-cell disease presents with a 3-day history of increasing pain and swelling over the distal humerus where there is exquisite tenderness. She is pyrexial, has a raised ESR and WCC. Her X-ray shows changes suggestive of a bone infarct.

❑   3.   A patient known to have AIDS and with a low CD4 count, presents with a chronically painful and swollen ankle that has been discharging milky fluid via two sinuses for the past 2 weeks. The ankle is neither particularly hot nor inflamed.

❑   4.   A 2-year-old presents with a reluctance to walk following her first day back at playgroup after recovering from a nasty chesty cold. All movements of her left hip are painful.

❑   5.   A film producer working in a small African town fell backwards into a sewage pit and sustained an open-fracture dislocation of his ankle. It was reduced in the township and placed in a temporary splint. He elected to fly home for treatment. On arrival in A&E 36 hours later he was septic with an acutely painful, swollen and red lower limb.

1.33   Tourniquets

- ❏ A   may be applied safely for up to 3 hours at a time
- ❏ B   should not be applied to cause a pressure exceeding 300 mmHg
- ❏ C   can cause focal demyelination of the peripheral nerve
- ❏ D   usually produce an axonotmesis
- ❏ E   are suitable for procedures under local anaesthesia

1.34   Pulse oximeters

- ❏ A   only sense changes in arterial blood
- ❏ B   are unaffected by carboxyhaemoglobin
- ❏ C   are accurate to 0.5% above 90% oxygen saturation
- ❏ D   may not indicate adequate ventilation
- ❏ E   may not give accurate readings in hypovolaemic shock
- ❏ F   are inaccurate under anaesthesia
- ❏ G   produce false-negative results with chronic lung disease

1.35   Theme: Appropriate antibiotics

- A   Flucloxacillin
- B   Fusidic acid
- C   Gentamicin
- D   Cefradine
- E   Amoxicillin
- F   Metronidazole

From the list above choose the most appropriate antibiotic for the following infections. Each may be used once, more than once, or not at all.

- ❏ 1.   A breast-feeding woman notices a painful fluctuant swelling in her left breast.

- ❏ 2.   A 3-year-old boy presents to A&E with a painful, swollen finger which is red.

- ❏ 3.   A 75-year-old male, 5 days post-TURP presents with rigors and loin pain.

1.36   The Nd–YAG laser

❏   A   has very little tissue penetration
❏   B   is principally used for tattoo removal
❏   C   has a role in the palliation of oesophageal carcinoma
❏   D   should be used in a designated 'Laser Controlled Area'
❏   E   user requires compulsory eye protection

1.37   T-tubes

❏   A   should be removed after 5 days
❏   B   are usually made from polyvinyl chloride
❏   C   cause an intense fibrous reaction
❏   D   are not affected by bile acids
❏   E   are used less frequently with the advent of ERCP
❏   F   should be brought out through the abdominal wound

1.38   Keloid scars

❏   A   are more common in pigmented skin
❏   B   occur within the limits of the surgical wound
❏   C   are most common on the flexure surfaces of the limbs
❏   D   may be re-excised with good results
❏   E   may respond to pressure dressing
❏   F   can be prevented by subcuticular sutures

1.39   Theme: Antibiotics

A   Co-amoxiclav
B   Erythromycin
C   Aminoglycosides
D   Cephalosporins
E   Polymyxins
F   Tetracyclines
G   Fusidic acid

For each of the statements below select the most likely antibiotic/class of antibiotics from the list above. Each option may be used once, more than once, or not at all.

❏   1.   Is effective against both aerobic and anaerobic bacteria.

❏   2.   May be used in the treatment of legionnaire's disease.

1.40   General host factors predisposing to wound infection include

- ❏ A   hypoxia
- ❏ B   pyrexia
- ❏ C   jaundice
- ❏ D   hypercalcaemia
- ❏ E   anaemia

1.41   Pulmonary tuberculosis

- ❏ A   is predominantly caused by *Mycobacterium tuberculosis bovis*
- ❏ B   is usually transmitted by ingestion of infected milk
- ❏ C   is rising in incidence in Western countries
- ❏ D   induced hypersensitivity reaction is mediated by B lymphocytes
- ❏ E   Gohn focus refers to involved regional lymph nodes
- ❏ F   Gohn complex refers to the combination of the Gohn focus and involved regional lymph nodes
- ❏ G   Gohn focus is usually subpleural in location

1.42   Actinomycosal infection

- ❏ A   is most commonly found in the groin
- ❏ B   is most commonly due to *Actinomyces propionibacterium*
- ❏ C   usually produces positive cultures at 48 hours
- ❏ D   produces a characteristic discharge containing sulphur granules
- ❏ E   is caused by Gram-negative obligate anaerobic bacteria

1.43   Human immunodeficiency virus (HIV) infection

- ❏ A   is caused by a retrovirus
- ❏ B   may be diagnosed by Western blotting
- ❏ C   is present in high titre in the blood of asymptomatic carriers
- ❏ D   risk of seroconversion following a needlestick injury from an HIV-positive patient is approximately 1 in 25
- ❏ E   is more infectious following a needlestick injury than hepatitis B

1.44   In hydatid disease

- ❏ A   the causative bacteria is *Echinococcus granulosus*
- ❏ B   humans are accidental intermediate hosts
- ❏ C   the normal intermediate host is the dog
- ❏ D   hepatic lesions are often asymptomatic
- ❏ E   diagnosis is made on needle aspiration of suspected lesions

1.45   Sterilisation of surgical equipment

❑   A   chemical sterilisation is appropriate for equipment unsuitable for exposure to steam
❑   B   2% glutaraldehyde can be used for plastic equipment
❑   C   dry-heat sterilisation may be appropriate for equipment that is not well penetrated by steam
❑   D   steam-heat autoclaving is effective for rapid sterilisation of instruments

1.46   Theme: Adverse drug reactions

A   Atenolol
B   Cisplatin
C   Glyceryl trinitrate
D   NSAIDs
E   Vincristine

For each of the adverse effects below, select the single most likely causative agent from the list above. Each of the above may be used once, more than once, or not at all.

❑   1.   Hypotension

❑   2.   Nephrotoxicity if patient not on a regimen of hydration and diuresis

❑   3.   Peptic ulceration

❑   4.   Bronchospasm

❑   5.   Bradycardia

1.47   *Clostridium difficile* infection

❑   A   may be adequately treated with a single dose of oral metronidazole
❑   B   is usually diagnosed by Gram staining of the faeces
❑   C   may be adequately treated with oral vancomycin
❑   D   should be followed up by stool culture from asymptomatic patients
❑   E   may lead to colonic perforation

1.48   Theme: Skin lesions

A   Cyst
B   Papule
C   Plaque
D   Macule
E   Hamartoma
F   Papilloma
G   Teratoma

For each of the definitions described below, select the most likely skin lesion from the list of options above. Each option may be used once, more than once, or not at all.

❏   1.   Elevated area

❏   2.   Flat lesion

❏   3.   Fluid-filled tumour

❏   4.   Overgrowth of normal constituents

❏   5.   Overgrowth of epithelial tissue

1.49   *Clostridium difficile*

❏   A   infection has been increasing in incidence during the past 10 years
❏   B   infection is only caused by antibiotic treatment
❏   C   infection is most commonly caused by gentamicin
❏   D   induced diarrhoea typically starts within a week of commencing antibiotics
❏   E   spores may be found in dust

1.50   Actinomycosis infection

❏   A   is very sensitive to penicillin treatment
❏   B   is frequently found in association with other bacteria
❏   C   is produced by Gram-negative rods
❏   D   may mimic inflammatory bowel disease
❏   E   usually resolves with antibiotics when associated with abscess formation

1.51   In viral hepatitis

❏   A   persistence of hepatitis B surface antigen indicates an increased risk of developing chronic liver disease

❏   B   chronic hepatitis B infection increases the risk of developing gallbladder carcinoma

❏   C   hepatitis C virus accounts for about 90% of cases of post-transfusion hepatitis

❏   D   the acute illness of hepatitis C virus is generally less severe than that of hepatitis B virus infection

1.52   Theme: Commensal bacteria in different organs

A   *Bacteroides fragilis*
B   *Gardnerella vaginalis*
C   *Streptococcus viridans*
D   *Neisseria meningitidis*
E   *Pneumocystis carinii*
F   *Staphylococcus aureus*
G   Sterile

For each of the below, please select the single most appropriate option from above. Each of the above may be used once, more than once, or not at all.

❏   1.   Cerebrospinal fluid

❏   2.   Colon

❏   3.   Upper respiratory tract

❏   4.   Bile

❏   5.   Bladder

1.53   Rectal anastomosis

❏ A   below the peritoneal reflection has a higher leak rate compared with those above the reflection
❏ B   fashioned by the double-layered technique, this is superior to the single-layered technique
❏ C   using staples has a significantly lower clinical leak rate than a hand-sewn anastomosis
❏ D   has a higher radiological than clinical leak rate
❏ E   fashioned using non-absorbable suture materials give superior functional results

1.54   A preparation of 10 ml of 0.5% bupivacaine heavy with 1 in 200,000 adrenaline (epinephrine)

❏ A   is isobaric
❏ B   contains 5 mg of bupivacaine
❏ C   contains 500 mg of adrenaline
❏ D   contains 8% dextrose
❏ E   is suitable for intravenous injection

1.55   The risk of overwhelming postsplenectomy sepsis may be reduced by

❏ A   HiB vaccination
❏ B   hepatitis B vaccination
❏ C   poliomyelitis vaccination
❏ D   prophylactic metronidazole
❏ E   pneumococcal vaccination

1.56   *Echinococcus granulosus*

❏ A   the mature form is found in dogs
❏ B   the cyst stage is found in humans
❏ C   causes epilepsy
❏ D   causes anaphylaxis
❏ E   causes peritonitis
❏ F   carries a risk for hepatocellular carcinoma
❏ G   is a cestode (tapeworm)

1.57   Theme: Organisms and the infections they cause

   A   Liver abscess
   B   Oesophagitis
   C   Endocarditis
   D   Pneumonia
   E   Osteomyelitis in a 1-year-old child

For each of the organisms listed below select the single most appropriate infection given above. Each of the above may be used once, more than once, or not at all.

❏   1.   *Haemophilus influenzae*

❏   2.   *Escherichia coli*

❏   3.   *Candida albicans*

❏   4.   *Staphylococcus aureus*

1.58   Theme: Classification of organisms

   A   Fungal
   B   Protozoal
   C   Bacterial
   D   Viral

For each of the organisms listed below, select the correct group of organisms it belongs to from the list above. Each option may be used once, more than once, or not at all.

❏   1.   *Aspergillus* spp.

❏   2.   *Nocardia asteroides*

❏   3.   *Listeria monocytogenes*

❏   4.   Varicella zoster

1.59   Baseline investigations for a patient with major burns include

❏   A   glycosylated haemoglobin
❏   B   arterial blood gases
❏   C   CXR
❏   D   AXR
❏   E   thoracic CT

1.60   Theme: Appropriate antibiotic treatment

A   Gentamicin
B   Clindamycin
C   Flucloxacillin
D   Vancomycin
E   Benzylpenicillin
F   Clarithromycin
G   Teicoplanin

For each of the pathogens below select the most appropriate antibiotic from the list above. Each of the above may be used once, more than once, or not at all.

❏   1.   *Clostridium difficile*

❏   2.   *Klebsiella pneumoniae*

1.61   In immunity and infection

❏   A   interferons are a family of glycoproteins which are released from virally infected cells
❏   B   natural killer cells are circulating lymphocytes capable of destroying virally infected cells without prior sensitisation
❏   C   the cytotoxic activity of natural killer cells is greatly reduced by the presence of interferon
❏   D   natural killer cells have no role in the destruction of malignant cells
❏   E   adaptive immunity, unlike innate immunity, is found only in higher animals

1.62   Immunocompromised patients

❏ A   have no impairment of wound healing
❏ B   have no increased complication rate following minor surgery
❏ C   with HIV infection have a high incidence of anorectal sepsis
❏ D   with HIV infection should not undergo surgery for anorectal
         abscesses
❏ E   may develop pyomyositis which may present as an abscess

1.63   HIV

❏ A   is less infectious than hepatitis B
❏ B   patients should be barrier-nursed
❏ C   risk for surgeons can be decreased by vaccination
❏ D   risk for surgeons is greater with a solid- than with a hollow-
         needlestick injury
❏ E   risk is greater for pathologists than for surgeons

1.64   Theme: Benign lesions of skin and lymphatics

A   Pilomatrixoma
B   Cylindroma
C   Ganglion
D   Cystic hygroma
E   Syringoma

For each tissue of origin listed below, select the correct benign lesion from the list above. Each option may be used once, more than once, or not at all.

❏   1.   Lymphatic channels

❏   2.   Apocrine gland

❏   3.   Synovial sheath

❏   4.   Eccrine gland

❏   5.   Hair follicle

1.65   Organs normally colonised by commensal bacteria include the

❏   A   oropharynx
❏   B   peritoneal cavity
❏   C   lung parenchyma
❏   D   retina
❏   E   aqueous humour

1.66   Toxins produced by *Staphylococcus aureus* include

❏   A   verotoxin
❏   B   hyaluronidase
❏   C   toxic-shock toxin
❏   D   haemolysin
❏   E   enterotoxin
❏   F   collagenase

1.67   In necrotising fasciitis

❏   A   the skin initially appears normal
❏   B   antibiotic therapy and hyperbaric oxygen do not limit the spread
❏   C   a bold and wide excision of the necrotic fascia, skin and muscle
         should be carried out without delay
❏   D   mortality from systemic infection and sepsis is high
❏   E   high doses of intravenous benzylpenicillin are indicated

1.68   Monopolar surgical diathermy

❏   A   utilises an alternating current of 400 Hz
❏   B   requires a patient plate electrode of at least 20 cm^2
❏   C   may be used for 'cutting' tissue
❏   D   may be safely applied through ordinary surgical forceps
❏   E   produces a local heating effect up to 1000 °C
❏   F   is safer than bipolar diathermy
❏   G   should not be used in patients with pacemakers
❏   H   produces burn injuries that are usually partial thickness

1.69   Techniques applicable to the diagnosis of bacterial infections are

❏   A   agar culturing
❏   B   immunocytochemistry
❏   C   PCR (polymerase chain reaction)
❏   D   Gram staining
❏   E   antibody detection in the serum

1.70   Theme: Microbiology following skin trauma

A   *Staphylococcus aureus*
B   *Streptococcus pyogenes*
C   *Pasteurella multocida*
D   *Streptococcus milleri*
E   *Pseudomonas aeruginosa*

For each of the clinical scenarios listed below, select the most likely offending pathogen from the list of bacteria above. Each option may be used once, more than once, or not at all.

❏   1.   Carbuncles

❏   2.   Infected dog bites

❏   3.   Cellulitis

❏   4.   Styes

❏   5.   Infected human bites

❏   6.   Infected leg ulcers

1.71   Gram stain is used to

❏   A   classify bacteria
❏   B   show bacterial morphology
❏   C   detect bacteria in a tissue specimen
❏   D   distinguish bacteria from parasites
❏   E   visualise the malarial parasite

1.72 ***Pseudomonas aeruginosa* is effectively treated by**

- ❏ A ticarcillin
- ❏ B ampicillin
- ❏ C phenoxymethylpenicillin
- ❏ D piperacillin
- ❏ E flucloxacillin

1.73 **Theme: Classification of organisms**

A Fungal
B Protozoal
C Bacterial
D Viral

For each of the organisms listed below, select the correct group of organisms from the list above. Each option may be used once, more than once, or not at all.

- ❏ 1. *Cryptosporidium* spp.

- ❏ 2. *Mycobacterium tuberculosis*

- ❏ 3. *Pneumocystis carinii*

- ❏ 4. *Cryptococcus neoformans*

- ❏ 5. *Histoplasmosis* spp.

1.74 **Toxoplasmosis**

- ❏ A is sexually transmitted
- ❏ B is a zoonosis
- ❏ C is a common complication of transplantation
- ❏ D is an epidemic disease
- ❏ E can be treated with metronidazole
- ❏ F is a cytomegalovirus
- ❏ G is associated with cervical lymphadenopathy

2.1 In acute inflammation, neutrophils

- ❏ A actively migrate into tissues
- ❏ B migrate in response to bradykinin
- ❏ C migrate in response to components of complement
- ❏ D have an average life-span of 10 days in the tissues
- ❏ E respond to colony-stimulating factors

2.2 Theme: Selection of drains for surgical procedures

A Sump
B Corrugated
C Suction
D Tube drain
E None

For each of the operations below, select the single most appropriate drain from the list above. Each of the above may be used once, more than once, or not at all.

- ❏ 1. Thyroidectomy

- ❏ 2. Primary inguinal hernia repair

- ❏ 3. Total hip replacement

- ❏ 4. Appendicectomy

2.3 In resuscitation

- ❏ A gelatins may cause anaphylaxis
- ❏ B colloid is adequate for intestinal fluid replacement
- ❏ C it is best to use whole blood in haemorrhaging trauma cases
- ❏ D Haemaccel contains potassium and calcium
- ❏ E normal saline contains 132 mmol/l of sodium

2.4   The following cells can regenerate:

❏   A   cardiac muscle cells
❏   B   peripheral nerve cells
❏   C   Schwann cells
❏   D   mucosal cells
❏   E   renal tubular cells

2.5   Theme: Anticoagulant treatment regimens

A   Warfarin to maintain an INR of 2.0–3.0
B   Unfractionated heparin 5000 IU subcutaneously bd
C   Unfractionated heparin intravenously to maintain an APTT ratio of 2.5–3.5
D   Tinzaparin 3500 U/kg o.d.
E   Tinzaparin 175 U/kg o.d.

For each of the clinical scenarios listed below, select the most appropriate anticoagulation regimen to initiate treatment from the list of options above. Each option may be used once, more than once, or not at all.

❏   1.   A 34-year-old woman with factor V Leiden deficiency but no previous history of venous thrombosis is admitted for correction of her hallux valgus. A previous hallux valgus procedure was complicated by excessive bleeding.

❏   2.   A 67-year-old woman develops a popliteal vein thrombosis 5 days after a total hip replacement.

❏   3.   A 45-year-old man takes warfarin for a prosthetic mitral valve and attends the ward 3 days before an elective pancreatectomy.

2.6   Nutritional status may be estimated from

❏   A   triceps muscle circumference
❏   B   body mass index
❏   C   serum lymphocyte transferrin
❏   D   hand-grip strength
❏   E   serum albumin

2.7 In a healthy adult male weighing 70 kg

❑ A   the body water content is 75%
❑ B   the plasma volume is approximately 5 litres
❑ C   approximately 1.5 litres of water are lost daily from the lungs
❑ D   the intracellular fluid volume is approximately two-thirds of the total body water
❑ E   the daily potassium requirement is approximately 3.5–5.0 mmol/kg

2.8 Theme: Investigations for DVT

A   Clinical examination
B   Doppler ultrasound (Duplex)
C   Impedance plethysmography
D   Phlebography
E   Radio-iodine-labelled fibrinogen scan

For each of the statements below, select the correct investigation from the list of options above. Each option may be used once, more than once, or not at all.

❑   1.   Indicates the extent and degree of fixity of thrombus.

❑   2.   Is contraindicated in the presence of severe peripheral vascular disease.

❑   3.   Has a 50% false-positive rate.

❑   4.   Lower limb incisions can give false positives.

❑   5.   Has a risk of inducing hepatitis.

2.9 Wound healing

❑ A   type I collagen predominates in the early stages of wound healing
❑ B   epithelial regeneration occurs to cover the surface
❑ C   tensile strength is associated with collagen content
❑ D   collagen undergoes remodelling at the end of the first week
❑ E   is unaffected by radiotherapy

2.10   In wound healing

- ❏ A   sutured surgical wounds heal by secondary intention
- ❏ B   fibroblasts are responsible for wound contraction
- ❏ C   copper deficiency delays wound healing
- ❏ D   hyperbaric oxygen significantly accelerates wound healing
- ❏ E   is delayed by azathioprine

2.11   Hypertrophy involves an

- ❏ A   increase in tissue size
- ❏ B   increase in cell size
- ❏ C   increase in cell number
- ❏ D   increase in the number of mitoses

2.12   Complications of TPN include

- ❏ A   hypocalcaemia
- ❏ B   hypercalcaemia
- ❏ C   hypokalaemia
- ❏ D   hypophosphataemia
- ❏ E   hyperuricaemia

2.13   Potential sequelae of terminal ileal resection include

- ❏ A   vitamin B_{12} deficiency
- ❏ B   folic acid deficiency
- ❏ C   iron deficiency
- ❏ D   gallstones
- ❏ E   pernicious anaemia
- ❏ F   diarrhoea

2.14   Asplenic patients are at a particularly increased risk of overwhelming sepsis from

- ❏ A   anaerobic bacteria
- ❏ B   *Streptococcus pneumoniae*
- ❏ C   *Neisseria meningitidis*
- ❏ D   *Haemophilus influenza*
- ❏ E   *Bacteroides fragilis*
- ❏ F   fungi

2.15 Theme: Sites of drug action in the kidney

A   Distal convoluted tubule
B   Proximal convoluted tubule
C   Ascending loop of Henle
D   Descending loop of Henle
E   Collecting ducts

For each of the drugs below, select the most likely site of action from the list of options above. Each option may be used once only, more than once, or not at all.

❏   1.   Furosemide (frusemide)
❏   2.   Amiloride
❏   3.   ADH
❏   4.   Aldosterone

2.16 Enteral route of nutrition

❏   A   may cause bacterial overgrowth in the gut
❏   B   reduces stress ulceration
❏   C   is less expensive than the parenteral route
❏   D   decreases the incidence of cholestasis by promoting biliary flow
❏   E   may be commenced immediately after GI surgery

2.17 Postoperative hypoxaemia

❏   A   is especially common in patients after upper abdominal surgery
❏   B   may account for some cases of postoperative confusion
❏   C   occurs episodically with regional anaesthesia
❏   D   can persist for up to 3 days postoperatively
❏   E   is less common with narcotic infusions compared to bolus doses

2.18 Following coronary artery bypass grafting:

❏   A   mortality is 50% at 5 years
❏   B   the incidence of endocarditis is increased
❏   C   aspirin should be given routinely
❏   D   warfarin should be given for life
❏   E   coronary artery stenting is a contraindication

2.19   Macrophages

- ❏   A   are derived from the bone marrow
- ❏   B   have phagocytic properties
- ❏   C   are important in humoral immunity
- ❏   D   can form megaloblasts
- ❏   E   are characteristically found in granulomas

2.20   A 200-ml bolus of Haemaccel

- ❏   A   produces a sustained (5 minutes) rise of 2 cm H_2O in a dehydrated patient
- ❏   B   produces an initial rise and fall in CVP in a dehydrated patient
- ❏   C   can produce the same intravascular expansion as 1 litre of normal saline
- ❏   D   producing a sustained CVP rise of more than 4 cm H_2O may indicate overfilling
- ❏   E   may produce anaphylactic shock

2.21   Theme: Nutrition

- A   Nasogastric feeding
- B   Postoperative jejunostomy feeding
- C   Parenteral nutrition
- D   Omega fatty acid feed
- E   Elemental diet

Select the most appropriate nutritional approach for each of the cases below. Each option may be used once only, more than once, or not at all.

- ❏   1.   A 30-year-old motorcyclist has sustained a severe head injury. He is comatose, but showing signs of slow recovery.

- ❏   2.   A 63-year-old man had a 3-stage oesophagectomy for mid-oesophageal squamous-cell carcinoma yesterday. The procedure is expected to be curative, but the patient lost 20% of his weight in the 3 months prior to the operation.

2.22 Side-effects of steroids include

❏ A avascular necrosis of bone
❏ B pancreatitis
❏ C hepatotoxicity
❏ D depression
❏ E bone marrow suppression

2.23 A 5% dextrose intravenous infusion

❏ A is isotonic on administration
❏ B remains within the extracellular intravascular space for at least 1 hour
❏ C is a good mode of resuscitation in the shocked patient
❏ D may give rise to type II respiratory failure
❏ E contains 60 kcal (~251 J)/l

2.24 Glomerular filtration rate (GFR)

❏ A declines with age
❏ B may be measured with inulin clearance
❏ C may be estimated by creatinine clearance
❏ D is unaffected by a protein-rich meal
❏ E decreases during pregnancy

2.25 Metabolic acidosis is seen in

❏ A vomiting
❏ B hyperaldosteronism
❏ C diabetic ketoacidosis
❏ D renal failure
❏ E hyperparathyroidism
❏ F septic shock

2.26 Respiratory acidosis may be seen in

❏ A pneumonia
❏ B crushing chest injury
❏ C excessive mechanical ventilation
❏ D pulmonary embolus (small)
❏ E head injury
❏ F tracheostomy

2.27   Hyponatraemia may occur

- ❏   A   with excess steroids
- ❏   B   in burns
- ❏   C   in fever
- ❏   D   in renal failure
- ❏   E   following TURP
- ❏   F   in intestinal obstruction
- ❏   G   in pyloric stenosis

2.28   Prolonged irrigation with glycine during a transurethral prostatectomy may cause

- ❏   A   clotting abnormality
- ❏   B   coma
- ❏   C   hypokalaemia
- ❏   D   hypocalcaemia
- ❏   E   metabolic alkalosis

2.29   Concerning wound healing

- ❏   A   most skin wounds regain their preinjury strength with time
- ❏   B   wound strength returns to 80% of preinjury strength by 3 months in uncomplicated cases
- ❏   C   the small bowel regains most of its strength by 10 days
- ❏   D   type III collagen is stronger than type I collagen
- ❏   E   there is a lag phase lasting 6 weeks following injury

2.30   With regard to postoperative complications

- ❏   A   the commonest cause of hyponatraemia is increased renal sodium loss
- ❏   B   hypoxia may occur only in the first 24 h after surgery
- ❏   C   cold, clammy peripheries may be seen in septic shock
- ❏   D   pneumonia should be suspected if tachypnoea, pyrexia and tachycardia appear during the first 24 h
- ❏   E   myocardial infarction is more common in postoperative patients with uncontrolled hypertension

2.31 Haemolytic anaemia

- ❏ A is characteristically microcytic
- ❏ B may lead to gallstones
- ❏ C causes elevated urine urobilinogen levels
- ❏ D causes elevated serum haptoglobin levels
- ❏ E is associated with a conjugated hyperbilirubinaemia

2.32 In fluid replacement for bleeding secondary to trauma

- ❏ A excessive crystalloid administration is associated with adult respiratory distress syndrome (ARDS)
- ❏ B initial volume expansion is more quickly achieved with crystalloid rather than colloid
- ❏ C colloid administration prevents a fall in haematocrit level
- ❏ D stored blood has a high pH
- ❏ E blood is the fluid of choice to correct an ongoing haemorrhage and hypotension

2.33 Third-space fluid loss in the perioperative period

- ❏ A is related to the degree of tissue injury
- ❏ B can be up to 15 ml/kg per h
- ❏ C has a fluid composition similar to interstitial fluid
- ❏ D is best replaced by dextrose–saline
- ❏ E includes losses from enterocutaneous fistulas

2.34 In laparoscopic surgery

- ❏ A the optimal insufflation gas is nitrogen
- ❏ B insufflation pressures up to 20 mmHg are acceptable
- ❏ C the spring-loaded shield of the Veress needle prevents damage to the bowel
- ❏ D venous return to the heart is reduced
- ❏ E shoulder-tip pain following surgery indicates intra-abdominal injury

2.35 Median sternotomy:

- ❑ A is a non-muscle-cutting procedure
- ❑ B is contraindicated in patients receiving heparin therapy
- ❑ C is the usual approach for thymectomy
- ❑ D usually involves opening the right pleura
- ❑ E may be used for surgery on a retrosternal goitre

2.36 Fine-needle aspiration cytology (FNAC)

- ❑ A will allow differentiation between invasive and *in situ* carcinoma
- ❑ B is useful to diagnose metastases
- ❑ C sample usually undergoes Gram staining
- ❑ D excludes malignancy if the result is classed as C2
- ❑ E can be used to diagnose thyroid lumps

2.37 Cytotoxic T cells

- ❑ A act via specific antigen receptors
- ❑ B are lymphocytes that are able to kill virally infected cells after prior sensitisation
- ❑ C do not have a role in graft rejection
- ❑ D play a major role in the protection of body surfaces
- ❑ E are involved in atopic dermatitis

2.38 The following conditions may be associated with a microcytic anaemia:

- ❑ A β-thalassaemia
- ❑ B carcinoma of the rectum
- ❑ C hereditary haemochromatosis
- ❑ D menorrhagia
- ❑ E chronic renal failure

2.39 Fresh-frozen plasma

- ❑ A must be thawed on the ward or in the operating theatre
- ❑ B contains albumin
- ❑ C may cause a severe transfusion reaction
- ❑ D contains immunoglobulins
- ❑ E is the blood product of choice for replacing fibrinogen

2.40   Theme: Wounds

A   Sterile
B   Clean
C   Clean-contaminated
D   Contaminated
E   Dirty

For each of the clinical scenarios listed below, select the most likely classification of wound from the list above. Each option may be used once, more than once, or not at all.

❏   1.   The small bowel has been entered but without significant spillage of contents.

❏   2.   Non-infected biliary tract has been entered.

❏   3.   A man presents to A&E 6 hours after sustaining a circular-saw wound to his leg.

❏   4.   A 67-year-old patient with motor neurone disease undergoes a tracheostomy.

❏   5.   An infected genitourinary tract has been entered.

❏   6.   A scalpel incision has been made for a ganglion excision.

❏   7.   A woman has sustained a crush wound to a leg.

2.41   In haemophilia

❏   A   mucosal membrane bleeding is the hallmark of haemophilia A
❏   B   female carriers of haemophilia A have no bleeding tendency
❏   C   haemophilia B is inherited as an autosomal recessive trait
❏   D   haemophilia B is a deficiency in factor IX
❏   E   pseudotumours may complicate intramuscular bleeds in patients with haemophilia A

2.42   Folate deficiency occurs in

- ❏ A   methotrexate therapy
- ❏ B   alcoholism
- ❏ C   pregnancy
- ❏ D   ileal resection
- ❏ E   Cushing's syndrome
- ❏ F   short-bowel syndrome

2.43   DVT

- ❏ A   occurs in 30% of surgical cases without surgical prophylaxis
- ❏ B   remains undetected in 50% of cases
- ❏ C   extends above the popliteal vein in 40% of cases
- ❏ D   incidence is increased in protein C deficiency
- ❏ E   is decreased in antithrombin III deficiency

2.44   Splenic rupture

- ❏ A   can occur as an isolated abdominal injury
- ❏ B   occurs as a complication of infectious mononucleosis
- ❏ C   with an avulsion of the splenic pedicle seen on ultrasound may be treated with conservative management
- ❏ D   is more commonly associated with lower rib fractures
- ❏ E   occurs most frequently 6 weeks following trauma

2.45   Chronic iron deficiency anaemia

- ❏ A   produces a right shift of the oxygen dissociation curve
- ❏ B   elevates the total iron binding capacity (TIBC)
- ❏ C   produces a low PCO_2
- ❏ D   is associated with dysphagia
- ❏ E   can be associated with aspirin therapy

2.46   Fibrinolysis

- ❏ A   is augmented by epsilon-aminocaproic acid (EACA)
- ❏ B   is inhibited by tranexamic acid
- ❏ C   is associated with protein C deficiency
- ❏ D   tPA is the commonest activator
- ❏ E   may be activated by factor XII

2.47   Vitamin B$_{12}$

❑   A   involved in red cell maturation process
❑   B   is involved in platelet synthesis
❑   C   is stored longer than vitamin C
❑   D   is the same as intrinsic factor
❑   E   is absorbed maximally in the duodenum

2.48   The following interfere with blood cross-matching and compatibility tests:

❑   A   Dextran-40
❑   B   aspirin
❑   C   clopidogrel
❑   D   warfarin
❑   E   Haemaccel

2.49   Human albumin solution

❑   A   is the most effective agent for acute volume replacement
❑   B   may induce hyponatraemia
❑   C   is useful in managing chronic liver disease
❑   D   must be stored at 4 °C
❑   E   is subject to a virus-inactivating procedure during manufacture

2.50   Autologous transfusion of precollected blood

❑   A   carries no risk of a transfusion reaction
❑   B   is useful in patients with multiple alloantibodies
❑   C   is a safe technique in all patients
❑   D   can supply up to 10 units of blood
❑   E   UK guidelines prohibit its use in patients with viral hepatitis

2.51   In the coagulation cascade

❑   A   synthesis of factors II, VII, IX and X is vitamin K dependent
❑   B   the intrinsic pathway includes factor VII
❑   C   fibrinogen cleaves prothrombin to yield thrombin
❑   D   factor VIII is synthesised mainly in the vascular endothelium
❑   E   antithrombin III deficiency predisposes to bleeding
❑   F   factor V deficiency predisposes to bleeding

2.52   Disseminated intravascular coagulation

- ❑ A   may present with thrombosis
- ❑ B   should be considered in septic patients with a rising platelet count
- ❑ C   is present in patients with raised fibrin degradation products
- ❑ D   is associated with adenocarcinoma of the bowel
- ❑ E   sometimes require fresh-frozen plasma and platelet transfusion

2.53   The treatment of acute haemolytic transfusion reaction includes

- ❑ A   removing the intravenous cannula from the patient
- ❑ B   fluid restriction to avoid pulmonary oedema
- ❑ C   furosemide (frusemide)
- ❑ D   1 litre of 20% mannitol
- ❑ E   insertion of a central line in an oliguric patient

2.54   The following conditions may be associated with a raised mean cell volume:

- ❑ A   dietary iron deficiency
- ❑ B   vegan diet
- ❑ C   alcoholic liver disease
- ❑ D   recovery from acute haemorrhage
- ❑ E   chronic haemolytic anaemia

2.55   Prolongation of the activated partial thromboplastin time (APTT)

- ❑ A   usually occurs with low-molecular-weight heparin treatment
- ❑ B   occurs after warfarin treatment
- ❑ C   indicates adequacy of thromboprophylaxis with subcutaneous heparin
- ❑ D   is usual in patients receiving intravenous heparin
- ❑ E   may indicate a lupus anticoagulant

2.56   Petechial haemorrhages are seen in

- ❑ A   scurvy
- ❑ B   fat embolus
- ❑ C   vitamin K deficiency
- ❑ D   von Willebrand's disease

2.57   In a patient presenting for elective laparoscopic cholecystectomy taking warfarin and aspirin for atrial fibrillation and who has an INR of 3

❑   A   the warfarin should be continued intraoperatively
❑   B   the aspirin should be stopped on the day before surgery
❑   C   INR is a measurement of APTT
❑   D   is at an excessive risk and should not have the operation
❑   E   the patient should be given vitamin K and fresh-frozen plasma to correct the INR

2.58   In the assessment of a patient's need for perioperative transfusion

❑   A   cardiac output increases sharply when the haemoglobin falls below 10 g/dl
❑   B   blood volume is approximately 40 ml/kg in adults
❑   C   elderly patients with a haemoglobin of 4.8 g/dl should urgently receive six units of packed cells
❑   D   crystalloids are a suitable replacement for acute bleeding in young patients with a 15% intravascular blood volume loss
❑   E   men tolerate haemodilution better than women

2.59   Signs of acute haemolytic transfusion reaction include

❑   A   agitation
❑   B   pain at the cannula site
❑   C   hypertension
❑   D   coagulopathy
❑   E   oliguria

2.60   Platelet count

❑   A   of <50 x 10^9/l is likely to cause spontaneous bleeding of the colon
❑   B   may be elevated in patients with an adenocarcinoma
❑   C   characteristically falls after splenectomy
❑   D   may be influenced by phlebotomy technique
❑   E   may be decreased in patients with an adenocarcinoma of the colon

2.61 Regarding coagulation factors

- ❑ A the principal site of synthesis is the vascular endothelium
- ❑ B tissue-factor expression by tumours may predispose to thrombosis
- ❑ C protein C has anticoagulant activity
- ❑ D protein S has anticoagulant activity
- ❑ E factor VII is a component of the extrinsic pathway

2.62 Immune-mediated transfusion reactions

- ❑ A must be due to ABO incompatibility if haemolysis occurs
- ❑ B may be due to a secondary antibody response
- ❑ C affect more than 10–20% of red cell or platelet transfusions
- ❑ D may be due to plasma-protein antigens
- ❑ E may be due to white cell antigens

2.63 Possible complications of blood transfusion include

- ❑ A graft-versus-host disease
- ❑ B an increased risk of recurrent malignancy
- ❑ C pancreatic endocrine insufficiency
- ❑ D life-threatening thrombocytopenia
- ❑ E T-cell leukaemia

2.64 The following are recognised sequelae of a massive blood transfusion:

- ❑ A hyperkalaemia
- ❑ B hypocalcaemia
- ❑ C dilutional thrombocytopenia
- ❑ D adult respiratory distress syndrome (ARDS)
- ❑ E hyperthermia

2.65 Cardiopulmonary bypass

- ❑ A is often associated with thrombocytosis
- ❑ B is often associated with platelet dysfunction
- ❑ C is usually combined with induced hyperthermia
- ❑ D does not affect coagulation factor levels
- ❑ E vitamin K is administered at the end of a bypass to neutralise remaining circulating heparin

2.66 The prothrombin time

- ❏ A measures the activity of the extrinsic coagulation pathway
- ❏ B is not usually prolonged in liver disease
- ❏ C is prolonged in haemophilia A
- ❏ D can be expressed as the INR when monitoring warfarin dosage
- ❏ E is prolonged in vitamin K malabsorption

2.67 The following increase the risk of perioperative venous thrombosis:

- ❏ A sickle-cell disease
- ❏ B adenocarcinoma of the ovary
- ❏ C antithrombin III deficiency
- ❏ D increased age
- ❏ E ulcerative colitis

2.68 Warfarin

- ❏ A impairs the recycling of vitamin K
- ❏ B inhibits the synthesis of fibrinogen
- ❏ C is best monitored by the APTT
- ❏ D does not affect the bioavailability of antibiotics
- ❏ E requires 24 hours to become effective

2.69 Aspirin

- ❏ A may be a useful antithrombotic agent following splenectomy
- ❏ B causes inhibition of cyclo-oxygenase for 24 hours
- ❏ C should be discontinued 48 hours before surgery to restore haemostasis
- ❏ D carries little risk of upper gastrointestinal bleeding

2.70 Low-molecular-weight heparins

- ❏ A have a mean molecular weight of 15 kDa
- ❏ B have a longer half-life than unfractionated heparins
- ❏ C act predominantly on factor Xa
- ❏ D have a low bioavailability after subcutaneous injection
- ❏ E are predominantly eliminated by the kidney

2.71   von Willebrand's disease

❏   A   is a sex-linked disorder
❏   B   is the commonest inherited bleeding disorder in surgical practice
❏   C   is associated with haemarthroses
❏   D   manifests as a prolonged APTT and bleeding time
❏   E   affected individuals may benefit from preoperative desmopressin

2.72   In the investigation of bleeding disorders

❏   A   bleeding time may be prolonged in patients receiving aspirin
❏   B   fibrinogen concentration is increased in sepsis
❏   C   bleeding time correlates well with the severity of surgical bleeding
❏   D   fibrinogen levels increase in disseminated intravascular coagulation (DIC)
❏   E   thrombin time is reduced in patients receiving heparin therapy

2.73   The haematological consequences of splenectomy include

❏   A   a thrombocytosis peaking between 3 and 4 months
❏   B   increased circulating Howell–Jolly bodies
❏   C   a reduction in circulating sideroblasts
❏   D   a leucocytosis within hours after operation
❏   E   reduced platelet adhesiveness

2.74   Human albumin solution

❏   A   may induce hypernatraemia
❏   B   is most commonly used for acute volume replacement
❏   C   is stored at room temperature
❏   D   is manufactured as a bacterial recombinant protein
❏   E   may be useful in the treatment of ascites in chronic liver disease

2.75   Acute haemolytic transfusion reaction

❏   A   are most severe if group O cells are transfused into a group-A recipient
❏   B   may present with loin pain
❏   C   are usually due to ABO typing errors
❏   D   may cause haemoglobinuria
❏   E   are clinically similar to the effects of bacterially contaminated blood

2.76   Theme: Analgesia

A   Nerve block
B   Baclofen
C   Dexamethasone
D   Tricyclic antidepressants
E   Non-steroidal anti-inflammatory agent
F   Intramuscular morphine sulphate
G   Opioid patient-controlled analgesia
H   Intermittent intramuscular pethidine

For each patient described below select the most appropriate type of analgesia. Each of the above may be used once, more than once, or not at all.

❑   1.   A 60-year-old woman complains of severe aching right hypochondrial pain 3 months after surgery for a Duke's D adenocarcinoma of the colon. Her LFTs are abnormal and ultrasound of her abdomen shows hypoechoic lesions.

❑   2.   A 13-year-old haemophiliac postappendicectomy patient complains of pain that is not responding to oral analgesia.

❑   3.   A 50-year-old man on long-term steroid therapy for asthma has carcinoma of the prostate that is invading the sacral plexus. He is now complaining of shooting pains in his right leg.

❑   4.   A 35-year-old man is admitted to A&E with a sudden onset of right loin pain radiating to the groin. Urinalysis demonstrates microscopic haematuria.

2.77   After lateral hemisection of the L5 segment of the spinal cord there is an ipsilateral

❑   A   loss of pain in the foot
❑   B   loss of fine touch in the foot
❑   C   loss of ankle jerk
❑   D   wasting of the quadriceps muscle
❑   E   Babinski sign

CHAPTER 3: TRAUMA

3.1   In severe burns

❏ A   only inhalational injury causes respiratory problems
❏ B   pulse and BP are useful indicators of fluid resuscitation
❏ C   urine sodium <20 mmol/l indicates adequate resuscitation
❏ D   partial-thickness burns usually result in skin anaesthesia
❏ E   the threshold for referring to a burns unit is 40% of total body
         surface area

3.2   Burns

❏ A   can result in water loss of 100 ml/m^2 per h from the body surface
❏ B   of the partial-thickness type are characteristically painless
❏ C   that are full-thickness are typically red, mottled and very painful
❏ D   causing partial-thickness injury do not require fluid resuscitation
❏ E   involving an inhalational injury should be transferred to a burns unit

3.3   Theme: Peripheral nerves of the upper limb

A   Radial nerve
B   Median nerve
C   Ulnar nerve at the elbow
D   Posterior interosseous nerve
E   Anterior interosseous nerve
F   Superficial branch of the ulnar nerve
G   Deep branch of the ulnar nerve

For each patient with nerve compression symptoms, select the nerve most
likely to be involved. Each option may be used once, more than once, or
not at all.

❏ 1.   A 23-year-old long-distance cyclist notices difficulty in writing
         after a race. There is weakness of finger adduction and abduction
         but normal sensation in the hand. Froment's sign is positive.

❏ 2.   A 30-year-old right-handed woman complains of pain and
         clumsiness after playing the piano. She has weak thumb- and
         index-finger flexion, but no sensory deficit.

❏ 3.   An 18-year-old weight-lifter develops paraesthesia in the ulnar
         two digits of his right hand. On examination, there is sensory
         loss in the little and ring fingers, but no motor loss.

3.4   Partial-thickness (second degree) burns typically cause

❏   A   loss of sensation
❏   B   hyperkalaemia
❏   C   blistering
❏   D   a wet appearance

3.5   Theme: Upper limb fractures

A   Neck of the humerus
B   Scaphoid
C   Smith's fracture
D   Colles' fracture
E   Supracondylar fracture of the humerus
F   Acromioclavicular joint disruption
G   Olecranon fracture

Match the statements below to the most appropriate fracture from the list above. Each option may be used once only, more than once, or not at all.

❏   1.   Treatment is with a collar and cuff.

❏   2.   Internal fixation is frequently necessary.

❏   3.   Treatment is with a broad arm sling.

❏   4.   Results in a dinner-fork deformity.

3.6   Compartment syndrome

❏   A   may produce cyanosis of the limb
❏   B   produces pallor of the limb
❏   C   produces numbness
❏   D   may cause severe pain
❏   E   can be excluded by a palpable distal pulse

3.7 **A previously healthy, 70 kg, male trauma victim has suffered an estimated blood loss of 2 litres (30–40% blood loss). Which of the following statements apply to this patient?**

❑ A   tachycardia, but unchanged systolic blood pressure
❑ B   unchanged systolic blood pressure, but increasing diastolic blood pressure
❑ C   reduced systolic blood pressure and narrow pulse pressure
❑ D   negligible urinary output
❑ E   widened pulse pressure
❑ F   unchanged respiratory rate

3.8 **Fat embolism**

❑ A   is associated with a petechial rash
❑ B   can be caused by closed fractures
❑ C   is associated with osteoporosis
❑ D   is a complication of long bone fractures
❑ E   produces fat in the sputum
❑ F   typically infarcts in the inferior mesenteric artery
❑ G   may be treatable with steroids

3.9 **Theme: Lower limb injuries**

A   Common peroneal nerve
B   Femoral nerve
C   Saphenous nerve
D   Tibial nerve
E   Sural nerve

For each of the statements below, select the most likely nerve from the list above. Each option may be used once, more than once, or not at all.

❑ 1.   A 42-year-old man undergoes a laminectomy whilst positioned on his lateral side during the operation. Postoperatively he complains of numbness over his medial malleolus.

❑ 2.   A 26-year-old footballer sustains an injury to his right knee during a game. He complains of a loss of sensation on the dorsal aspect of his foot and he is unable to dorsiflex and evert his foot.

3.10   Theme: Brachial plexus injuries

A   Upper brachial plexus
B   Lower brachial plexus
C   Radial nerve in the axilla
D   Axillary nerve
E   Radial nerve in the spiral groove
F   Long thoracic nerve
G   None of the above

For each of the cases below, select the most likely site of injury from the list of options above. Each may be used once, more than once, or not at all.

❏   1.   A rugby player presented to the A&E department following the successful reduction of a dislocated shoulder on the touchline. On examination, he had a full range of shoulder movements but there was some loss of sensation over the lower aspect of the deltoid muscle.

❏   2.   A scaffolder was brought into the A&E department having fallen from a height of 10 feet (~3 m). He had regained consciousness but did not recollect the accident. An accompanying workmate said he had managed to slow his fall by grabbing a scaffolding pole with his right hand. He was haemodynamically stable. The fingers of his right hand were hyperextended at the metacarpophalangeal joints and flexed at the interphalangeal joints.

❏   3.   Two days after the elective repair of an aortic aneurysm a patient complained to his consultant of difficulty in drinking from a cup. On examination he was found to have a left wrist drop associated with weakness of the grip of the left hand. There was some loss of sensation over the base of the thumb.

❏   4.   On review in the outpatient clinic following a left mastectomy with axillary clearance, a 50-year-old woman was noted to have marked protrusion of the inferior angle of the scapula.

3.11   Theme: Peripheral nerve injury

    A   Femoral nerve
    B   Common peroneal nerve
    C   Deep peroneal nerve
    D   Superficial peroneal nerve
    E   Sural nerve
    F   Tibial nerve
    G   Saphenous nerve

Choose the most appropriate option from the above list. Each option may be used once only, more than once, or not at all.

❑   1.   A 28-year-old man sustains a varus injury to his left knee whilst skiing. He notices loss of sensation over the front and anterior half of the leg and dorsum of the foot.

❑   2.   A 32-year-old motorcyclist is involved in an RTA and sustains a severe laceration 6 cm above the ankle on the lateral aspect of his leg. He is unable to evert his foot and has noticed some numbness over the dorsum of the foot and medial four toes.

3.12   The PASG (pneumatic antishock garment)

❑   A   reduces mortality from penetrating chest injuries when applied early
❑   B   raises systolic pressure by increasing peripheral resistance and myocardial afterload
❑   C   is indicated for splinting and control of pelvic fractures with continuing haemorrhage and hypotension
❑   D   is contraindicated when diaphragmatic rupture is suspected
❑   E   reduces the requirement for volume replacement

3.13   The catabolic phase of the metabolic response to trauma is characterised by

❑   A   decreased urine output
❑   B   increased sodium output
❑   C   gluconeogenesis
❑   D   negative nitrogen balance
❑   E   thrombocytosis

3.14 Theme: Chest injury management

A Oral analgesia
B Oral analgesia and admission
C Chest drain

For each of the scenarios listed below, select the most likely treatment from the list above. Each option may be used once only, more than once, or not at all.

❏ 1. A young footballer sustains a fractured 4th rib. His chest X-ray is normal.

❏ 2. An elderly man sustains a fractured 4th rib. His chest X-ray is normal.

❏ 3. A 23-year-old man is involved in a road traffic accident. He sustains a fractured 4th rib, fractured left femur and a pneumothorax.

3.15 Open 'sucking' chest wounds

❏ A are associated with a defect in the chest wall of more than twice the diameter of the trachea
❏ B should be treated by insertion of a chest drain through the wound
❏ C are commonly caused by blunt chest trauma
❏ D may initially be treated by applying an occlusive dressing sealed on three of its four sides
❏ E usually require surgical repair for definitive treatment

3.16 Haemorrhagic shock

❏ A increase catecholamine secretion by the adrenal cortex
❏ B causes the oxygen–haemoglobin dissociation curve to shift to the left
❏ C stimulates aortic baroreceptors
❏ D produces a decrease in ventilation–perfusion mismatch
❏ E causes an increase in tidal ventilation
❏ F causes a decrease in atrial pressure and subsequent reduction in ADH secretion

3.17   Theme: Sensation of lower limb

A   Sural nerve
B   Ilioinguinal nerve
C   Lateral cutaneous nerve of the thigh
D   Medial cutaneous nerve of the thigh
E   Peroneal nerve
F   Branch of the infrapatellar nerve
G   Iliohypogastric nerve
H   Saphenous nerve
I   Tibial nerve

For each of the statements below, select the most likely option from the list above. Each option may be used once, more than once, or not at all.

❏   1.   A 36-year-old woman, who wears tight trousers, complains of pain on the lateral aspect of her thigh. She has a triggerpoint medial to the anterior superior iliac spine.

❏   2.   A patient has a posterior lag of the knee with laxity of the medial collateral ligaments.

❏   3.   A patient reports numbness of the medial side of his leg following knee arthroscopy.

❏   4.   A patient reports numbness between the toes following varicose vein surgery.

3.18   In the immediate airway management of the multiple injured patient

❏   A   nasotracheal intubation may be considered for a spontaneously breathing, unconscious patient
❏   B   a cricothyroidotomy is indicated after failed endotracheal intubation
❏   C   the airway should be opened initially by extending the neck and performing a jaw thrust manoeuvre
❏   D   a nasopharyngeal airway is contraindicated in a base-of-skull fracture
❏   E   nasal prongs will provide adequate oxygen delivery to the patient

3.19   Theme: Spinal injuries

A   Cauda equina syndrome
B   Neurogenic shock
C   Cord transection at the C5 level
D   Hangman's fracture
E   C2 odontoid dens dislocation
F   A C1 Jefferson fracture
G   Lumbar wedge fracture

Match the statements below with the most appropriate spinal injury listed above. Each option may be used once only, more than once, or not at all.

❑   1.   This is caused by axial loading in a head injury leading to a 'blow out' fracture.

❑   2.   Diaphragmatic breathing will be present.

❑   3.   Can be detected on an X-ray by applying Steel's rule of three.

❑   4.   May require the use of vasopressors.

❑   5.   Will result in bladder signs and patchy motor weakness in the lower limbs.

❑   6.   Skull traction is contraindicated with this spinal injury.

❑   7.   Bradycardia will be present.

❑   8.   Flexion of the arms is preserved but extension is absent.

❑   9.   Grimaces to pain above, but not below, the clavicle.

3.20   Fractures of the frontobasal skull can cause

❑   A   anosmia
❑   B   visual field defects
❑   C   rhinorrhoea
❑   D   retroauricular ecchymoses
❑   E   periorbital ecchymosis

3.21 Theme: Cerebral pathology

A   CT head
B   Lumbar puncture
C   Skull X-rays
D   None of the above

For each of the clinical scenarios below, select the most appropriate investigation from the list above. Each option may be used once, more than once, or not at all.

❏   1.   A 25-year-old involved in an RTA develops increasing confusion and his GCS drops from 15 to 12.

❏   2.   A 45-year-old patient's GCS drops after a sudden onset headache.

3.22 Extradural haematoma

❏   A   is usually associated with a fracture
❏   B   is usually the result of damage to the anterior branch of the middle meningeal artery
❏   C   is typically biconcave on a CT scan
❏   D   is often limited by suture lines
❏   E   is frequently the result of a contre-coup injury

3.23 Tracheostomy

❏   A   may be complicated by tracheal stenosis
❏   B   has to be formally closed after use
❏   C   is a recognised cause of hypothyroidism
❏   D   is best placed at the first tracheal cartilage
❏   E   helps the cough reflex

3.24 The following anatomical differences in children make management of their airway more difficult than in adults

❏   A   a more caudally placed larynx
❏   B   smaller angle of the jaw
❏   C   a more U-shaped epiglottis
❏   D   relatively larger tongue
❏   E   larger head size compared to the body size

3.25   Theme: Peripheral nerve anatomy

A   Facial nerve
B   Lingual nerve
C   Ophthalmic nerve
D   Trochlear nerve
E   Cranial accessory nerve
F   Oculomotor nerve
G   Glossopharyngeal nerve
H   Cervical sympathetic trunk

For each of the patients below, select the nerve most likely to be involved from the list above. Each option may be used once, more than once, or not at all.

❑   1.   Two days after a left lower, wisdom tooth extraction, a fit 23-year-old man complains of a severe bleed from the left side of his tongue, which he has bitten. The tongue is insensitive to touch and taste stimuli on the left.

❑   2.   A fit 26-year-old man suddenly develops a persistent dry left eye, clouded vision, blunted taste sensation and an inability to empty food from the left vestibule.

❑   3.   A 25-year-old woman develops a left-sided ptosis and a dilated pupil.

❑   4.   A 25 year-old woman develops a left-sided ptosis and a constricted pupil.

❑   5.   A 40-year-old woman complains of clouding vision in her left eye after development of a rash over the left side of her forehead. She has burning pain over her left forehead and in her left eye, but no ptosis or diplopia. The corneal reflex is intact.

3.26   Post-traumatic stress disorder

❑   A   is usually delayed 4 weeks after the event
❑   B   the recollections are unpleasant
❑   C   the patient experiences flashbacks
❑   D   symptoms must last at least 1 month
❑   E   the patient usually seeks out situations similar to the traumatic event

3.27 The cauda equina

❏ A begins at lower border of L1
❏ B contains mainly motor fibres
❏ C begins at the subcostal plane
❏ D pain in the legs is a common feature of injury
❏ E injury typically causes a positive Babinski sign

3.28 Theme: Operative procedures in the resuscitation room

A Pericardiocentesis
B Tube chest drainage
C Needle thoracocentesis
D Emergency thoracotomy
E Venous cutdown
F Cricothyroidotomy
G Diagnostic peritoneal lavage
H Intraosseous infusion
I Central line placement
J Passage of a nasogastric tube
K Endotracheal intubation

For each clinical scenario described below, select the most appropriate procedure from the list above. Each option may be used once only, more than once, or not at all.

❏ 1. A patient with a systolic blood pressure of 60 mmHg following penetrating chest trauma, distended neck veins, reasonable bilateral air entry and central trachea.

❏ 2. A patient with a systolic blood pressure of 60 mmHg following blunt chest trauma, distended neck veins, no air entry on the right side and tracheal deviation to the left.

❏ 3. This is a prerequisite for diagnostic peritoneal lavage.

❏ 4. This is the recommended route for fluid replacement in children after peripheral cannulation fails.

3.29   Chronic subdural haematoma may cause

❑   A   anosmia
❑   B   rhinorrhoea
❑   C   air in the cranial cavity
❑   D   meningitis
❑   E   gait disturbance
❑   F   seizures

3.30   Theme: Trauma

A   Flail chest
B   Fracture of C3
C   Basal skull fracture
D   Fractured 1st rib
E   Ruptured diaphragm
F   Massive haemothorax
G   Jefferson's fracture
H   Cardiac tamponade
I   Hangman's fracture

For each of the statements in the list below, select the most appropriate option from the list above. Each option may be used once, more than once, or not at all.

❑   1.   Gas bubble is seen above the diaphragm on CXR.

❑   2.   Battle's sign is present.

❑   3.   Paradoxical breathing associated with pulmonary contusions.

❑   4.   Ring blow-out of C1.

❑   5.   Associated with major vessel injury.

❑   6.   Paralysis of the phrenic nerve occurs.

3.31   Spontaneous pneumothoraces

❏   A   produce increased breath sounds on the affected side
❏   B   produce increased resonance on the affected side of the chest
❏   C   cause trachea shift to the opposite side
❏   D   resolve, by volume, at a rate of 1% per week
❏   E   predominantly affect the right lung
❏   F   invariably require aspiration via either a large-bore cannula or chest drain
❏   G   are commoner in women

3.32   Signs of increased intracranial pressure include

❏   A   increased pulse rate
❏   B   increased BP
❏   C   neck stiffness
❏   D   bloody tap following lumbar puncture
❏   E   respiratory depression

3.33   Features of the crush syndrome include

❏   A   hyperkalaemia
❏   B   oliguria
❏   C   haemoglobinuria
❏   D   methaemoglobinaemia
❏   E   haemoconcentration

3.34   In blunt injury to the abdomen

❏   A   CT scan is of limited value in hollow viscus injury
❏   B   the liver is the commonest solid organ to be injured
❏   C   75% of patients have a diaphragm rupture
❏   D   retroperitoneal organs are rarely injured
❏   E   diagnostic peritoneal lavage is always indicated

3.35   Nerve injuries

❏   A   damage to the spinal accessory nerve causes winging of the scapula
❏   B   the axillary nerve contains fibres from C6 and C7
❏   C   radial nerve injuries cause wrist drop
❏   D   a positive Froment's test is associated with median nerve injury
❏   E   sciatic nerve injuries are associated with a high-stepping gait

3.36   Theme: Anatomy of the cerebral vasculature

 A Posterior cerebral artery
 B Posterior inferior cerebellar artery
 C Internal carotid artery
 D Middle meningeal artery
 E Vertebral artery
 F Basilar artery
 G Striate arteries
 H Middle cerebral artery

For each of the neurological abnormalities below, select the artery most likely to be affected from the list above. Each option may be used once, more than once, or not at all.

❑ 1. A 75-year-old man wakes one morning with a hemiparesis, and loss of discriminatory touch, movement and vibration, all on the left side. On protrusion, his tongue deviates to the right.

❑ 2. A 76-year-old man wakes one morning with absence of pain and temperature sensation over the right side of his body, dysarthria and dysphagia. There is also loss of pain and temperature sensation over the area of distribution of the left trigeminal nerve.

❑ 3. A 74-year-old man notices that he collides with objects on his right side, but he is able to read. His perimetry charts show that he has a complete right homonymous hemianopia with macular sparing.

❑ 4. A 76-year-old man suddenly collapses. When he recovers consciousness, he is found to have a complete right hemiparesis, complete right-sided anaesthesia, aphasia, and paralysis of his right lower facial musculature. There is also a right homonymous hemianopia.

3.37   Brain death is confirmed by

❑ A Glasgow Coma Scale score of 0
❑ B nystagmus when cold water is put into ear
❑ C absence of corneal reflex
❑ D absence of knee-jerk reflex
❑ E failure to breathe when given PO_2 of 12 kPa and PCO_2 of 7 kPa

3.38   Major traumatic injury should be suspected when

❏ A   there is a fall of more than 10 feet (~3 m)
❏ B   the victim is ejected from a vehicle
❏ C   there is an extrication time of 1 hour
❏ D   there is an impact velocity of 50 mph (~31 kph)
❏ E   death occurs in an occupant of the same vehicle

3.39   Theme: Anatomy of the brachial plexus and nerves of the upper arm

A   C5, C6, C7 roots of the brachial plexus
B   C8, T1 roots of the brachial plexus
C   Long thoracic nerve
D   Suprascapular nerve
E   Axillary nerve
F   Radial nerve
G   Ulnar nerve
H   Median nerve
I   Intercostobrachial nerve

For each patient with neurological abnormalities, select the single most likely site of nerve injury. Each option may be used once, more than once, or not at all.

❏   1.   A 3-day-old baby with a history of a difficult delivery followed by a floppy right arm. The arm is now held to the side, internally rotated and the forearm is pronated.

❏   2.   A 28-year-old man has lost the use of his left hand since falling from a tree and grabbing a branch to break his fall. Examination reveals a claw hand and left-sided Horner's syndrome.

❏   3.   A 55-year-old woman complains of aching and weakness in her right arm following a right mastectomy for breast carcinoma. Examination reveals winging of the right scapula on pressing against a wall.

❏   4.   A 20-year-old man has loss of abduction of the shoulder following an anterior dislocation of his right shoulder while playing rugby.

❏   5.   A 43-year-old man presents with a weak left arm since a drinking binge. He is unable to extend his wrist or elbow.

3.40   Theme: Operative procedures in the resuscitation room

   A   Pericardiocentesis
   B   Chest tube drainage
   C   Needle thoracocentesis
   D   Emergency thoracotomy
   E   Venous cutdown
   F   Cricothyroidotomy
   G   Diagnostic peritoneal lavage
   H   Intraosseous infusion
   I   Central line placement
   J   Passage of a nasogastric tube
   K   Endotracheal intubation

For each clinical scenario described below, select the most appropriate procedure from the list above. Each option may be used once only, more than once, or not at all.

❏   1.   The recommended route for fluid replacement in adults after peripheral cannulation fails.

❏   2.   The first procedure in a pulseless apnoeic patient who has been stabbed in the chest.

❏   3.   The second procedure in a pulseless apnoeic patient who has been stabbed in the chest.

❏   4.   Procedure required for a large haemothorax.

3.41   Tachycardia in response to haemorrhage may be absent in the following:

❏   A   hypothermia
❏   B   infants
❏   C   a patient with a pacemaker
❏   D   after administration of high-flow oxygen
❏   E   patients on β-blockers

3.42   Theme: Shock

    A   Cardiogenic shock
    B   Septic shock
    C   Neurogenic shock
    D   Hypovolaemic shock <15% volume loss
    E   Hypovolaemic shock 15–30% volume loss
    F   Hypovolaemic shock >40% volume loss

For each of the scenarios described below, choose the most appropriate type of shock from the list above. Each option may be used once, more than once, or not at all.

❑   1.   A motorcyclist was admitted to the A&E department having been thrown a distance of 30 feet (~10 m). He was wearing a helmet and had recovered consciousness at the scene. He remained confused. Pulse 40/min, respiratory rate 30/min, BP 75/60 mmHg. On catheterisation there was no urine output. Lateral cervical spine X-rays were suggestive of a fracture of C6.

❑   2.   A 25-year-old marathon runner was involved in a road traffic accident while out training. She was admitted to A&E with a pulse rate of 100, BP 75/60 mmHg, respiratory rate 30/min. Her abdomen was generally tender, peritoneal lavage was positive. There was no urine output.

❑   3.   A homeless man was found collapsed in a dark alleyway at 5 am on New Year's Day. He was unconscious and smelt of alcohol. On arrival in the A&E department his pulse was 110, BP 115/50 mmHg, he was apyrexial on admission, but his skin was noted to be flushed. During the secondary survey he was found to have sustained a penetrating abdominal injury.

3.43   Internal fixation should be used

❑   A   where fast healing is required
❑   B   where large forces are working in opposite directions
❑   C   in the multiply injured patient
❑   D   with compound fractures
❑   E   with pathological fractures

3.44   Theme: Burns in children

    A   1%
    B   4.5%
    C   7%
    D   9%
    E   14%
    F   18%

For each of the clinical scenarios regarding cutaneous burns in children listed below, select the most likely percentage of the total body surface area from the list above. Each option may be used once, more than once, or not at all.

❑   1.   Burns to all of the head and neck in an infant

❑   2.   Burns to all the anterior trunk (chest and abdomen)

❑   3.   Burns to all the male genitalia

❑   4.   Burns to all the posterior trunk (upper and lower back)

❑   5.   Burns to the whole anterior aspect of one lower limb

❑   6.   Burns to the whole aspect of one arm

❑   7.   Burns to the posterior aspect of both lower limbs

3.45   A surgical airway

❑ A   is indicated in fracture of the larynx
❑ B   is indicated in a large extradural haematoma
❑ C   is indicated in severe oropharyngeal haemorrhage
❑ D   may be performed by a needle through the thyrohyoid membrane
❑ E   may be complicated by oesophageal perforation

3.46   The early response to trauma (ebb phase) includes

❑ A   an increase in metabolic rate
❑ B   an increase in body temperature
❑ C   an increase in catecholamine levels
❑ D   decreased lactate levels
❑ E   increased glucose levels

3.47   Intraosseous infusion

❏   A   is routinely indicated in paediatric trauma
❏   B   can be used in children up to the age of 12 years
❏   C   is performed by the Seldinger technique
❏   D   is carried out by puncture on the surface of the tibia
❏   E   should be discontinued when other venous access has been
          obtained

**3.48   A cervical cord injury should be suspected in an unconscious
          patient if there is**

❏   A   grimacing to pain above the clavicle
❏   B   increased upper body tone
❏   C   priapism
❏   D   hypotension with bradycardia
❏   E   ability to extend the elbow

3.49   Theme: Neurotransmitters in the body

     A   Substance P
     B   Acetylcholine
     C   Adrenaline (epinephrine)
     D   Noradrenaline (norepinephrine)
     E   GABA

Select the most appropriate neurotransmitter from the list above for each
of the cases below. Each option may be used once only, more than once,
or not at all.

❏   1.   Is produced predominantly in the adrenal medulla.

❏   2.   Is an inhibitory neurotransmitter.

❏   3.   Is involved in neurogenic inflammation.

❏   4.   Predominant effect of this substance is peripheral
           vasoconstriction.

3.50   Following trauma, there is:

❏ A   increased muscle glycogen breakdown
❏ B   increased insulin secretion
❏ C   an elevation of blood glucose
❏ D   reduced excretion of excess water in the first 48 hours
❏ E   sodium conservation in the first 48 hours

3.51   Theme: Upper limb injuries

A   Axillary nerve
B   Median nerve
C   Ulnar nerve
D   Radial nerve

For each of the scenarios listed below, select the most likely nerve injury from the list above. Each option may be used once only, more than once, or not at all.

❏ 1.   A rugby player sustains a dislocation of his right shoulder. Clinical examination reveals an area of numbness over the badge area of his arm.
❏ 2.   A 6-year-old boy sustains a supracondylar fracture to his left humerus and is unable to oppose his thumb and index finger.

❏ 3.   A 10-year old boy falls off his bike dislocating his left elbow. Initially, there were no neurological signs. After joint relocation, the boy begins to complain of numbness in his little finger and is unable to grip anything.

3.52   Cerebrospinal fluid

❏ A   normally has a lower protein content than plasma
❏ B   flows between the third and fourth ventricles via the aqueduct of Sylvius
❏ C   is sterile
❏ D   is produced at a rate of 2 ml/h
❏ E   is produced by the arachnoid granulations

3.53   Cerebral blood flow

❏ A   fluctuates widely between a lying and a standing position
❏ B   is related to intracranial pressure
❏ C   is directly autoregulated to arterial PCO_2
❏ D   directly autoregulated to arterial PO_2
❏ E   is increased in the normal subject by the administration of mannitol

3.54   During fracture healing

❏ A   a vascular pannus is initially formed at the fracture site
❏ B   bone necrosis becomes apparent after 24–48 h
❏ C   osteoclasts lay down seams of uncalcified new bone
❏ D   the provisional callus is made up of woven bone
❏ E   woven bone is finally replaced with lamellar bone

3.55   Theme: Lower limb trauma

A   Anterior compartment syndrome
B   Posterior compartment syndrome
C   Arterial bleed
D   Traumatic nerve damage
E   DVT
F   Lateral compartment syndrome

For each of the scenarios listed below, select the most likely diagnosis from the list above. Each option may be used once only, more than once, or not at all.

❏ 1.   A motorcyclist rides into a lamp-post and is unable to bear weight on his left leg. Lachman's test is positive, but no bony injury is evident on X-ray. Passive dorsiflexion of the ankle causes considerable pain and the foot is cold and numb on palpation.

❏ 2.   Following an RTA, a patient sustained a displaced tibial fracture. He was admitted and an intramedullary nailing performed. He is now complaining of severe pain in the operated leg, especially on passive extension of the toes. He is also complaining of paraesthesia in the 1st web space.

3.56   Recognised features of cardiac tamponade include

❑ A   a 'globular' cardiac outline on CXR
❑ B   prominent heart sounds
❑ C   collapsed neck veins
❑ D   pulsus paradoxus
❑ E   hypertension
❑ F   Charcot's triad
❑ G   CVP may be normal

3.57   Regarding skin grafts

❑ A   split-skin grafts contain epidermis only
❑ B   split-skin grafts maintain their own blood supply
❑ C   thinner split-skin grafts are more likely to 'take' than thicker ones
❑ D   split-skin grafts result in greater contraction than full-thickness grafts
❑ E   minor degrees of bacterial contamination at the recipient site may inhibit a graft from 'taking'

3.58   Theme: Injury patterns following RTA trauma

A   Frontal-impact RTA
B   Side-impact RTA
C   Rear-impact RTA
D   Pedestrian in an RTA

For each of the traumatic injuries listed below, select the most likely scenario to produce the injuries from the list above. Each option may be used once, more than once, or not at all.

❑ 1. Pelvic compression fractures

❑ 2. Myocardial contusion

❑ 3. Lateral flail chest

❑ 4. Aortic transection

❑ 5. Lower limb fractures

3.59   Chronic subdural haematoma

❏   A   is usually produced by injury to the middle meningeal artery
❏   B   is rarely bilateral
❏   C   may not be present for several months
❏   D   usually produces papilloedema
❏   E   may occur after an apparently trivial injury

3.60   Absolute contraindication(s) to diagnostic peritoneal lavage (DPL) following abdominal trauma include

❏   A   early pregnancy
❏   B   an indication for laparotomy
❏   C   advanced cirrhosis
❏   D   known gastrointestinal malignancy
❏   E   previous abdominal operations

3.61   In the investigation of acute cervical spine injuries

❏   A   a good-quality lateral cervical spine film will identify approximately 70% of significant cervical spine injuries in adults
❏   B   an acceptable lateral cervical spine X-ray should include the upper border of T1
❏   C   normal AP, lateral and odontoid peg views effectively exclude significant cervical spine injury
❏   D   flexion and extension X-ray views are the best method of excluding ligamentous injury
❏   E   spinal cord injury without radiological abnormality is commoner in children than in adults
❏   F   if the C7–T1 junction is not visible on a lateral X-ray, a swimmer's view can be taken

3.62   Intervertebral disc collapse between L5 and S1

❏   A   would crush the L5 spinal nerve
❏   B   would impinge into the sacral segments of the cord
❏   C   usually causes pain to radiate over the medial malleolus
❏   D   would exaggerate the tendon reflex at the ankle
❏   E   may cause reduced sweating over the posterior aspect of the calf

3.63   Theme: Anatomy of intracranial haemorrhage/thrombosis

A   Cavernous venous sinus
B   External carotid artery
C   Middle meningeal artery
D   Sigmoid venous sinus
E   Internal carotid artery
F   Cerebral vein
G   Jugular vein
H   Cerebral artery

For each of the clinical scenarios below, select the vascular structure most likely to be involved from the list above. Each option may be used once, more than once, or not at all.

❏   1.   A collapsed 30-year-old woman is admitted with acute severe epistaxis. She had been complaining for some time previously of headache and diplopia, worse on looking to the left. On examination, she has a left-sided medial strabismus and pulsation of the left eye. Fresh red blood is gushing from her nose, her pulse is racing and her BP is dropping alarmingly. No signs of raised intracranial pressure are detectable.

❏   2.   A 12-year-old girl falls from her pony, hits her head on the trunk of a fallen tree and is knocked unconscious. She quickly recovers and feels well enough to continue the ride. That evening, she complains of headache and begins vomiting. Concerned by her increasingly detached behaviour, her father calls the doctor. She slowly drifts into unconsciousness. In A&E, she is found to be in a deep coma, with a bradycardia and mild papilloedema. Skull X-ray reveals a fracture over the left temple.

❏   3.   A 20-year-old male student comes to A&E complaining of morning headaches, which have remorselessly increased in severity and duration. Recently, his flatmate has noticed detached episodes in consciousness for which his friend has little or no recollection. Six weeks earlier the patient had bumped his head after an emergency stop whilst a passenger in his friend's car. He had hit his forehead on the windscreen, but was not knocked out and had dismissed the incident as minor. Whilst in A&E, he collapses and is unrousable. Examination reveals marked signs of raised intracranial pressure.

❏ 4. A 23-year-old man collapses whilst standing in a bus queue and is rushed to hospital without regaining consciousness. Examination confirms that he is deeply comatosed with severe signs of raised intracranial pressure, but no skull fractures.

❏ 5. A teenage girl with chronic sinusitis develops severe pain in her left eye and forehead. There is exophthalmos and oedema of the eyelids, cornea and root of her nose, associated with pyrexia, severe headache, and malaise. There is complete paralysis of all movements of the left eye.

3.64   Penetrating hepatic trauma

❏ A   can be managed conservatively in a stable patient
❏ B   may cause haemobilia
❏ C   is usually fatal
❏ D   causing excessive bleeding is best controlled by packing gauze swabs into the hepatic defect
❏ E   causing excessive bleeding may be controlled by Pringle's manoeuvre

3.65   In blunt head trauma

❏ A   the duration of post-traumatic amnesia correlates well with the degree of primary brain injury
❏ B   the duration of retrograde amnesia correlates well with the degree of primary brain injury
❏ C   depressed conscious level in a patient with a blood alcohol level over 300 mg/dl can safely be attributed to alcohol intoxication
❏ D   codeine phosphate analgesia must be avoided
❏ E   in a comatose patient with multiple injuries, haemodynamic stabilisation takes priority over evacuation of intracranial haematoma
❏ F   diffuse axonal injury is associated with wallerian degeneration

3.66   Theme: Cerebral injury

A   Subdural haematoma
B   Subarachnoid haemorrhage
C   Diffuse axonal injury
D   Extradural haematoma
E   Basal skull fracture
F   Intraventricular haemorrhage

For each of the patients below, select the form of cerebral injury from the list above which most closely matches the clinical scenario. Each option may be used once, more than once, or not at all.

❏   1.   A 28-year-old woman who was an unrestrained, front-seat car passenger hits the windscreen. She has an obvious broken nose and teeth. Bleeding from the nose, mouth and right ear is noted. She is conscious and has a GCS of 14.

❏   2.   A 40-year-old obese man presents with sudden onset of severe occipital headache.

❏   3.   An elderly man attends A&E having fallen a week before. He now has a fluctuating level of consciousness.

❏   4.   A 14-year-old girl fell off her bicycle. She had an initial loss of consciousness for 10 min, was then apparently normal for 1 hour, which was followed by a deteriorating level of consciousness.

3.67   The following are typical features of an acute extradural haematoma on CT scan:

❏   A   crescent-shaped haematoma
❏   B   haematoma crossing the suture line
❏   C   haematoma crossing the midline
❏   D   associated skull fracture
❏   E   decreased attenuation of the haematoma

3.68   Traumatic rupture of the thoracic aorta

❏ A   usually occurs just distal to the origin of the left subclavian artery
❏ B   is most common following an acceleration injury
❏ C   may cause a widened upper mediastinum and tracheal
           displacement
❏ D   is best demonstrated by CT scan
❏ E   is usually fatal
❏ G   can result in depression of the left mainstem bronchus

3.69   Theme: Radial nerve injury

A   Compression at the level of the elbow
B   Fracture at the level of the mid-humerus
C   Axillary compression
D   Laceration at the level of the wrist

For each of the scenarios listed below, select the most likely level of injury
from the list above. Each option may be used once only, more than once,
or not at all.

❏ 1. A 25-year-old man presents with weakness of the wrist and hand
         and paralysis of the triceps with an absent triceps reflex.

❏ 2. A 25-year-old man presenting with a wrist drop is unable to
         extend the metacarpophalangeal joints of the hand and has
         altered sensibility in the region of the anatomical snuff-box.

❏ 3. A 25-year-old man presents with failure to extend the
         metacarpophalangeal joints with weakness of thumb abduction
         and interphalangeal extension.

3.70   In the early assessment of severely injured patients

❏ A   hypotension must be assumed to be hypovolaemic in origin until
           proven otherwise
❏ B   a shorter neck facilitates orotracheal intubation
❏ C   tourniquets are to be encouraged for the control of blood loss
           from a limb
❏ D   a high-riding prostate is a contraindication to urethral
           catheterisation without a preceding urethrogram
❏ E   neck wounds penetrating the platysma should be explored in the
           A&E department

3.71   Diaphragmatic rupture from blunt trauma

❏   A   occurs most commonly to the right hemidiaphragm
❏   B   usually produces obvious initial CXR changes
❏   C   may cause abdominal visceral herniation that can be felt during the placement of a chest drain
❏   D   can be readily diagnosed by diagnostic peritoneal lavage (DPL)
❏   E   typically produces larger defects than penetrating injuries

3.72   Theme: Head injury

A   Extradural haematoma
B   Subdural haematoma
C   Base-of-skull fracture
D   Diffuse axonal injury
E   Concussion
F   Cerebral contusion

From the clinical scenarios below, select the one most likely pathology from the list above. Each option may be used once only, more than once, or not at all.

❏   1.   Prolonged coma, decerebrate posturing, no mass lesion on CT scan observed.

❏   2.   Bilateral 'black eyes' present.

❏   3.   Is typically associated with temporal bone fractures, headache, progression to coma, late unilateral pupil dilatation.

❏   4.   Brief loss of neurological function, confusion, double vision, headache and vomiting, usually all resolve rapidly – headaches and nausea may persist for a few weeks.

❏   5.   Transient loss of consciousness, return to consciousness, progression to coma occurs.

❏   6.   There is marked hearing loss, runny nose, sphenoid air–fluid level on X-ray.

❏   7.   Caused by the rupture of bridging veins. Skull fracture may not be evident, poor prognosis due to high incidence of associated brain damage.

3.73   Relating to soft tissue coverage

❏ A   composite grafts include skin, subcutaneous tissue and cartilage
❏ B   composite grafts maintain their own blood supply
❏ C   human epithelial cells can be grown in tissue cultures to provide
          sheets for grafting
❏ D   free flaps generally rely on blood supply from an artery of at
          least 3 mm in diameter
❏ E   advancement flaps depend on skin laxity to provide excess
          tissue when separated from their underlying structures

3.74   Gastrointestinal consequences of major burns include

❏ A   splanchnic vasodilatation
❏ B   acute gastric dilatation
❏ C   Cushing's ulcers
❏ D   paralytic ileus
❏ E   terminal ileal lymphoid hyperplasia

3.75   Theme: Tubes used in trauma

    A   Long, wide-bore central line
    B   Short, wide-bore intravenous cannula
    C   Urethral catheter
    D   Nasogastric tube
    E   Arterial line
    F   Cuffed endotracheal tube
    G   Guedel (oropharyngeal) airway

Select the most appropriate tube from the list above for each scenario or
definition below. Each option may be used once only, more than once, or
not at all.

❏ 1.   Reliable indicator of tissue perfusion in shock.

❏ 2.   Contraindicated in base-of-skull fractures.

❏ 3.   A definitive airway.

❏ 4.   The best route for giving fluids quickly.

❏ 5.   The best route for determining heart filling pressure.

❏ 6.   Will prevent aspiration of gastric contents.

3.76   In pelvic trauma

❑ A   pelvic fractures are usually isolated injuries
❑ B   haemorrhage is usually arterial in nature
❑ C   mortality of open pelvic fractures approaches 50%
❑ D   a single-view cystogram will exclude a bladder rupture
❑ E   pelvic vascular embolisation is the preferred operative approach
            for haemostasis
❑ F   penile meatal blood is an indication for retrograde
            urethrography
❑ G   retroperitoneal bleeding is unlikely
❑ H   external fixation can often control arterial bleeding

**3.77   Clinical indicators suggestive of acute inhalational injury
            include**

❑ A   dysphagia
❑ B   carbonaceous sputum
❑ C   oesophageal carbon deposits
❑ D   singeing of eyebrows
❑ E   subcutaneous emphysema

3.78   Acute traumatic diaphragmatic rupture

❑ A   is more frequent on the right side
❑ B   is often associated with mediastinal displacement
❑ C   may cause strangulation of abdominal viscera
❑ D   is usually treated surgically
❑ E   can often be treated conservatively

3.79   A femoral nerve injury would result in

❑ A   absence of the knee-jerk reflex
❑ B   anaesthesia over the anterior skin of the calf
❑ C   absence of the cremasteric reflex
❑ D   paraesthesia of the skin over the medial malleolus
❑ E   paraesthesia over the entire L2 dermatome

3.80   Theme: Patterns of injury

A   Fall from height
B   Rear car-seat passenger
C   Explosion
D   Trapped in house fire
E   Restrained front-seat passenger in rear-end car shunt
F   Fall into a canal

Select the most appropriate mechanism of injury from the list above, for the patterns of injury described below. Each option may be used once only, more than once, or not at all.

❑   1.   Multiple lacerations and deafness

❑   2.   Bilateral posterior hip dislocation and sternal fracture

❑   3.   Cervical neck sprain

❑   4.   Bilateral calcaneal fractures and C7 fracture

❑   5.   Pancreatic injury and lumbar spine fracture

3.81   Hyperbaric oxygen therapy

❑   A   can be used in the treatment of carbon monoxide poisoning
❑   B   can be applied with an anaesthetic breathing circuit
❑   C   may cause acute oxygen toxicity
❑   D   requires the use of a pressurised chamber
❑   E   typically consists of one 20-minute session

3.82   Traumatic chest injuries

❑   A   usually require surgery
❑   B   are associated with cardiac or major vascular injury in 10% of cases
❑   C   are responsible for 25% of trauma deaths
❑   D   producing sternal fractures may be associated with cardiac arrhythmias
❑   E   producing tracheal rupture are usually amenable to surgical repair with good outcome

3.83 Theme: Radiological signs in trauma

A   Anterior fat-pad sign
B   Posterior fat-pad sign
C   Apical capping
D   Talar shift
E   Loss of psoas shadow
F   Air–fluid level

For each of the conditions listed below, select the radiological sign that is most likely to be present on a plain film from the list above. Each option may be used once only, more than once, or not at all.

❏   1.   Traumatic thoracic aortic rupture

❏   2.   Unstable ankle

❏   3.   Retroperitoneal haemorrhage

❏   4.   Radial head fracture

3.84 During management of a multi-traumatised patient

❏   A   primary and secondary surveys should be repeated frequently to ascertain deterioration in patient status
❏   B   penile meatal blood is a contraindication to urethral catheterisation
❏   C   gastric tubes should not be passed transnasally if there is suspicion of a cribriform plate fracture
❏   D   skull X-rays are valuable in making immediate management decisions
❏   E   blood pressure is a good measure of actual tissue perfusion

3.85 Gunshot wounds to the abdomen

❏   A   should be managed non-operatively
❏   B   high-velocity bullets can result in tissue necrosis distant from the bullet track
❏   C   cause significant visceral injury in 40% of cases
❏   D   if an exit wound is absent, AXRs may help determine missile trajectory
❏   E   broad-spectrum antibiotics should be avoided to prevent organism resistance
❏   F   the mass of the bullet is more significant than its velocity

3.86   Tissue hypoxia secondary to chest trauma may result from

- ❏ A   pulmonary ventilation–perfusion mismatch
- ❏ B   hypocarbia
- ❏ C   hypovolaemia
- ❏ D   changes in the intrathoracic pressure relationships
- ❏ E   alveolar hypersensitivity

3.87   The primary survey of a seriously injured trauma patient includes

- ❏ A   airway maintenance with cervical spine control
- ❏ B   brief neurological examination
- ❏ C   abdominal assessment
- ❏ D   musculoskeletal assessment
- ❏ E   an assessment of pelvic stability
- ❏ F   control of external haemorrhage

3.88   Theme: Orthopaedic procedures

A   Intramedullary nail
B   Traction
C   Internal fixation with plate and screws
D   Debridement and external fixation
E   Amputation

For the fractures described below, select the most likely method of treatment from the list above. Each option may be used once only, more than once, or not at all.

- ❏ 1.   A 24-year-old male involved in an RTA presents with a severe closed head injury, flail chest and comminuted femoral shaft fracture. He is intubated for his head injury and a chest drain is inserted. He is now stabilised.

- ❏ 2.   A 30-year-old male involved in an RTA has a Grade IIIC open tibial fracture, complete loss of sensation in the sole of his foot and a tyre mark across his calf. At surgery his popliteal nerve is found to be crushed, shredded and divided.

- ❏ 3.   A 25-year-old man fell from a height, causing a haemopneumo-thorax, fractured left humerus and a closed comminuted fracture to the mid-shaft of the femur. A collar and cuff and a chest drain were used to stabilise the first two injuries.

3.89   Haemorrhage

❑ A   is defined as an acute or chronic loss of circulating blood
❑ B   the normal adult blood volume is approximately 7% of body weight
❑ C   the blood volume of obese patients is estimated by their ideal body weight
❑ D   the blood volume of children is approximately 15% of body weight
❑ E   tachycardia is the earliest measurable sign

3.90   Secondary survey of a severely injured patient

❑ A   only begins after the primary survey has been completed and resuscitation of life-threatening conditions has begun
❑ B   includes scoring on the Glasgow Coma Scale
❑ C   includes chest and pelvic X-rays
❑ D   does not include USS of the abdomen
❑ E   includes rectal examination
❑ F   includes urinary catheterisation

3.91   The Glasgow Coma Scale incorporates details on

❑ A   the best verbal response to stimulation
❑ B   peripheral reflex activity
❑ C   systolic blood pressure on arrival in the A&E department
❑ D   pulse rate following initial resuscitation
❑ E   eye opening to stimulation
❑ F   pupillary reflexes

3.92   Accepted diagnostic peritoneal lavage criteria indicating the need for laparotomy include

❑ A   catheter drainage of bile
❑ B   catheter aspiration of 5 ml of clear fluid
❑ C   lavage fluid exiting via a chest drain
❑ D   laboratory analysis of peritoneal lavage fluid (unspun) of 500 RBCs/mm^3
❑ E   laboratory analysis of peritoneal lavage fluid (unspun) of 500 WBCs/mm^3

3.93   In the treatment of spinal injuries

❑   A   IV naloxone has been shown to improve neurological recovery after spinal cord injury

❑   B   IV methylprednisolone given during the first 24 h significantly improves neurological recovery after spinal cord injury

❑   C   unstable thoracic spine fractures require operation as soon as the patient is haemodynamically stable

❑   D   fracture of the pedicles of the second cervical vertebra should initially be treated by in-line traction

❑   E   the initial neurological examination is a good predictor of prognosis

3.94   Theme: Knee injuries

A   Cruciate rupture
B   Osteoarthritis
C   Rheumatoid arthritis
D   Collateral ligament injury
E   Patella fracture

For each of the scenarios listed below, select the most likely injury from the list above. Each option may be used once only, more than once, or not at all.

❑   1.   A young footballer complains of an acutely swollen and painful knee. Aspiration reveals blood. There is no localised tenderness.

❑   2.   A middle-aged woman presents with a painful swollen knee after tripping and falling over. Aspiration reveals blood and fat globules.

❑   3.   A patient presents with tenderness on valgus and varus force.

3.95   The odontoid peg

❑   A   is connected to C1 by a transverse ligament
❑   B   is connected to the occiput by the alar ligament
❑   C   is seen on 'open mouth' view X-ray
❑   D   fracture causes a retropharyngeal haematoma
❑   E   has notochord remnant superiorly

3.96   Injury to the radial nerve in the radial (spiral) groove of the humerus causes loss of

❏   A   abduction of the thumb
❏   B   extension of the forearm
❏   C   supination
❏   D   cutaneous sensation over the dorsal surface of the first web space
❏   E   the brachioradialis tendon reflex

3.97   The following are complications of major burns:

❏   A   myoglobinuria
❏   B   hypoglycaemia
❏   C   hyponatraemia
❏   D   sepsis
❏   E   acute appendicitis

3.98   Theme: Chest trauma

A   Traumatic rupture of the thoracic aorta
B   Traumatic myocardial contusion
C   Cardiac tamponade
D   Tension pneumothorax
E   Massive haemothorax
F   Flail chest

For each of the traumatic conditions listed below, select the most appropriate major clinical signs from the list above. Each option may be used once, more than once, or not at all.

❏   1.   Restricted chest wall movement and rib crepitus

❏   2.   Shock associated with unilateral absent breath sounds and dullness to percussion

❏   3.   Tracheal displacement to the opposite side

❏   4.   Muffled heart sounds and pulsus paradoxus

❏   5.   Pleural capping and tracheal deviation to the right

❏   6.   Depression of the left main bronchus and obliteration of the aortopulmonary window on CXR

3.99   The posterior cord of the brachial plexus

❏   A   gives off the suprascapular nerve
❏   B   gives off branches to the shoulder joint
❏   C   supplies the deltoid muscle
❏   D   continues on as the radial nerve
❏   E   gives a supply to the coracobrachialis muscle

3.100   Signs of S1 nerve root compression include

❏   A   claw toes
❏   B   weakness of the extensor hallucis longus
❏   C   weakness of plantar flexion of the ankle
❏   D   weakness of ankle dorsiflexion
❏   E   enhanced ankle jerk reflex

3.101   Theme: Adult burns

A   1%
B   4.5%
C   7%
D   9%
E   14%
F   18%

For each of the statements below regarding adult cutaneous burns, select the correct percentage of the total body surface area from the list above. Each option may be used once, more than once, or not at all.

❏   1.   Burns to all the head and neck

❏   2.   Burns to all the anterior trunk (chest/abdomen)

❏   3.   Burns to all the male genitals

❏   4.   Burns to all the posterior trunk (upper and lower back)

❏   5.   Burns to the whole anterior aspect of one lower limb

❏   6.   Burns to the whole anterior aspect of one arm

❏   7.   Burns to the whole posterior aspect of both lower limbs

3.102 After damage to the ulnar nerve at the elbow, there is

❏ A anaesthesia over the skin of the thenar eminence
❏ B loss of abduction of the index finger
❏ C loss of adduction of the wrist
❏ D loss of flexion of the little finger
❏ E claw hand

3.103 Traction injury of the upper trunk of the brachial plexus results in

❏ A loss of medial rotation of the arm
❏ B paralysis of the deltoid muscle
❏ C loss of cutaneous sensation over the lateral surface of the arm
❏ D loss of supination
❏ E extension of the forearm

3.104 Theme: Shock

A Cardiogenic shock
B Neurogenic shock
C Spinal shock
D Haemorrhagic shock
E Septic shock

For each of the scenarios listed below, select the most appropriate type of shock from the list above. Each option may be used once only, more than once, or not at all.

❏ 1. Warm peripheries, tachycardia, onset several hours after trauma

❏ 2. Warm peripheries, bradycardia, onset immediately after trauma

❏ 3. Cold peripheries, tachycardia, develops rapidly after trauma

❏ 4. Cold peripheries, pulmonary oedema

3.105   Theme: Spinal trauma

A   Right posterior column
B   Spinothalamic tract
C   Corticospinal tract
D   Cerebral
E   Left posterior column
F   Medulla
G   Cauda equina
H   Cervical cord injury

For each of the clinical presentations below, select the most likely neurological injury from the list above. Each option may be used once, more than once, or not at all.

❏   1.   A young man is admitted after a high-velocity traffic accident. He is unconscious with flaccid areflexia and flaccid anal sphincter. He has diaphragmatic breathing and priapism.

❏   2.   A woman is admitted after having been hit by a car when crossing a busy road. She is complaining of pain between her shoulders. She is found to have lost position sense of her left toes and vibration sensation of her left foot.

CHAPTER 4: INTENSIVE CARE

4.1 **Common causes of an EMD (electromechanical dissociation) or pulseless electrical activity (PEA) arrest include**

- ❏ A hypovolaemia
- ❏ B electric shock
- ❏ C tension pneumothorax
- ❏ D hypoxia
- ❏ E cardiac tamponade

4.2 **Theme: Lung segments**

A Apical
B Superior lingular
C Lateral basal (left)
D Medial (right)
E Medial (left)
F Inferior lingular

For each of the statements below, select the most likely lung segment to be affected from the list above. Each option may be used once, more than once, or not at all.

- ❏ 1. A 3-year-old child has an inhaled a foreign body.

- ❏ 2. A 67-year-old presents with tuberculosis.

- ❏ 3. A 27-year-old presents with pneumonia.

- ❏ 4. A 20-year-old footballer has been kicked in the mouth and inhaled a tooth.

- ❏ 5. A patient presents with a past history of TB, CXR on preoperative assessment.

- ❏ 6. A patient has postoperative aspiration with formation of a pulmonary abscess.

4.3   Nutritional support

❑ A   cannot adequately be delivered except intravenously
❑ B   requirements are calculated according to the Harris–Benedict
         equation multiplied by a stress factor
❑ C   delivered enterally maintains the intestinal mucosa, thereby
         reducing bacterial translocation
❑ D   should only be used in elderly patients
❑ E   may result in metabolic complications
❑ F   can be delayed in obese individuals
❑ G   increases the risk of wound dehiscence

4.4   Myocardial blood flow

❑ A   is approximately 250 ml/min at rest
❑ B   is increased by pain
❑ C   the right coronary artery typically supplies one-third of the blood
         to the left ventricular muscle
❑ D   is dependent on arterial pressure
❑ E   occurs during systole

4.5   Theme: Cardiovascular physiology

    A   Atrial contraction (atrial systole)
    B   Isometric ventricular contraction
    C   Ventricular ejection
    D   Isometric ventricular relaxation
    E   Passive ventricular filling

For each of the events listed below, select the correct part of the cardiac
cycle from the list above. Each option may be used once, more than once,
or not at all.

❑ 1.   Closure of the mitral valve

❑ 2.   Opening of the aortic valve

❑ 3.   Second heart sound

❑ 4.   The Q wave

4.6   The pathophysiological effects of intermittent positive-pressure ventilation (IPPV) include

❑   A   reduced splanchnic blood flow
❑   B   decreased cardiac output
❑   C   hepatic failure
❑   D   hypotension
❑   E   pneumothorax
❑   F   lowered intracranial pressure

4.7   Cardiac index is defined as

❑   A   cardiac output/body surface area
❑   B   stroke volume × heart rate
❑   C   mean arterial pressure × systemic vascular resistance
❑   D   cardiac output/body weight
❑   E   cardiac output/heart rate

4.8   Respiratory insufficiency should be considered with

❑   A $PaO2$ 15 kPa on 40% O_2
❑   B $PaCO_2$ of 5 kPa on 40% O_2
❑   C   the inability to clear secretions
❑   D   a patient with confusion, agitation, drowsiness
❑   E   poor analgesia following abdominal surgery

4.9   Left coronary artery supplies

❑   A   majority of the left ventricle
❑   B   majority of the left atrium
❑   C   SA node in most cases
❑   D   AV node in most cases
❑   E   part of the right ventricle

4.10   Heart rate

❑   A   decreases on inspiration
❑   B   increases with pressure on the eyeball
❑   C   decreases with sleep
❑   D   increases after a meal
❑   E   decreases with pressure on the SA node

4.11   Theme: Structures in the transthoracic plane (of Louis)

A   Trachea
B   Superior vena cava
C   Mediastinal parietal pleura
D   T4 vertebra
E   Left brachiocephalic vein
F   Left pulmonary artery
G   Vagus nerve
H   2nd costal cartilage
I   Ascending aorta
J   Thoracic duct
K   Oesophagus
L   Left main bronchus

For each of the statements below, select the most likely option from the list above. Each option may be used once, more than once, or not at all.

❑   1.   Gives off a branch that ascends between the trachea and oesophagus.

❑   2.   Gives attachment to prevertebral fascia.

❑   3.   Has a vestigial ligamentous attachment.

❑   4.   Has a compound articulation with a secondary cartilaginous joint.

4.12   Central venous pressure

❑   A   affects atrial natriuretic peptide secretion
❑   B   affects antidiuretic hormone secretion
❑   C   regulates stroke volume
❑   D   depends on the tone of peripheral veins and venules
❑   E   is increased in congestive cardiac failure

4.13   The following are features of early septic shock:

❑   A   raised diastolic pressure
❑   B   bradycardia
❑   C   lymphopenia
❑   D   peripheral vasodilatation
❑   E   hypothermia
❑   F   neutropenia

4.14 Indications for enteral feeding include

- ❑ A severe diarrhoea
- ❑ B paralytic ileus
- ❑ C proximal small bowel fistula
- ❑ D large bowel obstruction
- ❑ E gastrocolic fistula

4.15 Pulmonary functional residual capacity is

- ❑ A equal to vital capacity minus the maximum inspiratory capacity
- ❑ B measured by the helium dilution technique
- ❑ C decreased in asthma
- ❑ D decreased in emphysema
- ❑ E decreased in pulmonary fibrosis

4.16 Nitrogen balance is positive

- ❑ A during the first 3 days following major surgery
- ❑ B in sepsis
- ❑ C during growth
- ❑ D whilst ACTH levels are high
- ❑ E immediately following exercise
- ❑ F following bone fractures

4.17 A high JVP is associated with

- ❑ A fluid overload
- ❑ B pericardial effusion
- ❑ C congestive cardiac failure
- ❑ D pulmonary hypertension
- ❑ E SVC obstruction

4.18 In atrial fibrillation, the following are acceptable treatments:

- ❑ A digoxin 0.25–0.5 mg orally, if no urgency
- ❑ B verapamil 5–10 mg intravenously
- ❑ C amiodarone 5 mg/kg IV infusion over 20 minutes
- ❑ D isoprenaline 2 mg/kg infusion over 2 minutes
- ❑ E phentolamine 10 mg/ml in 20 minutes

4.19   Theme: Respiratory physiology

A   Compliance
B   Functional residual capacity
C   PEEP
D   Vital capacity
E   Tidal volume
F FEV_1
G   Dead space
H   Shunt
I   West's zones
J   Starling resistor
K   Minute volume

For each of the definitions below, select the most appropriate term from the list above. Each option may be used once, more than once, or not at all.

❑   1.   This is the volume change per unit pressure change – a measure of distensibility.

❑   2.   Theoretical regions of lung tissue that demonstrate different effects of gravity on the regional alveoli and corresponding pulmonary circulation.

❑   3.   Equals the sum of residual volume and expiratory reserve volume.

❑   4.   This is the volume forcibly exhaled from full inspiration in 1 s.

❑   5.   An amount of venous blood that bypasses ventilated alveoli.

❑   6.   The volume of inspired air that takes no part in gas exchange.

❑   7.   Model of a length of collapsible tubing in a rigid box used to demonstrate the effects of gravity on regional pulmonary circulation.

❑   8.   The largest volume that can be expired after a maximal inspiration.

4.20   Theme: Structures in the transthoracic plane (of Louis)

A   Trachea
B   Superior vena cava
C   Mediastinal parietal pleura
D   T4 vertebra
E   Left brachiocephalic vein
F   Left pulmonary artery
G   Vagus nerve
H   2nd costal cartilage
I   Ascending aorta
J   Thoracic duct
K   Oesophagus
L   Left main bronchus

For each of the statements below, select the most likely option from the list above. Each option may be used once, more than once, or not at all.

❏   1.   Crosses the midline.

❏   2.   Has a bifurcation located in the plane.

❏   3.   Meet in the midline.

❏   4.   Receives the azygos vein.

4.21   Concerning the first rib, the

❏   A   scalenus medius is attached to the scalene tubercle
❏   B   subclavian artery passes posterior to the 1st thoracic nerve root
❏   C   subclavian vein passes across the 1st costochondral joint
❏   D   sympathetic trunk lies anterior to the neck
❏   E   subclavian vein and artery are separated by the scalenus anterior

4.22   In respiratory alkalosis

❏   A   carpopedal spasm may be corrected by rebreathing into a bag
❏   B   tetany occurs due to changes in calcium–protein binding
❏   C   there is a lowering of the plasma carbonic acid concentration
❏   D   there is an elevated HCO_3^- concentration in plasma
❏   E   the PCO_2 <5 kPa

4.23   Gas embolus is recognised in

❑   A   hydrogen peroxide wound irrigation
❑   B   criminal abortion
❑   C   varicose vein surgery
❑   D   central line insertion
❑   E   *Clostridium perfringens* infection

4.24   Risk of postoperative renal failure is increased in patients with

❑   A   preoperative sepsis
❑   B   preoperative jaundice
❑   C   preoperative hypertension
❑   D   benign prostatic hypertrophy

4.25   ARDS

❑   A   frequently causes no CXR changes
❑   B   produces hyaline fibrosis
❑   C   leads to increased alveolar permeability
❑   D   may occur secondary to septicaemia
❑   E   is commonly managed in a general-ward setting

4.26   Diaphragm

❑   A   descends after section of the phrenic nerve
❑   B   is attached to the lower six costal cartilages
❑   C   receives a sensory supply through the phrenic nerve
❑   D   has the oesophagus piercing the right crus
❑   E   has crura pierced by splanchnic nerves

4.27   The following are increased in acute renal failure:

❑   A   respiratory rate
❑   B   blood pH
❑   C   potassium
❑   D   arterial PCO_2
❑   E   plasma HCO_3^-

4.28   Nitric oxide

❏   A   is increased in endotoxic shock
❏   B   causes vasodilatation of smooth muscle
❏   C   is synthesised from inhaled nitrogen
❏   D   causes platelet aggregation
❏   E   is produced from protein metabolism in sepsis

4.29   In acute renal failure

❏   A   fluid resuscitation is rarely required
❏   B   acute cortical necrosis heralds a poor prognosis
❏   C   systemic infection characteristically complicates the illness
❏   D   pain control with NSAIDs should be stopped
❏   E   dialysis should be commenced early

4.30   Functional residual capacity (FRC)

❏   A   is increased in the elderly
❏   B   is measured by a helium dilution technique
❏   C   represents approximately <50% of vital capacity
❏   D   falls following abdominal surgery
❏   E   is the sum of the residual volume and expiratory reserve volume
❏   F   is reduced in asthma
❏   G   is increased in fibrosing alveolitis

4.31   When inserting an intercostal drain in the 5th intercostal space, the following structures are encountered:

❏   A   pectoralis major
❏   B   serratus anterior
❏   C   visceral pleura
❏   D   parietal pleura
❏   E   internal intercostal muscle
❏   F   transversus abdominis

4.32   In the heart, the right ventricle

❏   A   is the most likely chamber to be injured in a stabbing
❏   B   is the most anterior heart chamber
❏   C   is best visualised by transoesophageal echo
❏   D   is supplied by the right coronary artery
❏   E   receives no blood from the lungs

4.33 Complications of an ascending aortic dissection include

- ❑ A mitral valve rupture
- ❑ B aortic regurgitation
- ❑ C cardiac tamponade
- ❑ D acute myocardial infarction
- ❑ E pulmonary embolus
- ❑ F haemothorax

4.34 Atrial fibrillation may cause

- ❑ A mitral stenosis
- ❑ B stroke
- ❑ C mesenteric infarction
- ❑ D gangrene of the toes
- ❑ E dyspnoea
- ❑ F pulmonary embolism

4.35 The following actions may have a direct positive inotropic effect on the heart:

- ❑ A isoprenaline infusion
- ❑ B GTN infusion
- ❑ C intravenous calcium
- ❑ D intravenous furosemide (frusemide)
- ❑ E digoxin

4.36 The following cause an increase in the heart rate:

- ❑ A complete cardiac denervation
- ❑ B intravenous adenosine
- ❑ C intravenous adrenaline (epinephrine)
- ❑ D salbutamol
- ❑ E metronidazole

4.37 Causes of ARDS (adult respiratory distress syndrome) include

- ❑ A sepsis
- ❑ B fat embolism
- ❑ C acute pancreatitis
- ❑ D acute renal failure
- ❑ E burns

4.38   Theme: Ventilation

A   PEEP
B   CPAP
C   Intermittent mandatory ventilation
D   High-frequency jet insufflation
E   Pressure-controlled ventilation
F   Volume-controlled ventilation
G   Minute-volume divided ventilation
H   Reversed I:E ratio

For each of the statements below, select the most appropriate mode of ventilation from the list above. Each option may be used once, more than once, or not at all.

❑   1.   Application of positive airway pressure throughout all phases of spontaneous ventilation.

❑   2.   Can be used to improve oxygenation in respiratory failure in addition to PEEP.

❑   3.   With a tidal volume of up to 150 ml, cycled at 60–600/min, ventilation is often delivered via a cannula inserted through the cricothyroid membrane.

❑   4.   Ventilator mode best used to provide a fixed tidal volume.

❑   5.   Ventilation best used to expand poorly compliant lungs.

❑   6.   May be used to reduce FiO_2 requirement and improve oxygenation.

❑   7.   A preset minute volume is delivered by the ventilator, but the patient is allowed to breathe spontaneously between ventilator breaths.

4.39   Tracheostomy

❑   A   is uncomplicated by thyroid disease
❑   B   may be needed for bronchial toilet
❑   C   is straightforward in people with a short neck
❑   D   will increase anatomical dead space
❑   E   increases the ventilation–perfusion mismatch

4.40 Indications for intubation and ventilation include

- ❏ A inability to control the airway
- ❏ B PCO_2 >5 kPa
- ❏ C poor bronchial toilet
- ❏ D PaO_2 <10 kPa
- ❏ E GCS <8

4.41 Hazards of artificial ventilation include

- ❏ A basal atelectasis
- ❏ B surgical emphysema
- ❏ C hypotension
- ❏ D cerebral oedema
- ❏ E acute gastric dilatation

4.42 100% oxygen treatment may be administered by

- ❏ A CPAP circuit
- ❏ B normal face-mask
- ❏ C endotracheal tube
- ❏ D resuscitation bag with reservoir
- ❏ E nasal specula

4.43 Paralysis of the left hemidiaphragm

- ❏ A may be caused by section of the cord below C6
- ❏ B may be caused by section of the left phrenic nerve alone
- ❏ C causes flattening of the diaphragm during inspiration
- ❏ D causes paradoxical movement
- ❏ E increases intrathoracic pressure on the left
- ❏ F may occur with carcinoma of the bronchus

4.44 Inspiration involves

- ❏ A descent of the hemidiaphragms
- ❏ B reduction of the vertical dimension of the chest
- ❏ C upward/forward movement of the first rib
- ❏ D contraction of the intercostal muscles
- ❏ E long thoracic nerve of Bell (n. to the serratus anterior)

4.45   Theme: Renal failure

A   Oliguria
B   Hypercalcaemia
C   Acute tubular necrosis
D   Cortical necrosis
E   Hyperkalaemia
F   Prerenal renal failure
G   Hypertension
H   Pulmonary oedema
I   Pelviureteric junction obstruction

For each of the statements below, select the most appropriate diagnosis from the list above. Each option may be used once, more than once, or not at all.

❏   1.   A 29-year-old man is trapped in a car involved in an RTA, and sustains a prolonged period of hypotension. He is oliguric on admission and becomes anuric over the next few hours. He requires dialysis for 6 days, and over the next 4 days his renal function gradually returns to normal.

❏   2.   An 80-year-old man with a bowel perforation required 3 litres of crystalloid to correct his blood pressure and improve perfusion. As his haemoglobin was 8 g/dl preoperatively, he was transfused with three units of packed cells over 4 hours. During the final unit, he became hypoxic and confused.

❏   3.   A 35-year-old woman is admitted with a lacerated liver and perforated duodenum. Her urine output was initially 12 ml/h but following 2 litres of saline and 2 units of blood, it increased to 110 ml/h.

4.46   In the immediate postoperative period following an anterior resection there is an increased

❏   A   urinary sodium loss
❏   B   secretion of ADH
❏   C   urea production
❏   D   urine osmolality
❏   E   glomerular filtration rate

4.47 **Well-recognised causes of hypertension in the postoperative period are**

- ❑ A urinary retention
- ❑ B pain
- ❑ C isofluorane
- ❑ D epidural analgesia
- ❑ E acute tubular necrosis
- ❑ F sepsis

4.48 **Heat loss during laparotomy may be minimised by**

- ❑ A humidification of inspired gases
- ❑ B lavage with warm saline
- ❑ C maintaining the environmental temperature at 20 °C
- ❑ D use of a heated blanket set at 35 °C
- ❑ E use of a heat-reflecting blanket

4.49 **Hypokalaemia**

- ❑ A produces peaked T waves on ECG
- ❑ B causes the heart to arrest in diastole
- ❑ C is seen in metabolic acidosis
- ❑ D may occur following extensive muscle trauma
- ❑ E may be seen in pancreatic fistulas
- ❑ F may be seen in pyloric stenosis

4.50 **Complications of arterial lines include**

- ❑ A arteriovenous fistulas
- ❑ B anaemia
- ❑ C aneurysm
- ❑ D gangrene
- ❑ E heart block

4.51 **In the management of respiratory disorders**

- ❑ A $PaCO_2$ is increased in type I respiratory failure
- ❑ B $PaCO_2$ is reduced in type I respiratory failure
- ❑ C acute left ventricular failure reduces $PaCO_2$
- ❑ D oxygen saturation is always a good guide to tissue oxygenation
- ❑ E acidosis may occur with a high HCO_3^- concentration

4.52 Angiotensin II

❏ A stimulates renin release
❏ B inhibits aldosterone release
❏ C is a weak arteriolar vasoconstrictor
❏ D is converted from angiotensin I in the lung
❏ E is released by hypovolaemia

4.53 Drugs known to cause renal failure include the following:

❏ A mannitol
❏ B β-blockers
❏ C thyroxine
❏ D ciprofloxacin
❏ E vancomycin

4.54 Theme: Anatomy of the heart

A Right coronary artery
B Coronary sinus
C Membranous interventricular septum
D Moderator band
E Septal cusp of the tricuspid valve
F Anterior cusp of the mitral valve
G Muscular interventricular septum
H Interatrial septum
I Sulcus terminalis
J Left atrial appendage
K Oblique pericardial sinus
L Infundibulum

For each of the statements below, select the most likely option from the list above. Each option may be used once, more than once, or not at all.

❏ 1. Is connected to the largest papillary muscle.

❏ 2. Lies posterior to the left atrium.

❏ 3. Is the location of the bundle of His.

❏ 4. Is the location of the atrioventricular node.

4.55   Physiological responses to a loss of circulating blood volume include

❑   A   peripheral venular vasoconstriction
❑   B   peripheral arteriolar vasoconstriction
❑   C   reduced resistance to blood flow
❑   D   transcapillary refilling
❑   E   haemoconcentration
❑   F   tachycardia

4.56   The following suggest that respiratory failure is chronic rather than acute:

❑   A   plasma HCO_3^- of 39 mmol/l
❑   B PaO_2 of 9 kPa
❑   C PaO_2 of 7 kPa
❑   D   arterial pH 7.2
❑   E   the presence of a hypoxic respiratory drive

4.57   Acute renal failure

❑   A   is drug induced in 75% of cases
❑   B   occurs in approximately 30% of critically ill patients
❑   C   may produce little histological change
❑   D   is usually the result of damage to the proximal tubule
❑   E   carries an overall mortality rate of 10%

4.58   Central venous pressure (CVP)

❑   A   is affected by the Valsalva manoeuvre
❑   B   is elevated in right ventricular failure
❑   C   is normal in septic shock
❑   D   accurately reflects cardiac output
❑   E   is raised in hypertension

4.59   The oxygen–haemoglobin dissociation curve is displaced to the left by

❑   A   an increase in pH
❑   B   anaemia
❑   C   a fall in PCO_2
❑   D   pyrexia
❑   E   a fall in 2,3-DPG

4.60   In shock

- ❏ A   septic shock produces a high SVR and high CO
- ❏ B   cardiogenic shock produces a low SVR and low CO
- ❏ C   neurogenic shock produces a low SVR and high CO
- ❏ D   anaphylactic shock produces a very low lactic acid level
- ❏ E   septic shock produces a low SVR and high CO

4.61   Changes in cellular metabolism associated with shock include

- ❏ A   accumulation of lactic acid
- ❏ B   increased ATP production
- ❏ C   passage of sodium into cells
- ❏ D   passage of potassium into cells
- ❏ E   lysosomal fragmentation
- ❏ F   increased ketone production

4.62   The management of severe anaphylactic shock may include

- ❏ A   airway maintenance and oxygen
- ❏ B   intravenous fluids
- ❏ C   intra-arterial adrenaline (epinephrine)
- ❏ D   nebulised bronchoconstrictors
- ❏ E   β-blockers

4.63   Theme: Vascular resistance

- A   Increased peripheral vascular resistance
- B   Increased pulmonary vascular resistance
- C   Decreased peripheral vascular resistance
- D   No change in peripheral vascular resistance
- E   No change in pulmonary vascular resistance

Select from the list above, the most appropriate description for each of the cases below. Each option may be used once only, more than once, or not at all.

- ❏ 1. Septic shock
- ❏ 2. Oral calcium-channel blockers
- ❏ 3. Hypoxia
- ❏ 4. Bilateral below-knee amputations

4.64   Theme: Surface/radiological anatomy of the thorax

    A   5th intercostal space
    B   Left sternoclavicular joint
    C   Right sternoclavicular joint
    D   Right pulmonary artery
    E   Manubriosternal joint
    F   4th rib
    G   1st left costal cartilage
    H   1st right costal cartilage
    I   3rd intercostal space

For each of the statements below, select the most likely landmark from the list above. Each option may be used once, more than once, or not at all.

❑   1. Bifurcation of the brachiocephalic artery

❑   2. Horizontal fissure of the right lung

❑   3. Left ventricle

4.65   Signs of pulmonary thromboembolism may include

❑   A   ECG pattern of $S_1Q_3T_3$
❑   B   elevated arterial PCO_2
❑   C   mismatched defects on ventilation–perfusion lung scan
❑   D   pleural effusion on CXR
❑   E   obstruction in the pulmonary circulation on pulmonary angiography

4.66   Adult respiratory distress syndrome (ARDS)

❑   A   is occasionally due to pulmonary oedema of cardiac origin
❑   B   promotes superoxide-induced parenchymal damage
❑   C   does not affect pulmonary ventilation–perfusion matching
❑   D   is associated with discrete pulmonary nodules on X-ray

4.67   Features of ARDS include

❑   A   interstitial and alveolar oedema
❑   B   granulomas
❑   C   hyaline membrane formation
❑   D   glandular hyperplasia
❑   E   interstitial fibrosis

4.68   Theme: Pathological chest conditions

A   Pulmonary cysts
B   Bronchogenic cysts
C   Aspergilloma
D   Malignant mesothelioma
E   Idiopathic mediastinal fibrosis

For each of the clinical scenarios listed below, select the most likely lesion from the list above. Each of the options may be used once, more than once, or not at all.

❏   1.   Mycelial mass present with cellular debris.

❏   2.   Affects both visceral and parietal pleura.

❏   3.   Connected to the airways and therefore contain air.

❏   4.   Is thought to have an autoimmune aetiology.

❏   5.   Usually closely related to the trachea, hilum or oesophagus.

4.69   Multiple organ dysfunction syndrome (MODS)

❏   A   outcome is improved by the use of pulmonary artery catheters
❏   B   only occurs after major trauma
❏   C   may involve inflammatory mediators
❏   D   when treated aggressively has a universally excellent outcome
❏   E   survival is increased with the administration of endotoxin antibodies

4.70   A CT scan section through the manubriosternal joint will demonstrate

❏   A   the bifurcation of the brachiocephalic artery
❏   B   the commencement of the aortic arch
❏   C   T4 vertebral body
❏   D   the bifurcation of the trachea
❏   E   the thoracic duct crossing the midline

4.71   Bleeding from the middle meningeal artery following head injury

❏   A   the posterior branch is mainly affected
❏   B   results in an extradural haematoma
❏   C   may produce ipsilateral pupillary constriction
❏   D   is usually caused by a trivial incident
❏   E   typically causes a biconvex-shaped lesion on CT

4.72   The left lung has

❏   A   10 bronchopulmonary segments
❏   B   3 lobes
❏   C   3 bronchial openings
❏   D   2 pulmonary veins
❏   E   an arterial supply from the aorta

4.73   Theme: Trauma and shock

A   Neurogenic shock
B   Septic shock
C   Cardiogenic shock
D   Hypovolaemic shock

For each of the scenarios listed below, select the most likely diagnosis from the list above. Each option may be used once only, more than once, or not at all.

❏   1.   A 20-year-old man was walking across the road when he was hit by an oncoming car. He sustained a severe laceration to his scalp and some bruising was noted over his right eye. His Glasgow Coma Scale on admission to the A&E department was 12. He was maintaining his own airway. His blood pressure on admission was 70/40 mmHg with a tachycardia of 110/min. Severe pain was noted on springing of his pelvis with some perineal bruising.

❏   2.   A 60-year-old man who had a myocardial infarction 5 years ago was brought into the A&E complaining of epigastric pain. He appeared slightly dyspnoeic and icteric. He was noted to have a BP of 90/50 mmHg and a pulse of 100/min with warm peripheries. ECG and CXR were normal.

4.74   In the base of the skull the

❏   A   foramen magnum transmits the basilar artery
❏   B   foramen spinosum transmits the VIIth cranial nerve
❏   C   foramen rotundum transmits the maxillary nerve
❏   D   foramen ovale transmits the greater petrosal nerve
❏   E   foramen lacerum transmits the mandibular nerve

4.75   Main bronchial airways

❏   A   the left bronchus is longer than the right
❏   B   the right main bronchus has a wider diameter than the left
❏   C   aspiration pneumonitis is more common in the right lower lobe than the left
❏   D   the left main bronchus divides before entering the lung
❏   E   foreign bodies more commonly lodge in the right than the left main bronchus

4.76   The recurrent laryngeal nerve

❏   A   supplies the cricothyroid muscle
❏   B   partially supplies the trachea
❏   C   lies alongside the inferior thyroid artery
❏   D   should be retracted during tracheostomy to avoid damage
❏   E   runs between the oesophagus and trachea in the neck
❏   F   supplies the mucous surface of the vocal cords

4.77   The external jugular vein

❏   A   receives a branch from the retromandibular vein
❏   B   lies anterior to the scalenus anterior
❏   C   joins the subclavian vein
❏   D   has no valves
❏   E   pierces the deep cervical fascia

4.78   When dissecting the left main bronchus the following structures may be encountered:

❏   A   phrenic nerve
❏   B   vagus nerve
❏   C   recurrent laryngeal nerve
❏   D   azygos vein
❏   E   aorta

4.79   The right coronary artery

❏   A   originates in the anterior aortic sinus
❏   B   is overlain by the right atrial appendage
❏   C   supplies the sinoatrial node
❏   D   lies on the infundibulum of the right ventricle
❏   E   anastomoses with branches of the left coronary artery

4.80   Theme: Anatomy of the lungs and airways

A   Left main bronchus
B   Right main bronchus
C   Transthoracic plane
D   Left pulmonary artery
E   Left pulmonary vein
F   Trachea
G   Lobes of the lungs
H   Bronchial artery

For each of the statements below, select the most likely option from the list above. Each option may be used once, more than once, or not at all.

❏   1.   Is separated from the arch of the aorta by the vagus nerve.

❏   2.   Lies behind the left brachiocephalic vein.

❏   3.   Is the most anterior structure in the hilum.

❏   4.   Lies anterior to the oesophagus in the inferior mediastinum.

❏   5.   Bifurcates outside the lung.

4.81   The right atrium

❏   A   forms the right border of the heart
❏   B   lies in front of the left atrium
❏   C   has the coronary sinus opening above the septal cusp of the tricuspid valve
❏   D   has a posterior wall formed by the interatrial septum
❏   E   has the sinoatrial node medial to the sulcus terminalis

4.82   The diaphragm

❏ A   has a left crus attached to the L3 vertebra
❏ B   is pierced by the splanchnic nerves
❏ C   has an arterial supply from the abdominal aorta
❏ D   has a lateral arcuate ligament overlain by the kidney
❏ E   is related to the suprarenal glands

4.83   When dissecting the right main bronchus the following structures may be encountered:

❏ A   the right phrenic nerve
❏ B   the right vagus nerve
❏ C   the right recurrent laryngeal nerve
❏ D   the hemizygos nerve
❏ E   the azygos vein

4.84   Branches of the subclavian arteries supply the

❏ A   thyroid gland
❏ B   breast
❏ C   rectus abdominis muscle
❏ D   brainstem
❏ E   diaphragm

4.85   The hilum of the left lung

❏ A   has the phrenic nerve lying anterior
❏ B   has the vagus nerve lying posterior
❏ C   contains upper and lower lobe bronchi
❏ D   is separated from the aortic arch by the vagus nerve
❏ E   has the pulmonary artery anterior to the main bronchus

4.86   Cardiopulmonary bypass

❏ A   may produce mild postoperative neuropsychological problems
❏ B   is a recognised cause of pancreatitis
❏ C   is complicated by a severe stroke in 10% of cases
❏ D   causes a thrombocythaemia
❏ E   produces elevated cortisol levels

4.87   Theme: Cardiorespiratory physiology

A   Cardiac output of 2 litres
B   Metabolic acidosis
C   Low MCV
D   Shift of the O_2 dissociation curve to the right
E   Shift of the O_2 dissociation curve to the left
F   Normal blood volume is only maintained owing to aldosterone
G   Packed cell volume of 40%

Select the most appropriate answer from the list above for each of the cases below. Each option may be used once only, more than once, or not at all.

❑   1.   A 45-year-old RTA victim has lost 2 litres blood, has a fractured pelvis and a ruptured spleen. He is grossly hypotensive.

❑   2.   A 38-year-old woman has long-standing menorrhagies.

❑   3.   A 52-year-old man suffers from chronic bronchitis and is retaining CO_2.

4.88   The following factors increase cardiac output:

❑   A   standing from a lying position
❑   B   eating
❑   C   rapid arrhythmias
❑   D   long-term acclimatisation at altitude
❑   E   late pregnancy
❑   F   histamine

4.89   Perioperative myocardial infarction

❑   A   most commonly occurs on day 1 postoperatively
❑   B   is more common in patients with previous infarction
❑   C   is unaffected by the degree of anaesthetic monitoring
❑   D   has a mortality of 50–70%
❑   E   is rare in patients with no previous history of coronary heart disease

4.90 The functional residual capacity (FRC)

- ❏ A can be measured using the helium dilution technique
- ❏ B is the tidal volume plus the expiratory reserve volume
- ❏ C is approximately 60% of vital capacity
- ❏ D is decreased when supine
- ❏ E is approximately 2.5 litres in a healthy adult male

4.91 Lung spirometry is able to measure

- ❏ A total lung capacity
- ❏ B FEV_1
- ❏ C residual volume
- ❏ D the FEV_1:FVC ratio
- ❏ E the peak expiratory flow rate

4.92 Pulse oximetry

- ❏ A provides a direct indication of arterial PO_2
- ❏ B has a linear relationship with oxygen carriage
- ❏ C is inaccurate in the presence of high levels of carbon monoxide
- ❏ D indicates adequate tissue oxygen delivery if readings are over 95%
- ❏ E indicates adequate ventilation if readings are over 95%

4.93 Central tendon of the diaphragm is pierced by the

- ❏ A oesophagus
- ❏ B vagus nerve
- ❏ C inferior vena cava
- ❏ D greater splanchnic nerves
- ❏ E right phrenic nerve
- ❏ F aorta
- ❏ G azygos vein

4.94 The aortic arch

- ❏ A lies anterior to the brachiocephalic veins
- ❏ B gives attachment to the pretracheal fascia
- ❏ C arches directly over the right pulmonary artery
- ❏ D arches above the manubriosternal joint
- ❏ E is covered by pleura

4.95   The left phrenic nerve

❑   A   carries sympathetic fibres to the diaphragm
❑   B   lies on the fibrous pericardium
❑   C   innervates the peritoneum
❑   D   originates from the C5 segment of the spinal cord
❑   E   enters the chest anterior to the subclavian vein

4.96   The surface of the right lung is indented by the

❑   A   trachea
❑   B   oesophagus
❑   C   superior vena cava
❑   D   right ventricle
❑   E   subclavian vein

4.97   Theme: The denervated heart

A   Lack of parasympathetic stimulation
B   Release of catecholamines
C   Increased venous return
D   Transplant rejection
E   Hypersensitivity of SA node to catecholamines
F   Decreased baroreceptor activity

For each of the heart rhythms listed below, select the most likely cause from the list of options above. Each option may be used once only, more than once, or not at all.

❑   1.   Resting tachycardia

❑   2.   Tachycardia in response to exercise

❑   3.   Ventricular fibrillation

4.98   Theme: Blood gases

    A   Metabolic acidosis
    B   Metabolic alkalosis
    C   Respiratory acidosis
    D   Respiratory alkalosis
    E   Chronic respiratory acidosis
    F   Normal acid–base balance

For each of the sets of results below, choose the most likely diagnosis from the list of options above. Each option may be used once only, more than once, or not at all.

	pH	PO_2 (kPa)	PCO_2 (kPa)	HCO_3^- (mmol/l)
❏ 1.	7.6	10.2	5.8	32
❏ 2.	7.3	8.0	8.2	28
❏ 3.	7.2	14.0	3.5	12
❏ 4.	7.4	12.0	5.2	22

4.99   The trachea

❏   A   is palpable
❏   B   bifurcates behind the manubriosternal joint
❏   C   has a left main bronchus more vertical than the right
❏   D   has a left main bronchus that branches outside the hilum
❏   E   is innervated by the recurrent laryngeal nerve

CHAPTER 5: NEOPLASIA: TECHNIQUES AND OUTCOME OF SURGERY

5.1 **The following tumours and related markers have been correctly paired:**

- ❑ A teratoma and α-fetoprotein
- ❑ B parathyroid tumours and calcitonin
- ❑ C choriocarcinoma and β-hCG
- ❑ D serous ovarian cancer and CA-125
- ❑ E prostate carcinoma and alkaline phosphatase
- ❑ F cervical cancer and squamous-cell carcinoma antigen

5.2 **The following are suggestive of a good prognosis in malignant melanoma:**

- ❑ A male sex
- ❑ B low Breslow thickness
- ❑ C the presence of ulceration
- ❑ D older age
- ❑ E mucosal primary site
- ❑ F truncal primary site
- ❑ G white ethnicity

5.3 **Theme: Audit**

A Outcome
B Incident review
C Criterion
D Strategic

For each of the situations below select the most likely answer from the list above. Each option may be used once, more than once, or not at all.

- ❑ 1. Assessment of trauma patients who are brought into the A&E department unconscious and hypotensive, to evaluate whether colloid fluids were given.

- ❑ 2. The use of emergency IVU.

5.4   In devising a suitable screening test for malignant cancer, the

❏ A   test should have high specificity
❏ B   test should have high sensitivity
❏ C   tumour should be of anaplastic type
❏ D   tumour should have a short latent phase
❏ E   test should be well accepted by the population
❏ F   natural history of the disease should be adequately understood

5.5   Malignant melanoma

❏ A   spreads via the bloodstream if lymph nodes are palpable
❏ B   may be excised with a 1-cm excision margin for a Breslow
         thickness 0.75 mm
❏ C   skin metastases may regress spontaneously
❏ D   resection of lymph nodes increases survival by 50%
❏ E   originating in the neck and trunk are more frequently associated
         with the male sex

5.6   The following are malignant:

❏ A   mucosal hamartoma
❏ B   sarcoma
❏ C   melanoma
❏ D   adenoma
❏ E   Krukenberg tumour
❏ F   Zollinger–Ellison syndrome
❏ G   Barrett's oesophagus

5.7   In the management of early breast cancer

❏ A   axillary dissection prolongs survival
❏ B   mastectomy is associated with significantly higher survival rates
         than conservative surgery
❏ C   postoperative radiotherapy reduces the incidence of local
         recurrence
❏ D   adjuvant tamoxifen reduces mortality in postmenopausal
         patients
❏ E   systemic chemotherapy has improved local control but not
         overall survival

5.8   Theme: Consent for surgical treatment

A   Yes, surgery can proceed
B   No, surgery cannot proceed
C   Apply to make the child a ward of court
D   Obtain consent from wife
E   Obtain consent from patient

For each of the situations below, select the most likely answer from the list above. Each option may be used once, more than once, or not at all.

❑   1.   A 24-year-old man found unconscious by the road side is brought in by ambulance. It is evident that the patient's condition is rapidly deteriorating because of an expanding extradural haematoma and he is unable to give consent. His wife had been contacted and is at the hospital but has expressed her refusal to allow him to be operated on. Would you proceed against her wishes?

❑   2.   A member of an extreme religious sect has brought in his 11-year-old son with generalised peritonitis from a perforated appendix. His condition deteriorates and he needs a laparotomy which both parents adamantly refuse, saying that he will recover through the fervent prayers of members of his sect. Despite repeated attempts by the surgical team to persuade the parents of this child, they refuse to give consent for the surgical treatment that the surgeon deems to be essential. What option is available to the surgeon?

❑   3.   A 70-year-old severely psychiatrically ill woman is undergoing compulsory psychiatric treatment having been sectioned under the Mental Health Act. She has a fall in the psychiatry unit and sustains a fracture of the neck of her right femur for which she is referred for surgical treatment The orthopaedic surgeon is of the opinion that internal fixation of the fracture is her best management, in agreement with her psychiatrist. Her psychiatric state does not allow her to give informed consent for surgery. What process should follow?

❑   4.   A 63-year-old man with a brain tumour refuses any surgery and expresses his wish formally in writing. He is judged to be competent mentally. The following day he enters into a coma and his wife who was abroad arrives at his bedside and demands that surgical treatment is commenced. Can surgery proceed?

5.9   Aggressiveness of a malignant melanoma is suggested by

- ❑   A   lymphadenopathy
- ❑   B   bleeding
- ❑   C   satellite lesions
- ❑   D   flat lesions
- ❑   E   amelanotic lesions

5.10   Malignancy

- ❑   A   is the second highest cause of mortality in the UK
- ❑   B   testicular tumours usually spread to inguinal lymph nodes
- ❑   C   prostatic carcinoma spreads to the vertebrae, bypassing the lungs
- ❑   D   prostatic tumours are most commonly adenocarcinomas
- ❑   E   osteosarcoma spreads to the lungs via the thoracic duct

5.11   β-Naphthylamine is a known cause of

- ❑   A   small-cell carcinoma of the lung
- ❑   B   bladder cancer
- ❑   C   breast cancer
- ❑   D   adenocarcinoma of the stomach
- ❑   E   chemical pneumonitis
- ❑   F   lymphoma

5.12   Theme: Death and the law

   A   Coroner
   B   Any medical practitioner
   C   Registrar of births and deaths
   D   Coroner's officer
   E   Medical practitioner who attended during previous 14 days

For each of the statements below, select the most likely answer from the list above. Each option may be used once, more than once, or not at all.

- ❑   1.   Certify death.

- ❑   2.   Issue immediate death certificate.

- ❑   3.   Call an inquest.

- ❑   4.   Send information concerning the cause of death to the Office of Population Censuses and Surveys.

5.13 Ductal carcinoma *in situ* (DCIS) of the breast

❏ A usually presents as a palpable mass
❏ B can be distinguished from invasive carcinoma on fine-needle aspiration cytology (FNAC)
❏ C accounts for around 17% of screen-detected breast cancers
❏ D is generally curable by total mastectomy
❏ E is associated with axillary node metastases in 20% of cases
❏ F is radioresistant

5.14 The following factors indicate a poor prognosis in breast cancer:

❏ A involvement of the internal mammary nodes
❏ B tubular type
❏ C abundance of oestrogen receptors
❏ D high histological grade (III)
❏ E age over 50 years at presentation

5.15 Theme: Cancer therapy options

A Radiotherapy and steroids
B Hormonal manipulation
C Systemic chemotherapy
D Surgical resection

For each of the clinical scenarios listed below, select the most appropriate management options from the list above. Each option may be used once, more than once, or not at all.

❏ 1. Recurrent non-Hodgkin's lymphoma

❏ 2. Isolated pulmonary metastasis from colorectal cancer

❏ 3. Residual anal squamous-cell carcinoma (SCC) after local radiotherapy

❏ 4. Metastatic prostatic carcinoma not involving bone

❏ 5. Diffuse intracranial metastatic melanoma

good or bad?.

5.16   Prognostic indicators in breast cancer include

❏   A   an affected 1st-degree relative
❏   B   inflammatory carcinoma
❏   C   oestrogen-receptor positivity
❏   D   presence of involved internal thoracic nodes
❏   E   presence of an involved supraclavicular node

5.17   Patients suitable for conservative breast surgery include those with

❏   A   lobular carcinoma
❏   B   ductal carcinoma *in situ*
❏   C   a tumour of 5 cm diameter
❏   D   a tumour with proven metastases
❏   E   tumours in separate quadrants
❏   F   diffuse malignant microcalcifications
❏   G   previous radiotherapy to the breast

5.18   Staging of malignant tumours

❏   A   helps to establish prognosis
❏   B   includes details of locoregional and distant sites
❏   C   can be made solely on the basis of a histological specimen
❏   D   may be altered by response to irradiation treatment
❏   E   takes into account the local anatomy for individual primary
             tumour sites

5.19   Which of the following have malignant potential:

❏   A   Bowen's disease
❏   B   solar keratosis
❏   C   keratoacanthoma
❏   D   Spitz naevus
❏   E   molluscum contagiosum
❏   F   basal-cell papilloma

5.20   Concerning cutaneous naevi

❏   A   junctional activity is a prominent feature of intradermal naevi
❏   B   junctional naevi have a high malignant potential
❏   C   compound naevi have both junctional activity and intradermal
             components
❏   D   halo naevi have a predilection to infiltrate nerves

5.21   Lobular carcinoma *in situ* (LCIS)

❑   A   usually presents as a discrete breast lump
❑   B   has a comedo variant
❑   C   progresses to invasive lobular carcinoma in almost all cases if
            left untreated
❑   D   has a characteristic mammographic appearance
❑   E   occurs exclusively in postmenopausal women

5.22   Theme: Malignant melanoma

    A   Superficial spreading melanoma
    B   Acral lentiginous melanoma
    C   Lentigo maligna melanoma
    D   Nodular melanoma
    E   Amelanotic melanoma

For each of the scenarios given below, select the correct type of cutaneous
malignant melanoma from the list above. Each option may be used once,
more than once, or not at all.

❑   1.   Occurs within a Hutchinson's melanotic freckle.

❑   2.   Has a predilection for sites with thick epidermis such as the sole
            of the foot.

❑   3.   Usually occurs on the face of elderly patients.

❑   4.   Is the commonest type of cutaneous malignant melanoma.

**5.23   Adenocarcinoma is the commonest type of primary malignancy
            to occur in the**

❑   A   bladder
❑   B   colon
❑   C   bronchus
❑   D   prostate
❑   E   uterine cervix

5.24   Oncogenes

❑ A   are normal components of cellular molecular physiology
❑ B   code for proteins involved in cell division
❑ C   such as the v-*erbB2* product are overexpressed in colon cancer
❑ D   such as mutated K-*ras* are present in up to 60% of colorectal
         cancers
❑ E   are expressed during embryogenesis

5.25   Lung tumour resection

❑ A   is precluded by cavitation of the tumour
❑ B   is contraindicated if ipsilateral lymph nodes are involved
❑ C   is curative in 50% of adenocarcinomas
❑ D   can be complicated by postoperative atrial fibrillation
❑ E   is indicated in oat-cell carcinoma

5.26   Theme: Histological tumour types

A   Hamartoma
B   Neuroendocrine tumour
C   Neoplastic polyp
D   Stromal tumour

For each of the tumours/polyps listed below, select the correct histological
type they belong to from the list above. Each option may be used once,
more than once, or not at all.

❑   1.   Villous adenoma

❑   2.   Peutz–Jeghers polyp

❑   3.   Juvenile polyp

❑   4.   Carcinoid tumour

❑   5.   Insulinoma

❑   6.   Leiomyosarcoma

❑   7.   Glucagonoma

5.27 Tumour suppressor genes include:

- [ ] A *erb2*
- [ ] B K-*ras*
- [ ] C *myc*
- [ ] D retinoblastoma gene (*RB1*)
- [ ] E *TP53*
- [ ] F *BRCA1*

5.28 α-Fetoprotein levels can be raised in

- [ ] A nephroblastoma
- [ ] B hepatocellular carcinoma
- [ ] C colonic carcinoma
- [ ] D biliary tumours
- [ ] E congenital adrenal hyperplasia
- [ ] F pure seminoma of the testicle
- [ ] G pregnancy

5.29 The following have a significant metastatic potential:

- [ ] A colonic adenoma
- [ ] B cholangiocarcinoma
- [ ] C lipoma
- [ ] D chondroma
- [ ] E adenocarcinoma
- [ ] F fibroadenoma
- [ ] G basal-cell carcinoma

5.30 Squamous-cell carcinoma of the skin

- [ ] A is associated with chemical exposure
- [ ] B may be locally destructive
- [ ] C can be treated with radiotherapy
- [ ] D can be treated with topical chemotherapy
- [ ] E is associated with albinism
- [ ] F can be found in a Marjolin's ulcer
- [ ] G most lesions are preceded by actinic keratoses

5.31   Theme: Tumour markers

A   α-Fetoprotein
B   β-hCG
C   Carcinoembryonic antigen (CEA)
D   Paraproteins
E   Acid phosphatase

For each of the tumours listed below, select the most appropriate serum marker from the list above. Each option may be used once, more than once, or not at all.

❑   1. Choriocarcinoma

❑   2. Hepatoma

❑   3. Prostatic carcinoma

❑   4. Colorectal cancer

❑   5. Multiple myeloma

5.32   The mammary gland

❑   A   is mainly supplied by the lateral thoracic artery
❑   B   predominantly drains to the internal thoracic nodes
❑   C   partly lies on the external oblique muscle
❑   D   contains 5 main lactiferous ducts that drain separately at the nipple
❑   E   is a modified sebaceous gland

5.33   Renal carcinoma

❑   A   typically presents with haematuria, loin pain and mass
❑   B   when excised may cause regression of metastatic deposits
❑   C   may involve the renal vein
❑   D   is a recognised cause of solitary lung metastases
❑   E   is typically multifocal
❑   F   occurs mostly in the renal pelvis
❑   G   is generally radiosensitive

5.34   Bronchial carcinoma

❏ A   when associated with SIADH suggests irresectability
❏ B   can be cured at resection if the mediastinal lymph nodes are
         also removed
❏ C   is associated with *p53* mutations in 70% cases
❏ D   of the small-cell type is relatively radioresistant
❏ E   can cause hypokalaemia
❏ F   can cause hyponatraemia

5.35   Theme: Chemotherapy regimens

A   Malignant carcinoid
B   Colorectal carcinoma
C   Testicular seminoma
D   Breast carcinoma

For each of the tumour scenarios listed below, select the most appropriate
chemotherapeutic regimen from the list above. Each option may be used
once, more than once, or not at all.

❏   1.   Combination of 5-fluorouracil and folinic acid

❏   2.   Combination of cyclophosphamide, methotrexate and 5-
           fluorouracil

❏   3.   Combination of bleomycin, cisplatin and etoposide

5.36   Liver metastases

❏ A   originating from primary gastrointestinal tumours account for
         approximately 50% of cases
❏ B   are best imaged by unenhanced CT
❏ C   secondary to breast cancer are often amenable to surgical
         resection
❏ D   resection in colorectal cancer improves 5-year survival by 25%
❏ E   produce a rise in carcinoembryonic antigen levels following
         colorectal cancer resection

5.37   Anal cancer

❏   A   is predominantly an adenocarcinoma
❏   B   is associated with condyloma acuminata
❏   C   responds well to radiotherapy
❏   D   typically metastasises to the lungs
❏   E   is related to cytomegalovirus infection
❏   F   typically metastasises along the inferior mesenteric vessels
❏   G   is associated with AIDS
❏   H   most commonly presents with bleeding

5.38   Radiotherapy can be the sole primary treatment for

❏   A   adenocarcinoma of oesophagus
❏   B   gastric carcinoma
❏   C   vocal fold (T_1) tumour
❏   D   rectal carcinoma
❏   E   cystosarcoma phylloides breast tumour
❏   F   anal cancer

5.39   The following are premalignant conditions:

❏   A   familial adenomatous polyposis
❏   B   Paget's disease of the nipple
❏   C   acanthosis nigricans
❏   D   keratoacanthoma
❏   E   solar keratosis

5.40   Malignant ascites

❏   A   is a common feature of ovarian cancer
❏   B   should be drained as rapidly as possible
❏   C   may be treated with diuretics
❏   D   is rarely seen in pancreatic cancer
❏   E   may be treated using a Denver shunt

5.41 Colonic malignancy

- ❏ A has an improved prognosis if the mesenteric lymph nodes are uninvolved
- ❏ B villous adenomas have the greatest malignant potential of all adenomas
- ❏ C Dukes' B tumours have invaded as far as, but not through, the muscularis propria
- ❏ D approximately 30% of cases present with obstruction or perforation
- ❏ E may be screened usefully by CEA

5.42 Risk factors for colonic cancer include

- ❏ A smoking
- ❏ B vegan diet
- ❏ C family history of colon cancer
- ❏ D familial adenomatous polyposis
- ❏ E chronic ulcerative colitis
- ❏ F diverticulosis
- ❏ G alcohol

5.43 Carcinoma of the caecum commonly presents

- ❏ A with a right iliac fossa mass
- ❏ B with iron deficiency anaemia
- ❏ C with constipation ✗
- ❏ D with passage of frank blood per rectum
- ❏ E in people under 50 years of age

5.44 Papillary carcinoma of the thyroid

- ❏ A commonly metastases to the liver
- ❏ B is associated with endocrine tumours
- ❏ C is TSH-dependent
- ❏ D may present with hyperthyroidism
- ❏ E may be diagnosed by FNA cytology
- ❏ F is normally sensitive to radioactive iodine
- ❏ G should be treated with surgical resection if radioactive iodine treatment fails
- ❏ H the Hurthle-cell variant carries the best prognosis

5.45   The National Breast Screening Programme

❏ A   has led to a major increase in benign breast biopsies
❏ B   an interval cancer is one that is detected between screening mammograms
❏ C   screens women every 5 years
❏ D   is carried out on all women aged between 45 and 65 years of age
❏ E   has increased the proportion of T_0 disease
❏ F   a quarter of cancers detected are not palpable on physical examination

5.46   Screening

❏ A   prevents femoral neck fractures
❏ B   prevents death from cervical cancer
❏ C   reduces lung cancer mortality
❏ D   prevents death from medullary carcinoma of the thyroid
❏ E   prevents death from ovarian cancer

5.47   Malignant tumours may be distinguishable from benign tumours by the presence of

❏ A   a capsule
❏ B   higher mitotic rate
❏ C   metastasis
❏ D   oncogene activation
❏ E   loss of tumour-cell cohesion

5.48   Maxillary sinus carcinoma is associated with

❏ A   a chronic nasal foreign body
❏ B   facial pain
❏ C   trismus
❏ D   enophthalmos
❏ E   work in the hardwood-furniture industry
❏ F   anosmia
❏ G   proptosis

5.49 Alkylating agents

- ❑ A can cause myelosuppression
- ❑ B can be antibiotics
- ❑ C include cyclophosphamide
- ❑ D prevent spindle formation
- ❑ E do not cause hair loss

5.50 Neuroblastomas may arise from the

- ❑ A anterior root of the spinal cord
- ❑ B posterior root of the spinal cord
- ❑ C sympathetic chain
- ❑ D adrenal medulla
- ❑ E peripheral nerves

5.51 Prostate cancer

- ❑ A rarely invades the rectum because of Denonvilliers' fascia
- ❑ B presents with metastases in more than 70% of cases
- ❑ C commonly involves local lymph nodes
- ❑ D is commonly an adenocarcinoma
- ❑ E atypically arises in the peripheral zone of the gland
- ❑ F prostate specific antigen (PSA) >100 is diagnostic of prostate carcinoma
- ❑ G bony secondaries usually appear as lytic lesions on plain X-ray

5.52 Audit

- ❑ A is primarily concerned with outcome analysis
- ❑ B should be led by the audit department
- ❑ C can be a process of peer review
- ❑ D only concerns doctors
- ❑ E process refers to what is done to the patient

5.53 Serum carcinoembryonic antigen (CEA)

- ❑ A may be useful in the detection of colorectal cancer
- ❑ B is a glycoprotein
- ❑ C is raised in 90% of cases of colorectal cancer
- ❑ D has a mean half-life of 100 days
- ❑ E is elevated in some smokers

5.54   Common carcinogens and their associated malignancies include

❑ A   ultraviolet radiation and basal-cell carcinoma
❑ B   β-naphthylamine and gastric cancer
❑ C   asbestos and mesothelioma
❑ D   benzene and colonic cancer
❑ E   arsenic and lung cancer

5.55   Cancer registries

❑ A   would benefit from an increased hospital postmortem rate
❑ B   are only useful for retrospective studies
❑ C   are most useful at a local level
❑ D   can monitor 5-year survival rates
❑ E   have no value in cancer screening

5.56   Hamartomas

❑ A   may be present at birth
❑ B   arise at the vermilion border of the lip in Peutz–Jeghers syndrome
❑ C   are mass lesions
❑ D   contain a variety of normal tissue components
❑ E   grow autonomously
❑ F   grow rapidly in size

5.57   Adenomas

❑ A   are typically encapsulated
❑ B   can arise in transitional epithelial cells
❑ C   typically invade the basement membrane
❑ D   are typically annular lesions
❑ E   do not contain dysplastic cells

5.58   A $T_2N_1M_0$ tumour

❑ A   is equivalent to a Dukes' B classification
❑ B   is equivalent to a Manchester stage II breast carcinoma
❑ C   when applied to breast carcinoma indicates ipsilateral fixed
         axillary lymphadenopathy
❑ D   generally has a better prognosis than a $T_1N_2M_0$ tumour
❑ E   does not require adjuvant therapy

5.59   Oncogenes

❏   A   code for proteins involved in cellular regulatory processes
❏   B   in some cases encode for growth factors
❏   C   must be mutated for carcinogenesis to occur
❏   D   exhibit a high degree of evolutionary variability
❏   E   may be transmitted by viruses

5.60   The ability of neoplastic cells to metastasise depends upon

❏   A   tumour angiogenesis
❏   B   decreased cellular cohesion
❏   C   protease secretion
❏   D   reduced cellular adherence to the basement membrane
❏   E   increased production of E-cadherins

5.61   In the cell cycle

❏   A   DNA synthesis occurs during the M phase
❏   B   the cell is metabolically inactive in G_1 phase
❏   C   the M phase leads to the production of two haploid cells
❏   D   changes in regulatory mechanisms may cause neoplastic transformation
❏   E   tissue growth rate depends on the length of the S phase

5.62   Chemotherapy toxicity

❏   A   is reduced by combination with other chemotherapeutic agents
❏   B   may be increased in hepatic impairment
❏   C   may be treated by serotonin antagonists
❏   D   may present with epistaxis
❏   E   is associated with permanent hair loss
❏   F   is reduced with a higher creatinine clearance

5.63   Early complications of radiotherapy include

❏   A   infertility
❏   B   hypothyroidism
❏   C   bone marrow failure
❏   D   mouth ulcers
❏   E   hair loss
❏   F   diarrhoea
❏   G   osteitis

5.64   Known causes of gynaecomastia include

❑   A   bromocriptine
❑   B   cimetidine
❑   C   oral corticosteroids
❑   D   parathyroid gland tumours
❑   E   liver cirrhosis
❑   F   testicular teratomas
❑   G   adrenal gland tumours

5.65   Fibroadenomas

❑   A   develop from single breast cells
❑   B   should be assessed by fine-needle aspiration
❑   C   must be removed in patients over 40 years of age
❑   D   never develop into carcinoma
❑   E   bigger than 5 cm are known as phylloides tumours

5.66   Management of screen-detected breast lesions

❑   A   should undergo excision and frozen section to determine the best management
❑   B   needle localisation facilitates excision
❑   C   following excision the lesion should be sent for perioperative radiological assessment
❑   D   the double-dye technique is better than the guide-wire/needle technique for localisation
❑   E   excision is not always required

5.67   In the UICC TNM classification of breast cancer

❑   A   a T_1 lesion is 2 cm or less
❑   B   a T_4 lesion is larger than 5 cm
❑   C   an N_1 lesion has mobile ipsilateral axillary lymphadenopathy
❑   D   an N_3 lesion has fixed contralateral axillary lymphadenopathy
❑   E M_1 tumours would be Manchester stage IV

5.68   In terminal malignancy, bone pain may be reduced with

❑   A   radiotherapy
❑   B   NSAIDs
❑   C   prednisolone
❑   D   antidepressants
❑   E   a TENS machine

5.69   Obtaining informed consent for a surgical procedure

❑   A   involves reference to a patient's moral rights
❑   B   involves respect for patient autonomy
❑   C   requires only that the patient signs a consent form after an explanation of the procedure
❑   D   is unnecessary in a patient detained under Section 3 of the Mental Health Act
❑   E   on children capable of expressing an opinion requires acceptance of their views
❑   F   the use of invasive monitoring devices should be explained

5.70   Adjuvant chemotherapy for breast cancer

❑   A   single-agent chemotherapy has a significantly greater beneficial effect on survival than combination chemotherapy
❑   B   is most commonly given by intermittent injection
❑   C   is the treatment of choice for metastases
❑   D   has little role in the treatment of inflammatory cancers
❑   E   has a clinical response limited to premenopausal women

5.71   Oesophageal cancer

❑   A   has an overall 5-year survival of less than 10%
❑   B   has an overall 1-year survival of about 75%
❑   C   is associated with prominent lymphatic permeation
❑   D   is associated with β-naphthylamine exposure
❑   E   stenting is a valuable palliative option for upper-third tumours

5.72   Radiotherapy for breast cancer

❏   A   has been clearly shown to improve overall survival
❏   B   has been clearly shown to reduce local recurrence rates
             following conservative breast surgery
❏   C   should be applied to the axilla, if axillary clearance reveals three
             or more involved lymph nodes
❏   D   is the treatment of choice for the palliation of painful bone
             metastases
❏   E   generally includes an extra boost to the internal mammary chain
             lymph nodes for lateral tumours

5.73   The following are considered to be premalignant conditions:

❏   A   Barrett's oesophagus
❏   B   Paget's disease of the breast
❏   C   Peutz–Jeghers syndrome
❏   D   balanitis xerotica obliterans
❏   E   familial adenomatous polyposis

5.74   Malignant testicular tumours

❏   A   are mostly germ-cell tumours
❏   B   have a peak incidence between 20 and 40 years of age
❏   C   are falling in incidence
❏   D   teratomas are more radiosensitive than seminomas
❏   E   untreated, teratomas have a poorer prognosis than seminomas
❏   F   seminomas tend to present at an earlier age than teratomas

5.75   Known risk factors for male breast carcinoma include

❏   A   family history
❏   B   smoking
❏   C   testosterone antagonists
❏   D   Klinefelter's syndrome
❏   E   mumps orchitis

5.76   Interpretation of the results of screening programmes for cancer must allow for

❏   A   selection bias
❏   B   calculation bias
❏   C   detection bias
❏   D   length bias
❏   E   lead-time bias

5.77   In statistical analysis

❏   A   a type I error is finding results that are not statistically significant when the populations are identical
❏   B   a type II error is finding a statistically significant result when the populations are identical
❏   C   an unpaired *t*-test compares two groups on the assumption that the two populations are normally distributed
❏   D   parametric tests are used when data from population groups do not follow a Gaussian distribution
❏   E   non-parametric tests are less powerful than parametric tests

5.78   Colorectal carcinoma

❏   A   is thought to arise from pre-existing polyps in 35% of cases
❏   B   is more common following ureterosigmoidostomy
❏   C   is associated with abnormalities of chromosome 17
❏   D   breaching the bowel wall and spreading into the perirectal tissues and lymph nodes is classified as Dukes' C stage
❏   E   usually spreads in a longitudinal manner within the wall of the bowel

5.79   Contraindications to curative surgery in patients with non-small-cell lung cancer include

❏   A   malignant pleural effusion
❏   B   superior vena cava syndrome
❏   C   contralateral lung metastasis
❏   D   tumour less than 3 cm in diameter
❏   E FEV_1 less than 3 litres

5.80   In statistical analysis

❏   A   the mean of a set of values is the same as the standard error
❏   B   the median of a set of values is the same as the average
❏   C   standard deviation is a measure of the variability of a set of
        values
❏   D   parametric tests are used for the assessment of data that follows
        a non-Gaussian distribution
❏   E   the outcome of a rank or score (e.g. Ranson's score) cannot be
        Gaussian in distribution

**5.81   Relative indications for mastectomy rather than conservative
        breast excision include**

❏   A   larger breasts
❏   B   extensive ductal carcinoma *in situ* (DCIS)
❏   C   impalpable disease
❏   D   salvage surgery
❏   E   axillary lymph node involvement

**5.82   Oesophageal pathologies that may predispose to oesophageal
        carcinoma include**

❏   A   oesophageal webs
❏   B   pharyngeal pouches
❏   C   corrosive oesophagitis
❏   D   achalasia
❏   E   oesophageal varices
❏   F   hiatus hernia

5.83   Concerning malignant melanoma

❏   A   elective regional lymph node dissection has been clearly shown
        to increase survival
❏   B   *en bloc* excision of involved regional lymph nodes is
        recommended in the absence of distant spread
❏   C   it responds well to chemotherapy
❏   D   it has a 60–70% 5-year survival rate when associated with
        excision of solitary metastases
❏   E   it is highly radiosensitive
❏   F   sentinel node biopsy has no useful role

5.84   In colorectal cancer screening for low-risk groups

❏   A   faecal occult blood testing has never been shown to increase the detection of colorectal tumours confined to the bowel wall

❏   B   compliance rates in faecal occult blood-testing screening studies are of the order of 30–50%

❏   C   the optimal period between repeat testing has yet to be established

❏   D   patients should be on a high-roughage, meat-free diet for at least 24 hours prior to testing

❏   E   the Haemoccult faecal occult blood-testing technique relies on a transaminase reaction to produce a positive result

❏   F   the commonest cause for a positive test is an early adenocarcinoma

5.85   Carcinoid tumours

❏   A   of the small bowel often behave in a malignant fashion
❏   B   are usually slow growing
❏   C   prognosis is independent of the size of the primary
❏   D   produce the carcinoid syndrome by releasing catecholamines
❏   E   are associated with increased urinary 5-HIAA excretion

5.86   In the setting of clinical trials

❏   A   single-blinding refers to the patient not knowing which treatment he/she has received

❏   B   double-blinding refers to both the patient and their family not knowing which treatment the patient has received

❏   C   randomisation refers to a selection process in which treatment options are decided for individual patients

❏   D   participants can withdraw even after signing a consent

❏   E   using historical controls provides a more reliable group for comparison than a group randomised to control

5.87   Fibroadenomas of the breast

❏   A   contain both epithelial and stromal elements
❏   B   are macroscopically encapsulated lesions
❏   C   have a moderate to high risk of cancerous change
❏   D   capable of regressing spontaneously
❏   E   interfere with breast-feeding

5.88   When performing an incisional biopsy of a suspected large cutaneous squamous-cell carcinoma (SCC)

❏   A   tissue should be taken from the junction of abnormal and normal tissue

❏   B   tissue from the centre of the lesion is the most likely to yield a histological diagnosis

❏   C   multiple biopsies may be required to make a diagnosis

❏   D   a single, benign biopsy excludes a malignant lesion

5.89   Cutaneous squamous-cell carcinoma (SCC)

❏   A   is associated with xeroderma pigmentosum

❏   B   may complicate long-standing venous ulceration

❏   C   may regress to produce Bowen's disease

❏   D   has an increased incidence in renal transplant recipients

❏   E   metastasises to lymph nodes in approximately 15% of cases

❏   F   behaves more aggressively when found on the vulva

5.90   Theme: Testicular tumours

A   Teratoma
B   Seminoma
C   Choriocarcinoma

For each of the statements below, select the most likely testicular tumour type from the list above. Each option may be used once, more than once, or not at all.

❏   1.   Secrete α-fetoprotein (α-FP) in approximately 70% of cases.

❏   2.   Secrete β-hCG in less than 10% of cases.

❏   3.   Secrete either α-FP or β-hCG in about 90% of cases.

❏   4.   Secrete β-hCG in approximately 60% of cases.

❏   5.   Almost always secrete β-hCG.

5.91   The following tumours are related to smoking:

- ❑   A   squamous-cell carcinoma of the cervix
- ❑   B   acute myeloid leukaemia
- ❑   C   transitional-cell carcinoma of the bladder
- ❑   D   non-Hodgkin's lymphoma
- ❑   E   carcinoma of the larynx

5.92   The breast

- ❑   A   has an arterial supply derived from the axillary artery
- ❑   B   is drained by the internal thoracic vein
- ❑   C   has a nipple in the T3 dermatome
- ❑   D   drains 60% of its lymph via the axillary lymph nodes
- ❑   E   has a retromammary space over the pectoralis minor muscle

5.93   In axillary lymph node dissection

- ❑   A   the medial wall of the axilla is formed by the serratus anterior
- ❑   B   the clavipectoral fascia on the edge of the pectoralis major should be divided to enter the axilla
- ❑   C   inadvertent division of the thoracodorsal nerve may lead to a winged scapula
- ❑   D   level II nodes are those lying lateral to the pectoralis minor
- ❑   E   an anaesthetic patch on the upper medial arm is a recognised complication

5.94   The lymphatic drainage of the female breast

- ❑   A   crosses the midline
- ❑   B   crosses the diaphragm
- ❑   C   drains to interpectoral nodes
- ❑   D   drains into the subclavian vein
- ❑   E   drains to external mammary nodes

5.95   Theme: Thyroid cancer

A   papillary carcinoma
B   follicular carcinoma
C   medullary-cell carcinoma
D   anaplastic carcinoma
E   lymphoma
F   thyroid secondaries from another primary organ

For each of the statements below, select the correct thyroid carcinoma from the list above. Each option may be used once, more than once, or not at all.

❏   1.   Has early haematogenous and lymphatic spread.

❏   2.   Is usually very radiosensitive.

❏   3.   Accounts for 60% of thyroid carcinoma cases.

❏   4.   Is derived from parafollicular C cells.

❏   5.   Commonly metastasises to bone and lung, with lymphatic spread being unusual.

5.96   The following clinical features may be indicative of the development of a melanoma in a pre-existing mole:

❏   A   itching
❏   B   decreased pigmentation
❏   C   regularity
❏   D   subcutaneous crepitus
❏   E   satellite lesions

5.97   The following factors predict a good prognosis in malignant melanoma:

❏   A   male sex
❏   B   low Breslow thickness
❏   C   the presence of ulceration
❏   D   older age lesion on the trunk
❏   E   a mucosal primary site

5.98   Theme: Hormone-secreting tumours

A   Calcitonin
B   Erythropoietin
C   5-Hydroxytryptamine
D   Growth hormone
E   α-Fetoprotein
F   ACTH

For each of the tumours listed below, select the most likely hormone produced by the tumour from the list above. Each option may be used once, more than once, or not at all.

❑   1.   Testicular teratoma

❑   2.   Bronchial carcinoma

❑   3.   Medullary thyroid carcinoma

❑   4.   Carcinoid tumour

❑   5.   Hypernephroma

5.99   Cases that should be referred to the coroner include

❑   A   violent death
❑   B   death due to AIDS
❑   C   death due to unknown causes
❑   D   death due to notifiable disease
❑   E   death due to anaesthetic
❑   F   death due to self-neglect
❑   G   death while recovering from an anaesthetic
❑   H   cause of death related to former employment

5.100   Informed consent should include discussion about

❑   A   per rectal analgesia use
❑   B   exact identity of the surgeon
❑   C   alternative options
❑   D   possible failure
❑   E   explanation of the risk of anaesthetic

5.101   Standardised data for surgical waiting lists include

❏   A   date of referral from GP
❏   B   telephone number of patient
❏   C   diagnosis and treatment
❏   D   concomitant medical illness
❏   E   proof of invalidity benefit

5.102   Thrombophlebitis migrans is associated with

❏   A   carcinoma of the pancreas
❏   B   phlegmasia caerulae dolens
❏   C   bronchial carcinoma
❏   D   venous insufficiency
❏   E   diabetes
❏   F   Lyme disease

PRACTICE PAPER 1 –
MULTIPLE CHOICE QUESTIONS

Time allowed: 2 ½ hours

1   **Characteristic features of aortic stenosis include**

- ❏   A   angina
- ❏   B   exertional syncope
- ❏   C   hypertension
- ❏   D   a systolic murmur that radiates to the axilla
- ❏   E   bounding femoral pulse

2   **A patient-controlled analgesia (PCA) pump**

- ❏   A   has a lock-out system
- ❏   B   is useful in the treatment of confused elderly patients
- ❏   C   needs its syringe changing every 6 hours
- ❏   D   can be looked after by a healthcare support worker
- ❏   E   should give a variable bolus dose each time

3   **The following have an autosomal dominant inheritance pattern:**

- ❏   A   hereditary spherocytosis
- ❏   B   FAP (familial adenomatous polyposis)
- ❏   C   cystic fibrosis
- ❏   D   trisomy 21
- ❏   E   haemophilia

4   **Diazepam**

- ❏   A   antagonises GABA receptors
- ❏   B   is reversed by naloxone
- ❏   C   causes amnesia
- ❏   D   is broken down into active metabolites

5   **Extrapulmonary symptoms of sarcoid include**

- ❏   A   macroglossia
- ❏   B   lymphadenopathy
- ❏   C   splenomegaly
- ❏   D   candidiasis

6   **Sterilisation can be achieved by**

❏   A   immersion in chlorhexidine for 20 minutes
❏   B   boiling in water for 10 minutes
❏   C   β-radiation
❏   D   ethylene oxide
❏   E   immersion in 70% alcohol for 15 minutes

7   **The following are causes of hyperkalaemia:**

❏   A   metabolic acidosis
❏   B   blood transfusion
❏   C   Cushing's syndrome
❏   D   parathyroid adenoma
❏   E   Addison's disease

8   **Pseudomembranous colitis**

❏   A   is rare in children
❏   B   should be suspected if a patient develops profuse, watery, foul-smelling diarrhoea postoperatively
❏   C   may be treated with clindamycin
❏   D   may require antimotility agents for pain
❏   E   is caused by *Clostridium perfringens*
❏   F   may be treated with metronidazole

9   ***Bacteroides fragilis***

❏   A   is the commonest organism in the gastrointestinal tract
❏   B   causes Vincent's angina
❏   C   is responsible for most postappendicectomy wound infections
❏   D   is a facultative anaerobe
❏   E   is best treated by metronidazole

10   **Brain abscesses are a recognised complication of**

❏   A   middle ear infection
❏   B   bronchiectasis
❏   C   hypophysectomy
❏   D   cerebral tumour
❏   E   infective endocarditis

11   A surgeon dissecting behind the right main bronchus is likely to encounter the

❏   A   vagus nerve
❏   B   phrenic nerve
❏   C   recurrent laryngeal nerve
❏   D   hemiazygos nerve
❏   E   azygos vein

12   Atrophy of tissue

❏   A   can be the result of ischaemia
❏   B   is associated with fibrosis
❏   C   is a physiological process
❏   D   occurs during fetal development
❏   E   predisposes to malignant disease

13   Postoperative complications

❏   A   pulmonary embolus most commonly occurs at day 5
❏   B   respiratory tract infection is common
❏   C   wound infection usually occurs around day 10
❏   D   a pyrexia always indicates an underlying infection
❏   E   presence of bowel sounds excludes pseudo-obstruction

14   Split-skin grafts

❏   A   take better when thicker
❏   B   take easily on bone of the middle of the face
❏   C   are the best treatment for pressure sores
❏   D   are often harvested from the thigh or buttock
❏   E   can be stored in the fridge for future application on the ward

15   Postoperative analgesia

❏   A   intrathecal morphine is commonly used after intra-abdominal surgery
❏   B   patient-controlled morphine is an effective route for analgesia
❏   C   morphine is contraindicated in alcoholics
❏   D   is best given regularly during the first few days postoperatively
❏   E   may cause confusion in the elderly

16   **Cells involved in the wound-healing process include**

- ❏   A   fibroblasts
- ❏   B   megaloblasts
- ❏   C   megakaryocytes
- ❏   D   lymphocytes
- ❏   E   macrophages

17   **In the first 2 postoperative days after a major colonic resection the patient will have**

- ❏   A   a positive nitrogen balance
- ❏   B   an increased secretion of ACTH
- ❏   C   a decrease in the free fatty-acid concentration
- ❏   D   a decrease in sodium excretion in the urine
- ❏   E   an increased ADH secretion

18   **A rapid loss of 25% of the blood volume will**

- ❏   A   increase ADH levels
- ❏   B   activate the renin–angiotensin system
- ❏   C   stimulate thirst
- ❏   D   produce a fall in the blood glucose level
- ❏   E   produce hyperkalaemia

19   **The following deaths require a coroner's postmortem:**

- ❏   A   death of a patient with metastatic breast cancer
- ❏   B   death from MI during a clinical trial
- ❏   C   death of a patient 12 hours after surgery
- ❏   D   death of a patient involved in trauma
- ❏   E   death of a patient due to self-neglect

20   **Low-molecular-weight heparins**

- ❏   A   may be used alone to treat pulmonary embolus
- ❏   B   have a longer half-life than unfractionated heparin
- ❏   C   do not prolong the activated partial thromboplastin time
- ❏   D   are effective in thromboprophylaxis
- ❏   E   should not be used in pregnancy

21   Complications associated with massive blood transfusion include

❏   A   hypokalaemia
❏   B   hypothermia
❏   C   disseminated intravascular coagulation
❏   D   thrombocytopenia
❏   E   eosinophilia

22   When performing a pneumonectomy from the posterior approach

❏   A   the vagus nerve is in front of the lung root
❏   B   the phrenic nerve is in front of the lung root
❏   C   the azygos vein arches over the right main bronchus
❏   D   the oesophagus is behind the left atrium
❏   E   the arch of the aorta indents the oesophagus

23   Burns

❏   A   covering the front and back of the trunk cover an area of >30%
❏   B   of the full-thickness type are painless
❏   C   complicated by secondary infection are usually due to *Streptococcus pyogenes*
❏   D   fluid replacement should be with colloids only
❏   E   management would involve bladder catheterisation

24   Anterior compartment syndrome of the leg

❏   A   would characteristically cause paraesthesia in the 1st phalangeal cleft
❏   B   is associated with weakened plantar flexion
❏   C   would affect the posterior tibial artery
❏   D   would produce paraesthesia in the distribution of the superficial peroneal nerve
❏   E   may result in an ischaemic contracture

25   Fat embolism

❑   A   may occur after a femoral fracture
❑   B   arises from the bone marrow only
❑   C   can cause a V/Q mismatch
❑   D   frequently causes symptoms
❑   E   cannot be caused by closed fractures

26   The following X-rays are mandatory during the primary survey of a trauma victim:

❑   A   lateral skull
❑   B   plain supine abdomen
❑   C   chest
❑   D   pelvis
❑   E   femur if a femoral fracture is suspected

27   Diagnoses compatible with a high CVP and low BP include

❑   A   septic shock
❑   B   pulmonary embolism
❑   C   pericardial effusion
❑   D   tension pneumothorax
❑   E   neurogenic shock

28   Signs and symptoms suggestive of an anterior fossa fracture include

❑   A   visual disturbance
❑   B   rhinorrhoea
❑   C   anosmia
❑   D   pneumatocele
❑   E   bilateral 'black eyes'

29   Management of a 12-year-old child who has swallowed an open safety pin. It has been seen in the stomach on an abdominal film

❑   A   urgent gastroscopy and removal
❑   B   observation until pin passes per anus
❑   C   MRI
❑   D   laparotomy

30   Damage to the upper trunk of the brachial plexus produces

❏   A   anaesthesia over the scapula
❏   B   loss of arm abduction
❏   C   wasting of the lumbricals
❏   D   loss of sensation over the dorsum of the hand
❏   E   weakness of wrist extension

31   Non-union of fractures is caused by

❏   A   relative hypothermia of the fracture site
❏   B   separation of the fracture fragments
❏   C   interposition of tissue
❏   D   multiple bone fragments
❏   E   poor blood supply

32   Flail chest

❏   A   usually results from trauma associated with multiple rib fractures
❏   B   mainly produces ventilatory problems as a result of loss of abnormal local chest wall movement
❏   C   often requires artificial ventilation to prevent hypoxia
❏   D   patients should be monitored in an intensive therapy unit
❏   E   frequently requires thoracotomy in its management

33   Sequelae of major burns include

❏   A   reduced RBC survival
❏   B   disseminated intravascular coagulation
❏   C   myocardial suppression
❏   D   late thrombocytosis
❏   E   histamine release
❏   F   increased immunoglobulin production

34   Recognised features of a tension pneumothorax include

❏   A   hypertension
❏   B   absence of breath sounds on the affected side
❏   C   hyperresonance to percussion on the affected side
❏   D   distended neck veins
❏   E   tracheal deviation to the affected side

35   Penetrating lower chest wounds

❑   A   may be associated with false aneurysm formation
❑   B   are associated with a significant intra-abdominal organ injury in
          5% of lower chest stab wounds
❑   C   are associated with a significant intra-abdominal organ injury in
          60% of lower chest gunshot wounds
❑   D   can usually be managed without the use of chest drainage
❑   E   requiring pneumonectomy have a high mortality rate

36   In pelvic trauma

❑   A   mechanically unstable pelvic injuries involve at least two
          disruptions of the pelvic ring
❑   B   blood loss is best controlled by mechanical stabilisation of the
          pelvis
❑   C   acetabular fractures are best visualised on AP X-rays of the pelvis
❑   D   acetabular fractures are caused by anterior pressure on the pubic
          rami
❑   E   acetabular fractures require immediate surgical fixation

37   Concerning lung volumes and capacities

❑   A   the sum of the resting tidal volume and inspiratory reserve
          volume is the inspiratory capacity
❑   B   the total volume of both lungs is called the vital capacity
❑   C   the maximum ventilation volume is the functional residual
          capacity plus the inspiratory capacity
❑   D   the functional residual capacity can be measured with a
          spirometer
❑   E   the forced expiratory volume in 1 s is >70% of the vital capacity
          in a healthy adult

**38   Structures seen on the level of the manubriosternal joint
        include**

❑   A   lower border of T4 vertebra
❑   B   tracheal bifurcation
❑   C   left brachiocephalic vein
❑   D   descending aorta
❑   E   left subclavian artery
❑   F   oesophagus

39   Signs of L5 nerve root compression include

❏   A   weakness of the extensor hallucis longus
❏   B   allodynia in the L5 dermatome
❏   C   weakness of ankle dorsiflexion
❏   D   wasting of the extensor digitorum brevis
❏   E   loss of sensation in the S1 dermatome

40   The middle lobe of the right lung

❏   A   is separated from the lower lobe by the transverse fissure
❏   B   may be auscultated at the 5th intercostal space posteriorly
❏   C   is indented by the right atrium
❏   D   has a diaphragmatic surface
❏   E   has three bronchopulmonary segments

41   Recognised clinical features of hypokalaemia include

❏   A   muscle weakness
❏   B   tall, peaked T waves on ECG
❏   C   decreased digoxin toxicity
❏   D   bowel ileus
❏   E   polyuria

42   Adult respiratory distress syndrome (ARDS)

❏   A   is associated with an increase in lung compliance
❏   B   increases pulmonary vascular resistance
❏   C   causes a reduction in fibrin degradation products
❏   D   causes patchy alveolar infiltrates on the chest radiograph
❏   E   is associated with a low pulmonary capillary wedge occlusion
            pressure
❏   F   causes a refractory hypoxaemia
❏   G   can be treated with inhaled nitric oxide

43   Features of atrial fibrillation include

❏   A   prominent P waves
❏   B   regular pulse
❏   C   T-wave changes
❏   D   a regular heart rhythm
❏   E   conversion to sinus rhythm with carotid massage
❏   F   intolerance of warm weather

44   Coronary perfusion is decreased

❏   A   in hypoxia
❏   B   by ADH
❏   C   by α-stimulation
❏   D   by β-stimulation

45   In the cardiac cycle

❏   A   the 'a' wave of the JVP corresponds to the closure of the tricuspid valve
❏   B   all the ventricles and atria are relaxed together sometime in the cardiac cycle
❏   C   the 'a–c' interval of the JVP corresponds to PR interval on the ECG
❏   D   the descent of the 'v' wave corresponds to the opening of the mitral valve
❏   E   1st heart sound corresponds to the opening of the mitral, tricuspid valves
❏   F   2nd heart sound corresponds to aortic valve closure
❏   G   isovolumetric relaxation (isometric) occurs after aortic pulmonary valve closure
❏   H   QRS commences with the 1st heart sound
❏   I   myocardial cells all contract at the same time

46   Disseminated intravascular coagulation (DIC)

❏   A   is confirmed by elevated fibrinogen degradation products
❏   B   produces a characteristic raised platelet count
❏   C   is best managed with whole blood transfusion
❏   D   is associated with increased fibrinolysis
❏   E   may present with thrombosis

47   Essential components of total parenteral nutrition include

❏   A   emulsifiers
❏   B   nitrogen
❏   C   fibrinogen
❏   D   carbohydrate
❏   E   calcium

48   The thoracic duct

❏   A   lies on the posterior intercostal vessels
❏   B   has no valves
❏   C   runs through the thoracic inlet to the left of the oesophagus
❏   D   receives the right bronchomediastinal lymph trunk
❏   E   arches over the left suprapleural membrane

49   The right phrenic nerve

❏   A   originates from nerve roots C3, 4, 5
❏   B   is purely motor
❏   C   lies anterior to the scalenus anterior muscle
❏   D   gives off the right recurrent laryngeal nerve at the level of the
          right subclavian artery
❏   E   lies lateral to the right vagus nerve in the thorax

**50   Recognised complications of central venous line insertion
          include**

❏   A   arterial air embolism
❏   B   haemorrhage
❏   C   pneumothorax
❏   D   chylothorax
❏   E   venous air embolism

**51   The following can be measured (directly or indirectly) using
          Swan–Ganz catheterisation:**

❏   A   cardiac index
❏   B FiO_2
❏   C   left ventricular stroke work
❏   D   end tidal CO_2
❏   E   pulmonary artery occlusion pressure

**52   Agents clinically useful in the treatment of colorectal cancer
          include**

❏   A   cyclophosphamide
❏   B   5-fluorouracil (5-FU)
❏   C   vincristine
❏   D   folinic acid (leucovorin)
❏   E   irinotecan

53   Tumour markers

❑   A   may be useful in monitoring the response to anticancer treatment

❑   B   may yield prognostic information

❑   C   play an important role in the management of testicular germ-cell tumours

❑   D   are sufficiently sensitive for screening purposes in the majority of cases

❑   E   CA-125 is found in the normal ovary

❑   F   PSA is found in the normal prostate

54   Malignant tumours can be differentiated from benign on the basis of

❑   A   presence of a capsule

❑   B   metastases

❑   C   slow growth rate

❑   D   poor differentiation of cells

❑   E   cells of differing sizes

55   Mammography

❑   A   is diagnostically most useful in women in their twenties

❑   B   is currently employed to screen all women >50 years in the UK for breast carcinoma

❑   C   is unnecessary in patients with clinically obvious breast carcinoma

❑   D   is approximately 60% sensitive for the detection of breast carcinoma

❑   E   may lead to the detection of DCIS

❑   F   employing two views is superior

56   In the cell cycle

❑   A   RNA and proteins are synthesised during G_1 phase

❑   B   duplication of cellular DNA occurs during G_2 phase

❑   C   the average duration of the cell cycle is approximately 10 days

❑   D   mitosis occurs during the M phase

❑   E   tumour growth follows Gompertzian kinetics

❑   F   cytotoxic drugs act mainly on resting cells

57   Recognised complications of radiotherapy to the breast include

- ❑   A   lymphoedema of the arm
- ❑   B   telangiectasia
- ❑   C   pulmonary fibrosis
- ❑   D   intercostobrachial nerve injury
- ❑   E   nausea

58   Needle-aspiration cytology

- ❑   A   is able to differentiate invasive from *in situ* carcinoma
- ❑   B   is useful in the diagnosis of metastases
- ❑   C   routinely undergoes Gram staining
- ❑   D   can have 70–100% accuracy in distinguishing between benign and malignant cell populations

59   Consent for surgery must include information regarding

- ❑   A   risk of failure of the procedure
- ❑   B   risk of anaesthetic
- ❑   C   the use of rectal NSAIDs
- ❑   D   possibility of recurrence
- ❑   E   the fine detail of the operation

60   Thrombophlebitis migrans is associated with

- ❑   A   carcinoma of pancreas
- ❑   B   phlegmasia cerulae dolens
- ❑   C   bronchial carcinoma
- ❑   D   venous insufficiency
- ❑   E   diabetes
- ❑   F   Lyme disease

61   Tamoxifen

- ❑   A   increases the disease-free interval in carcinoma of the breast
- ❑   B   decreases the risk of contralateral breast cancer
- ❑   C   is used in premenopausal patients
- ❑   D   can cause endometrial cancer
- ❑   E   reduces mortality from breast cancer
- ❑   F   increases the risk of osteoporosis in postmenopausal women

62 Bone tumours

- ❏ A malignant primary bone tumours are rare
- ❏ B the commonest type is a metastasis from a primary malignant tumour at another site
- ❏ C Ewing's sarcoma has a good prognosis
- ❏ D benign bone tumours tend to occur in the elderly
- ❏ E primary malignant bone tumours usually run an indolent clinical course
- ❏ F are the leading cause of pathological fractures
- ❏ G osteosarcoma is the commonest malignant primary

63 In faecal occult blood test (FOBT) screening with Haemoccult

- ❏ A false-negatives may result from ingestion of animal haemoglobin
- ❏ B false-positives may result from ingestion of certain vegetables due to their folic acid content
- ❏ C screen-detected tumours are more likely to be at an earlier stage than symptomatic disease
- ❏ D it has been shown to lead to a 15–30% reduction in incidence in patients with colorectal cancer-specific mortality
- ❏ E approximately 40% of patients with a positive test will on investigation turn out to have a colorectal carcinoma

64 Which of the following statistical tests are examples of parametric tests:

- ❏ A paired *t*-test
- ❏ B unpaired *t*-test
- ❏ C Wilcoxon test
- ❏ D Mann–Whitney test
- ❏ E ANOVA test

65 Gastric cancer

- ❏ A is an adenocarcinoma in approximately 95% of cases
- ❏ B is associated with a previous partial gastrectomy
- ❏ C commonly causes anorexia and weight loss
- ❏ D presents with a palpable abdominal mass in approximately 50% of cases
- ❏ E outside Japan, only approximately 30% are diagnosed at an early stage

PRACTICE PAPER 1 –
EXTENDED MATCHING QUESTIONS

Theme: Skin lesions

    A   Central keratin plug
    B   Keratin pearl formation
    C   Intraepidermal (*in situ*) squamous carcinoma
    D   S-100 positive on immunohistochemical staining
    E   Palisading basal cells at the periphery of tumour islands
    F   Intraepithelial adenocarcinoma

For each of the lesions listed below, select the most appropriate characteristics from the list above. Each option may be used once, more than once, or not at all.

❑ **66** Malignant melanoma

❑ **67** Basal-cell carcinoma

❑ **68** Squamous-cell carcinoma

❑ **69** Bowen's disease

❑ **70** Keratoacanthoma

Theme: Local anaesthetic agents

    A   Bupivacaine
    B   Amethocaine
    C   Prilocaine
    D   Cocaine
    E   Cinchocaine
    F   Dibucaine
    G   None of above

For each scenario listed below, select the most appropriate local anaesthetic agent from the list of options above. Each option may be used once, more than once, or not at all.

❑ **71** This agent is commonly used for conjunctival anaesthesia.

❑ **72** This agent has previously caused deaths when used in Bier's blocks.

❑ **73** This agent causes sympathetic stimulation.

Theme: Operative management

    A   Carry on with surgery regardless
    B   Wait 6 months
    C   Wait 4 weeks
    D   Cancel surgery
    E   Conservative management
    F   Immediate surgery and intensive-care unit booking

For each of the clinical scenarios described below, select the most appropriate management plan from the list above. Each option may be used once, more than once, or not at all.

❑ **74** A 25-year-old woman is diagnosed with acute appendicitis at the beginning of the third trimester of her pregnancy.

❑ **75** A 25-year-old woman is diagnosed with acute appendicitis and is taking the oral contraceptive pill.

❑ **76** A 30-year-old woman is on your waiting list for a right inguinal hernia repair, but is on the oral contraceptive pill.

Theme: Mediastinal conditions

    A   Aortic dissection
    B   Carcinoma of the oesophagus
    C   Mallory–Weiss tear
    D   Marfan's syndrome
    E   Achalasia

For each of the scenarios described below, select the most likely diagnosis from the list above. Each option may be used once only, more than once, or not at all.

❑ **77** A tall, middle-aged woman presents complaining of a sudden onset of chest pain.

❑ **78** A 73-year-old man has anaemia, weight loss and difficulty swallowing.

❑ **79** A young man is complaining of violent retching after an alcoholic binge.

Theme: Mediastinal masses

    A   Superior mediastinum
    B   Anterior mediastinum
    C   Middle mediastinum
    D   Posterior mediastinum

For each of the pathologies listed below, select the correct part of the mediastinum in which they are found from the list above. Each option may be used once, more than once, or not at all.

❏   **80**   Thymic lesions

❏   **81**   Neural tumours

❏   **82**   Thyroid mass

❏   **83**   Lymphoma

❏   **84**   Bronchogenic cyst

Theme: Tumour type

    A   Adenocarcinoma
    B   Squamous-cell carcinoma
    C   Melanoma
    D   Sarcoma
    E   Lymphoma

Which of the above histological tumour types most clearly fits the clinical picture below? Each option may be used once, more than once, or not at all.

❏   **85**   Tumour arising in association with the Epstein–Barr virus

❏   **86**   Tumour arising within the quadriceps muscle

❏   **87**   Tumour arising in association with human papillomavirus types 16 and 18

❏   **88**   Tumour arising in Barrett's oesophagus

❏   **89**   Krukenberg tumour

Theme: Death certificates

    A   Report to the coroner
    B   Issue a death certificate
    C   Order a hospital postmortem
    D   Ask families for permission for a postmortem
    E   Ask the GP to issue a death certificate

For each of the situations below, select the most likely answer from the list above. Each option may be used once, more than once, or not at all.

❏   **90** A 20-year-old man was found emaciated in a derelict building, unwell. He was found to have 2 liver abscesses and be HIV-positive, and died 5 days after admission to hospital.

❏   **91** A 50-year-old man was admitted with jaundice secondary to cholangiocarcinoma. His tumour was resected, but the patient died 5 days later from an MI.

Theme: Paraneoplastic syndromes
⏐
    A   Multiple myeloma
    B   Pancreatic carcinoma
    C   Colon carcinoma
    D   Renal carcinoma
    E   Thymoma
    F   Lymphoma

For each of the clinical systemic manifestations below, select the tumour most likely to produce these effects from the list above. Each option may be used once, more than once, or not at all.

❏   **92** Myasthenia gravis

❏   **93** Polycythaemia

❏   **94** Hypercalcaemia

❏   **95** Hyperglycaemia

Theme: Mode of tumour spread

    A   Local invasion
    B   Blood-borne spread
    C   Transcoelomic spread
    D   Lymphatic spread

For each of the tumours below, select the predominant mode of spread from the list above. Each option may be used once, more than once, or not at all.

❏   **96** Seminoma of the testis

❏   **97** Cutaneous basal-cell carcinoma

❏   **98** Papillary thyroid carcinoma

❏   **99** Follicular thyroid carcinoma

❏   **100** Ovarian carcinoma

Theme: Multiple endocrine neoplasia (MEN) syndromes

    A   MEN I
    B   MEN IIA
    C   MEN IIB

For each option given below, select the most likely MEN syndrome from the list above. Each option may be used once, more than once, or not at all.

❏   **101** Submucosal neuromas

❏   **102** Pancreatic islet-cell adenomas

❏   **103** Marfanoid appearance

❏   **104** Pituitary hyperplasia

Theme: Arterial blood gas analysis/acid–base balance

A Metabolic acidosis
B Respiratory acidosis
C Metabolic alkalosis
D Respiratory alkalosis
E Compensated respiratory alkalosis

From the options above, select the most appropriate description of acid–base status from the list below. Each option may be used once, more than once, or not at all.

❑ **105** A 64-year-old man arrives collapsed at the A&E with a suspected leaking abdominal aortic aneurysm. Blood gases show a pH of 7.05, PCO_2 of 3.5 kPa, PO_2 of 12 kPa and a bicarbonate concentration of 7 mmol/l.

❑ **106** A 72-year-old man becomes confused on the ward 6 hours after major abdominal surgery. Blood gases show a pH of 7.24, PCO_2 of 8 kPa, PO_2 of 8 kPa, and bicarbonate concentration of 25 mmol/l.

❑ **107** A 70-year-old man with a 3-week history of vomiting has a blood gas picture demonstrating a pH of 7.56, PCO_2 of 7.2 kPa, PO_2 of 13 kPa and bicarbonate concentration of 45 mmol/l.

Theme: Heart murmurs

A Ejection systolic murmur
B Continuous systolic murmur
C Early diastolic murmur
D Machinery murmur
E Split second heart sound

For each of the abnormalities below, choose the most likely diagnosis from the list of options above. Each option may be used once only, more than once, or not at all.

❑ **108** VSD

❑ **109** ASD

❑ **110** Aortic regurgitation

Theme: Pelvic fracture

    A   Rotationally and vertically stable
    B   Rotationally unstable, vertically stable pelvic fracture
    C   Rotationally unstable, vertically unstable pelvic fracture

For each of the pelvic injuries below, select the correct classification of pelvic fracture from the list above. Each option may be used once, more than once, or not at all.

❏   **111** Lateral compression fracture

❏   **112** Open-book fracture

❏   **113** Vertical shear injuries

❏   **114** Isolated iliac wing fracture

❏   **115** Isolated pubic ramus fracture

Theme: Chest injury

    A   Aortic injury
    B   Pericardial injury
    C   Pneumothorax
    D   Flail segment
    E   Pulmonary contusions

For each of the scenarios below, select the most likely chest injury from the list of options above. Each option may be used once only, more than once, or not at all.

❏   **116** A young man with a penetrating chest injury is clinically well on admission, and has a normal chest film. However, he deteriorates whilst on the ward and has a tachycardia, hypotension and dyspnoea when you are asked to review him. His pulse is weak and his JVP is raised.

❏   **117** A cricketer is hit by a ball in the chest. He initially carries on with the game but then collapses, and is 'blue-lighted' to A&E. He is dyspnoeic, drowsy and has barely audible breath sounds.

Theme: Anatomy of the brachial plexus

    A   C7 root
    B   Posterior cord
    C   Upper trunk
    D   Middle trunk
    E   C6 root
    F   Medial cord
    G   Median nerve
    H   Anterior divisions

For each of the statements below, select the most likely option from the list below. Each option may be used once, more than once, or not at all.

❏   **118** Is formed by branches from two different cords.

❏   **119** Gives off the suprascapular nerve.

❏   **120** Has no contribution from anterior divisions.

❏   **121** Is formed from a single anterior division.

❏   **122** Is a direct continuation of the C7 root.

❏   **123** Innervates the entire flexor compartment of the upper limb.

❏   **124** Receives a grey ramus from the inferior cervical (or stellate) sympathetic ganglion.

❏   **125** Contributes a branch to the long thoracic nerve of Bell.

PRACTICE PAPER 2 –
MULTIPLE CHOICE QUESTIONS

Time allowed: 2 ½ hours

1   **Requirements for the design of a new theatre suite should include provisions for**

❏   A   a dedicated trauma theatre
❏   B   a separate theatre for infected cases
❏   C   a separate daytime emergency list
❏   D   fewer recovery staff at the start of lists

2   **The following block transmission in postsynaptic autonomic fibres:**

❏   A   suxamethonium
❏   B   hexamethonium
❏   C   bupivacaine
❏   D   guanethidine
❏   E   pentazocine
❏   F   fentanyl

3   **Viral hepatitis**

❏   A   hepatitis A is a RNA virus
❏   B   hepatitis B is a RNA virus
❏   C   hepatitis A has an incubation period of 2–5 days
❏   D   hepatitis A rarely causes fulminant hepatitis
❏   E   hepatitis A may give rise to a carrier state

4   **Infectious causes of abdominal pain in HIV-infected individuals include**

❏   A   cryptosporidium
❏   B   cytomegalovirus
❏   C   *Clostridium perfringens*
❏   D   Kaposi's sarcoma
❏   E   *Mycobacterium tuberculosis*

5   **Complications of epidural anaesthetic include**

❏   A   postdural puncture headache
❏   B   hypertension
❏   C   bradycardia
❏   D   urine retention
❏   E   hyperventilation

6 **A 50-year-old man with type I diabetes mellitus is scheduled for elective cholecystectomy**

❑ A   preoperative investigations should include U&E, FBC, CXR and ECG

❑ B   the best assessment of his normal diabetic control is random blood glucose

❑ C   should not receive insulin on the morning of surgery in case he becomes hypoglycaemic

❑ D   all blood glucose tests should be sent to the laboratory as bedside tests are too inaccurate

❑ E   the Alberti regimen may be applicable

7 **Diathermy**

❑ A   uses a low-current density for thermocautery

❑ B   using a high-frequency alternating current has less chance of causing ventricular fibrillation

❑ C   may cause accidental burns if the patient is near but not touching earth

❑ D   belongs to Class 3 of the International Electrotechnical Commission Standards

❑ E   cannot be used in a patient with a pacemaker

8 ***Streptococcus pyogenes***

❑ A   produces an erythrogenic toxin

❑ B   is α-haemolytic

❑ C   belongs to Lancefield group A

❑ D   is found in clusters

❑ E   is sensitive to tetracycline

❑ F   is associated with glomerulonephritis

9 **Correct pairings of the organ and predominant commensal bacterial flora include**

❑ A   skin and coliforms

❑ B   lower respiratory tract and streptococci

❑ C   oropharynx and streptococci

❑ D   large bowel and *Bacteroides fragilis*

❑ E   vagina and lactobacillus

10   Antibiotic prophylaxis in surgery

❑   A   IV antibiotics given 3 hours following a right hemicolectomy are effective in preventing infection
❑   B   some degree of contamination occurs in all operations
❑   C   with the exception of prolonged operations, single-dose prophylaxis is effective in most clinical situations
❑   D   prophylaxis should be used wherever the risk of wound infection is increased
❑   E   choice of the antibiotic antimicrobial spectrum is not important

11   Phagocytosis involves

❑   A   release of lysosomal products
❑   B   lymphocyte activation
❑   C   interleukin release
❑   D   hydrogen peroxide
❑   E   elastase release

12   Analgesia for a patient with incurable malignant disease

❑   A   morphine is more effective than pethidine
❑   B   morphine is addictive and so should not be given
❑   C   some opiate formulations allow the patient to have transdermal analgesia
❑   D   in terminal stages, morphine administration via an epidural catheter is most effective
❑   E   morphine may be administered in the patient's home

13   Pyrexia within 24 hours of surgery may be due to

❑   A   atelectasis
❑   B   pneumonia
❑   C   DVT
❑   D   wound infection
❑   E   urinary tract infections

14 DVT

- ❏ A may be prevented by the use of subcutaneous low-molecular-weight heparins
- ❏ B frequently occur after total hip replacement
- ❏ C are effectively diagnosed by Doppler ultrasound
- ❏ D are less common in obese patients
- ❏ E are more common in dehydrated patients

15 Acute retention of urine can be associated with

- ❏ A haemorrhoidectomy
- ❏ B multiple sclerosis
- ❏ C α-adrenoreceptor blockade
- ❏ D bladder tumours
- ❏ E constipation

16 Wound healing by secondary intention occurs

- ❏ A when the wound edges are opposed
- ❏ B when the wound breaks apart
- ❏ C when there is irreparable skin loss
- ❏ D at the same rate as healing by primary intention
- ❏ E when the wound becomes infected

17 Renal blood flow

- ❏ A may be reduced by 50% in acute renal failure
- ❏ B is normally kept constant by autoregulation
- ❏ C is higher in the medulla than in the cortex
- ❏ D is unaffected by hypertension

18 In closure of the abdomen following laparotomy

- ❏ A a layered closure technique is inferior to that of mass closure
- ❏ B monofilament suture causes less infection
- ❏ C peritoneum should be closed separately
- ❏ D use of continuous non-absorbable suture is satisfactory
- ❏ E suture:wound length ratio of <2:1 is ideal

19   Intravascular haemolysis

❏   A   seldom occurs after ABO-mismatched blood transfusion
❏   B   may occur after burns
❏   C   is common in autoimmune haemolytic anaemia
❏   D   may occur in disseminated intravascular coagulation
❏   E   may occur after mitral valve replacement

20   Platelet transfusion should be administered

❏   A   only to patients with a platelet count of <50 × 10⁹/l before ophthalmic surgery
❏   B   at a frequency of no more than two pools every 12 hours
❏   C   at least 36 hours preoperatively to correct thrombocytopenia
❏   D   to all immune thrombocytopenia patients requiring elective splenectomy
❏   E   to all hospital patients with a platelet count of <75 × 10⁹/l

21   Compartment syndrome

❏   A   commonly occurs with fractures of the proximal humerus
❏   B   may cause renal failure
❏   C   is associated with a relatively early onset of paraesthesia
❏   D   may cause cardiac arrest
❏   E   results in a tense swelling in the affected limb

22   Characteristic features of haemorrhagic shock include

❏   A   coma
❏   B   reduced urine output
❏   C   decreased peripheral vascular resistance
❏   D   bradycardia
❏   E   hypotension

23   Vascular access for the resuscitation of the shocked patient

❏   A   should include central venous access as a first-line measure
❏   B   is combined with blood sampling for crossmatch
❏   C   in children under 12 years of age may be via the intraosseous route
❏   D   is the first requirement in resuscitation
❏   E   is best achieved by the initial use of two large-bore cannulas
❏   F   longer cannulas allow for faster fluid delivery

24   **Chest X-ray features of a diaphragmatic rupture include**

❏   A   ipsilateral mediastinal shift
❏   B   loculated pneumothorax
❏   C   widening of the mediastinum
❏   D   pulmonary contusion
❏   E   pleural effusion
❏   F   upper rib fractures

25   **In paediatric trauma**

❏   A   damage to the internal organs is more frequently seen without overlying bone fractures
❏   B   hypothermia develops faster in children than in adults
❏   C   owing to the smaller mass, a linear force produces a greater force per unit area compared with adults
❏   D   rib fractures are suggestive of a large transference of energy
❏   E   hypovolaemic shock can occur in infants due to intracranial bleeding

26   **Signs of blood loss in an infant include**

❏   A   hypotension
❏   B   reduced capillary refill
❏   C   dulled response to pain
❏   D   reduced urine output
❏   E   bradycardia
❏   F   lethargy
❏   G   increased specific gravity of urine

27   **In the investigation of cardiac injury following penetrating thoracic trauma**

❏   A   CXR has a high sensitivity
❏   B   CXR has a high specificity
❏   C   ECHO has a high sensitivity
❏   D   ECHO has a high specificity
❏   E   a CT scan is the 'gold standard'
❏   G   ECGs have a high sensitivity

28   Compound fractures

❏ A   should not be treated by internal fixation
❏ B   treatment is influenced by soft tissue involvement
❏ C   cannot lead to compartment syndrome
❏ D   should be assumed to be contaminated
❏ E   primary wound closure may not be possible

29   'Open' or 'sucking' pneumothorax

❏ A   results from a chest wall defect that remains open
❏ B   causes air to pass preferentially through the chest wall with each respiratory effort
❏ C   impairs gaseous exchange but not ventilation
❏ D   is treated acutely by sealing the chest wall defect completely
❏ E   defects usually require definitive surgical closure

30   In a multitrauma patient

❏ A   the maximum rate of fluid administration is determined by the internal diameter of the cannula
❏ B   a minimum of four large-gauge cannulas should be inserted
❏ C   initial fluid replacement should be with blood
❏ D   hypovolaemic shock is treated with vasopressive agents
❏ E   hypothermia may produce cardiac dysrhythmias
❏ F   normal saline is the ideal fluid for initial resuscitation

31   Clinical signs of significant penetrating neck injury include

❏ A   an expanding haematoma
❏ B   dysphonia
❏ C   exophthalmos
❏ D   dysphagia
❏ E   haemoptysis

32   After damage to the common peroneal nerve there is

❏ A   failure of the foot to clear the ground on walking
❏ B   loss of cutaneous sensation over the sole of the foot
❏ C   weakness of inversion of the foot
❏ D   wasting of muscles in the anterior compartment of the calf
❏ E   collapse of the transverse arch of the foot

33   **With respect to inotropic agents**

- ❑ A   adrenaline (epinephrine) stimulates α- and β-receptors
- ❑ B   noradrenaline (norepinephrine) is predominantly a β-agonist
- ❑ C   dopexamine is a splanchnic vasodilator
- ❑ D   dobutamine increases systemic vascular resistance
- ❑ E   adrenaline may reduce renal blood flow at higher doses

34   **The sympathetic chain**

- ❑ A   lies on the heads of the ribs
- ❑ B   lies anterior to the posterior intercostal vessels
- ❑ C   lies medial to the splanchnic nerves
- ❑ D   receives white rami communicantes from all thoracic nerve roots
- ❑ E   passes into the abdomen behind the lateral arcuate ligament

35   **Acute circulatory failure with a high CVP and a low BP can be seen in**

- ❑ A   haemorrhage
- ❑ B   congestive cardiac failure
- ❑ C   septicaemia
- ❑ D   tension pneumothorax
- ❑ E   venous air embolism
- ❑ F   pulmonary embolism
- ❑ G   myocardial infarction
- ❑ H   fast atrial fibrillation

36   **The oxygen–haemoglobin dissociation curve**

- ❑ A   produces a left shift in metabolic acidosis
- ❑ B   produces a right shift with an increase in red cell 2,3-DPG
- ❑ C   produces a right shift with a pyrexia
- ❑ D   produces a left shift with hypercarbia
- ❑ E   produces a left shift with hypocapnia

37   Cardiac surgery

❏   A   is performed with controlled hypotension
❏   B   may be complicated by cardiac tamponade
❏   C   usually involves total circulatory arrest
❏   D   always requires a midline sternotomy incision
❏   E   revascularisation of ischaemic myocardium produces permanent resolution of angina

38   Pulmonary artery occlusion pressure

❏   A   may be used to exclude pulmonary oedema
❏   B   is low in cardiogenic shock
❏   C   may be useful for an aortic aneurysm repair
❏   D   is used routinely in the management of postoperative MI

39   The character of the JVP (jugular venous pressure) wave

❏   A   'a' wave refers to atrial contraction
❏   B   'c' wave refers to closure of the mitral and tricuspid valves
❏   C   'v' wave refers to a full atrium
❏   D   'v' wave occurs with and just after the carotid pulse
❏   E   'a' wave is absent in atrial fibrillation

40   Acute renal failure (ARF)

❏   A   may lead to elevated plasma Ca^{2+} and PO_4^{2-} levels
❏   B   carries an increased risk of GI tract bleeding
❏   C   is usually associated with urinary Na^+ excretion >20 mmol/l
❏   D   produces a urine osmolality >400 mOsm/l
❏   E   persisting for longer than 4 weeks, patients should undergo a renal biopsy

41   The catabolic phase of the metabolic response to injury

❏   A   is accompanied by increased energy expenditure
❏   B   is accompanied by a positive nitrogen balance
❏   C   varies in response to the severity of the trauma
❏   D   is most dramatic following multisystem trauma and extensive burns
❏   E   is prolonged by sepsis

42   Adult respiratory distress syndrome (ARDS)

❑   A   usually requires pulmonary biopsy for diagnosis
❑   B   increases pulmonary compliance
❑   C   increases physiological dead space
❑   D   produces an overall mortality of approximately 90%
❑   E   prognosis is independent of other organ complications

43   Left coronary artery supplies

❑   A   entire left ventricle   — *most*
❑   B   entire left atrium
❑   C   sinoatrial node in the majority of cases
❑   D   atrioventricular node in the majority of cases
❑   E   part of the right ventricle

44   The first rib

❑   A   has the scalenus anterior inserting into its tubercule
❑   B   has the subclavian vein overlying the vertebral transverse
         processes
❑   C   has the subclavian vein running behind the scalenus anterior
❑   D   is related to the pleura
❑   E   is related to the cervicothoracic ganglion
❑   F   is related to the upper two roots of the brachial plexus

45   The oesophagus

❑   A   is formed at the lower border of the cricoid cartilage
❑   B   passes through the central tendon of the diaphragm
❑   C   receives a sensory nerve supply from the phrenic nerve
❑   D   lies behind the right atrium
❑   E   is crossed anteriorly by the right main bronchus

46   The clavipectoral fascia is

❑   A   pierced by the basilic vein
❑   B   split to enclose the pectoralis major muscle
❑   C   pierced by the medial pectoral nerves
❑   D   overlain by the infraclavicular lymph nodes
❑   E   overlain by the C4 dermatome

47   The left brachiocephalic vein drains the

❏   A   cervical vertebrae
❏   B   bronchi
❏   C   intercostal spaces
❏   D   thoracic duct
❏   E   thyroid gland

48   Prognostic indicators for malignant melanoma include

❏   A   male sex
❏   B   ulceration
❏   C   presence of abnormal melanocytes adjacent to the tumour
❏   D   lymphatic invasion
❏   E   anatomical location

49   The following are malignant:

❏   A   lymphoma
❏   B   meningioma
❏   C   rhabdomyoma
❏   D   melanoma
❏   E   chondrosarcoma

50   Metastatic spread

❏   A   commonly occurs transluminally
❏   B   via the lymphatics is a common feature of basal-cell carcinoma
❏   C   via the lymphatics is a feature of osteosarcoma
❏   D   via the blood is a common feature of prostatic carcinoma
❏   E   to regional lymph nodes usually follows the pattern of venous drainage

51   Fat necrosis in the female breast

❏   A   is more common in premenopausal women
❏   B   is a recognised complication of breast trauma
❏   C   may present with a skin lump associated with skin tethering
❏   D   is characterised by branching microcalcification on mammography
❏   E   frequently mimics carcinoma clinically

52   Hypercalcaemia may be associated with

❑   A   carcinoma of the bronchus
❑   B   prolonged immobilisation
❑   C   hypoparathyroidism
❑   D   blood transfusion
❑   E   multiple myeloma
❑   F   renal insufficiency
❑   G   hyperthyroidism

53   Osteosarcoma

❑   A   produces an appearance of sunray spicules on plain X-ray
❑   B   most commonly affects the diaphysis of the long bones
❑   C   is commonest in the 30–40-year-old age group
❑   D   is associated with Paget's disease
❑   E   is a well-known sequelae of osteochondroma

54   Nipple discharge in females

❑   A   is usually abnormal
❑   B   occurs in duct ectasia
❑   C   is effectively treated by microdochectomy if only one duct is involved
❑   D   is bloodstained in intraductal papillomas
❑   E   is associated with fibroadenosis

55   Postmenopausal hormone replacement therapy (HRT)

❑   A   should be increased before surgery
❑   B   should contain oestrogen alone in those patients who have had a hysterectomy
❑   C   decreases the risk of breast cancer
❑   D   increases the risk of thrombosis
❑   E   protects against colorectal cancer

56   Testicular tumours in men aged 25–30 years

❏   A   are most commonly seminomas
❏   B   are removed by a trans-scrotal approach
❏   C   primarily metastasise to inguinal nodes
❏   D   increased risk of incidence is confined to the maldescended testis
❏   E   require a CT scan of the abdomen and thorax
❏   F   acid phosphatase is a useful marker
❏   G   can present as a painless lumps

57   The following skin lesions have malignant potential:

❏   A   squamous cell
❏   B   Merkel cell
❏   C   dermatofibroma
❏   D   Bowen's disease
❏   E   solar keratosis

58   Bronchial carcinoma

❏   A   has a lower incidence in the <50-year-old age group
❏   B   kills over 30,000 people a year in the UK
❏   C   is generally curable by resection
❏   D   can be treated by resection of the tumour and the affected mediastinal lymph nodes
❏   E   in the presence of malignant pleural effusion usually implies tumour inoperability
❏   F   may be caused by smoking in 50% of cases in the UK
❏   G   has a strong link between smoking and adenocarcinoma

59   Clinical audit in surgical practice

❏   A   needs to be surgeon-led
❏   B   patients must consent before inclusion
❏   C   may include altering clinical practice if findings suggest improvements can be made
❏   D   must include detailed clinical information on patients
❏   E   is more reliable if data collection is carried out prospectively

60   Familial adenomatous polyposis (FAP)

❏   A   is inherited via an autosomal recessive pattern
❏   B   is associated with abnormalities on chromosome 5
❏   C   has an incidence of about 1 in 500 live births
❏   D   arises as new mutations without a positive family history in
            approximately 30% of cases
❏   E   has a near lifetime risk of developing colorectal cancer of
            virtually 100%

61   In statistical analysis of clinical trial results

❏   A   the p value is a probability score, ranging from 0 to 100
❏   B   the p value for significance is traditionally set at 0.01
❏   C   if two means are compared, the null hypothesis is that the two
            populations have different means
❏   D   a p value of 0.001 is more significant than a p value of 0.01
❏   E   a higher p value increases the likelihood that differences are
            only due to chance

62   In patients with burns

❏   A   gastric ulcers may occur
❏   B   cystinuria may occur
❏   C   ARDS commonly develops
❏   D   carbonaceous sputum is indicative of inhalation injury
❏   E   partial-thickness burns are often pale and have a leathery
            appearance

63   Cerebrospinal fluid

❏   A   has the same pH as blood
❏   B   pressures normally lie between 20 and 25 cmH_2O in the supine
            position
❏   C   contains less glucose than blood
❏   D   contains less protein than blood
❏   E   contains less glucose than nasal mucus

64   Complications of total parenteral nutrition include

❏   A   pneumothorax
❏   B   air embolus
❏   C   fat embolus
❏   D   hypocalcaemia
❏   E   hypokalaemia
❏   F   obesity

65   Cancer of the rectum

❏   A   is always treated with preoperative radiotherapy
❏   B   radiotherapy reduces local recurrence
❏   C   surgery requires a distal 5-cm margin clearance
❏   D   when removed using total mesorectal excision technique
           improves prognosis
❏   E   removal of the whole rectum results in incontinence
❏   F   low advanced tumours can be removed by transanal endoscopic
           microsurgery

PRACTICE PAPER 2 –
EXTENDED MATCHING QUESTIONS

Theme: Microorganisms

- A *Escherichia coli*
- B *Streptococcus pneumoniae*
- C *Clostridium difficile*
- D *Staphylococcus aureus*
- E *Haemophilus influenzae*
- F *Clostridium perfringens*
- G None of the above

From the list above, choose the most common causative organism for the following infections. Each may be used once, more than once, or not at all.

❏ **66** Ludwig's angina

❏ **67** Vincent's angina

❏ **68** Postoperative diarrhoea

Theme: Hepatitis B

- A Raised titre of anti-HBs antibody
- B Low titre of anti-HBs antibody
- C Positive HBeAg in serum
- D HBsAg

For each of the statements below, select the most likely answer from the list above. Each option may be used once, more than once, or not at all.

❏ **69** Requires a surgeon to immediately cease performing all invasive procedures.

❏ **70** Signifies previous hepatitis B infection.

❏ **71** Is produced after successful hepatitis B vaccination, indicating immunity.

❏ **72** Indicates current acute or chronic infection.

Theme: Sterilisation techniques

    A   Ethylene oxide
    B   Hot air
    C   2% glutaraldehyde
    D   Dry saturated steam
    E   Little Sister II
    F   Low-temperature steam and formaldehyde
    G   Irradiation

Select the most appropriate method of sterilisation from the list above for each of the materials below. Each option may be used once, more than once, or not at all.

❏   **73** Air-tight container

❏   **74** Gastroscope

Theme: Anatomy of the heart

    A   Right coronary artery
    B   Coronary sinus
    C   Membranous interventricular septum
    D   Moderator band
    E   Septal cusp of the tricuspid valve
    F   Anterior cusp of the mitral valve
    G   Muscular interventricular septum
    H   Interatrial septum
    I   Sulcus terminalis
    J   Left atrial appendage
    K   Oblique pericardial sinus
    L   Infundibulum

For each of the statements below, select the most likely option from the list above. Each option may be used once, more than once, or not at all.

❏   **75** This is the location of the sinoatrial node.

❏   **76** Originates from the anterior aortic sinus.

❏   **77** Overlies the left coronary artery.

❏   **78** Drains into the right atrium.

Theme: Skin conditions

    A   Erysipelas
    B   Pyoderma gangrenosum
    C   Pyogenic granuloma
    D   Granuloma annulare
    E   Necrotising fasciitis

For each of the patients described below, select the most likely diagnosis from the list of options above. Each option may be used once, more than once, or not at all.

❏ **79** A 55-year-old woman developed acute spreading cellulitis on one thigh, 1 week after drainage of a perianal abscess. She became ill with rigors and fever, and the affected skin appeared blistered.

❏ **80** A 5-year-old child presents with a red nodule on his lower lips, which bleeds easily with contact.

Theme: Surface/radiological anatomy of the thorax

    A   5th intercostal space
    B   Left sternoclavicular joint
    C   Right sternoclavicular joint
    D   Right pulmonary artery
    E   Manubriosternal joint
    F   4th rib
    G   1st left costal cartilage
    H   1st right costal cartilage
    I   3rd intercostal space

For each of the statements below, select the most likely landmark from the list above. Each option may be used once, more than once, or not at all.

❏ **81** Hilum of the lung

❏ **82** Commencement of the superior vena cava

❏ **83** Lower border of the arch of the aorta

❏ **84** Termination of the thoracic duct

Theme: Statistics

    A   Wilcoxon test
    B   Paired *t*-test
    C   Unpaired *t*-test
    D   Chi-squared test

Which of the above are the most appropriate for the following cases? Each option may be used once, more than once, or not at all.

❏   **85** Na^+ and urea level pre- and postoperatively in the same individuals.

❏   **86** Non-Gaussian data.

❏   **87** Hypothesis that remaining nil by mouth preoperatively causes significant dehydration in children. Data comprising pre- and postoperative urea and electrolyte values is collected from 100 patients. The data is normally distributed.

❏   **88** Aspirin is thought to cause excessive bleeding following TURPs. You calculate a fall in haemoglobin for patients either taking or not taking aspirin. In both groups the data includes several patients who suffer massive haemorrhages, and who thus skew the distribution.

Theme: Acid–base balance/status

    A   Pulmonary embolus
    B   Acute renal failure
    C   Pyloric stenosis
    D   Flail chest

For each of the acid–base disturbance conditions described below, select the most likely diagnosis from the list above. Each option may be used once, more than once, or not at all.

❏   **89** Hypocapnia

❏   **90** Metabolic acidosis

❏   **91** Metabolic alkalosis

Theme: Drug classification

    A   Antimetabolites
    B   Alkylating agents
    C   Corticosteroids
    D   T-lymphocyte suppressor

For each of the drugs listed below, select the correct group of immuno-suppressive agents they belong to from the list above. Each option may be used once, more than once, or not at all.

❏   **92**   Cyclophosphamide

❏   **93**   Methylprednisolone

❏   **94**   Azathioprine

❏   **95**   Ciclosporin

❏   **96**   6-Mercaptopurine

Theme: Cardiac physiology

Select the most appropriate set of observations in the above table for each of the cases below. Each option may be used once only, more than once, or not at all.

	HR	SV	Pulse pressure (PP)
A	40	250	40
B	50	140	50
C	100	70	70
D	120	35	70
E	180	25	90
F	200	35	50

❏   **97**   A 25-year-old marathon runner is seen at preadmission clinic for elective surgery.

❏   **98**   A 40-year-old patient presents with uncontrolled hyperthyroidism.

❏   **99**   A fit 50-year-old patient undergoing laparoscopic cholecystectomy.

Theme: Shock

    A   Fat embolism
    B   Thromboembolism
    C   Cardiogenic shock
    D   Hypovolaemic shock

For each of the scenarios listed below, select the most likely diagnosis from the list above. Each option may be used once only, more than once, or not at all.

❑ **100** A 26-year-old man with a comminuted closed fracture of the femur shaft undergoes intramedullary nail fixation. Two days postoperatively, he develops a pyrexia, shortness of breath and a tachycardia.

❑ **101** A 72-year-old man with an underlying prostate carcinoma sustains a femoral shaft fracture. He undergoes intramedullary nail fixation. At day 6 postoperatively, he develops shortness of breath, hypotension and a tachycardia.

❑ **102** A 60-year-old man develops sudden back pain and is brought into A&E with a swollen, tense abdomen. He is tachycardic, with a low-volume pulse and low BP.

Theme: Dyspnoea

    A   Left tension pneumothorax
    B   Cardiac tamponade
    C   Left haemothorax
    D   Pulmonary embolus

For each of the descriptions listed below, select the most likely diagnosis from the list above. Each option may be used once only, more than once, or not at all.

❑ **103** A patient has distended neck veins, having been stabbed lateral to the trachea. Examination reveals decreased breath sounds, hyperresonant lung fields and tracheal deviation.

❑ **104** A patient presents with ECG changes in lead III, Q wave with inverted T and changes in lead I.

❑ **105** A patient has dullness to percussion of the left chest.

Theme: Peripheral nerve anatomy

    A Long thoracic
    B Median
    C Axillary
    D Radial
    E Musculocutaneous
    F Ulnar
    G Suprascapular
    H Medial pectoral
    I Thoracodorsal
    J Upper subscapular

For each of the patients listed below, select the nerve most likely to be involved from the list above. Each option may be used once, more than once, or not at all.

❏   **106** Whilst playing football, a young man dislocates his right shoulder. The dislocation is reduced soon after. Once the shoulder is pain-free, he notices that he cannot carry weights with his right arm and is unable to raise his arm from his side for more than a few degrees. Neurological examination reveals loss of abduction and blunted sensation over the skin covering the lateral part of the deltoid muscle. All reflexes are normal.

❏   **107** After a mastectomy, a 40-year-old woman loses the ability to fold her right arm behind her back and reach up to the opposite scapula.

❏   **108** A 15-year-old boy riding in the passenger seat of a car escapes any apparent injury after a head-on collision because he was wearing a seat belt. However, after the accident he found he was unable to raise his arm easily and has visited A&E twice with spontaneous dislocation of the shoulder.

❏   **109** A builder falls off scaffolding on to his right side, fracturing his right humerus. Because of the patient's shocked state and the pain, only a limited neurological examination is possible. This reveals an absence of the brachioradialis reflex, blunted cutaneous sensation over the first dorsal interosseous muscle and wrist drop.

❑ **110** After a radical mastectomy, a 41-year-old woman is unable to push a loaded supermarket trolley with her right arm. Her husband has noticed a deformity in her upper back on the right side that becomes more prominent when she pushes against resistance with the outstretched right arm.

Theme: 5-year survival rates of tumours

    A <5%
    B 5–10%
    C 25%
    D 50–60%
    E 70–75%
    F 90–95%
    G >95%

For each of the clinical scenarios listed below, select the most likely 5-year survival rate from the list above. Each option may be used once, more than once, or not at all.

❑ **111** Carcinoid of the vermiform appendix

❑ **112** Duke's A rectal cancer

❑ **113** Oesophageal cancer

❑ **114** Pancreatic carcinoma

❑ **115** Metastatic prostatic cancer

❑ **116** Duke's B rectal cancer

Theme: Nosocomial infection

A   *Streptococcus pyogenes*
B   *Legionella pneumophilia*
C   *Pseudomonas aeruginosa*
D   *Escherichia coli*
E   *Staphylococcus aureus* (MRSA)
F   *Proteus* spp.
G   *Pneumocystis carinii*
H   *Toxoplasma gondii*

From the list above choose the most common causative organism of the following infections. Each may be used once, more than once, or not at all.

❑   **117** A whole ward block of elderly patients is closed as a result of an outbreak of this organism.

❑   **118** Following investigation of wound infections in postoperative patients, a member of the ward staff was found to be the carrier of this pathogenic organism.

❑   **119** The microbiologist telephones you to say that a group of patients on the same ward with urinary catheters post-TURP have grown the same organisms in their urine, all resistant to trimethoprim.

❑   **120** An elderly woman attending for an elective surgical procedure has a productive cough. She has recently returned from a holiday in Spain and had nausea and, vomiting and diarrhoea.

Theme: Haemorrhagic shock

    A   Blood loss of 1.3 litres
    B   Blood loss of 1.7 litres
    C   Blood loss of 2.5 litres
    D   Blood loss of 0.75 litres
    E   Blood loss of 1 litre

For each of the above volumes of blood loss, select the most appropriate physiological change. Each option may be used once, more than once, or not at all.

❑   **121** Normal heart rate

❑   **122** Unconscious

❑   **123** Reduced systolic pressure

❑   **124** Confused and lethargic

❑   **125** Raised diastolic pressure

ANSWERS – CHAPTER 1:
PERIOPERATIVE MANAGEMENT 1

1.1   AB
Metastatic calcification is defined as 'calcification occurring in otherwise normal tissue', and mainly affects the vessels, kidneys, lungs and gastric mucosa. Renal calculi are more likely to occur in patients with hyper-parathyroidism. Squamous-cell carcinoma of the lung can produce parathyroid hormone and therefore cause hyperparathyroidism. Rheumatoid arthritis is not associated with metastatic calcification. Rheumatoid nodules are made up of collagen, fibroblasts and macrophages. Calcification does occur in atherosclerosis and old tuberculous lesions, but this is dystrophic calcification.

1.2   ABCD
Hyperglycaemia results in increased vascular osmolarity and all its consequences. Poorly controlled diabetics have an increased risk of infection with unusual organisms due to impairment of leucocyte phagocytic activity. There is no reported increased risk of haemorrhage.

1.3   Viral hepatitis
1. **D   Hepatitis D**
2. **B   Hepatitis B**
3. **E   Hepatitis E**
4. **B   Hepatitis B**

Hepatitis D is an incomplete RNA particle enclosed in a shell of HbsAg. Both hepatitis B and C may cause hepatocellular carcinoma. Hepatitis may be transmitted sexually, vertically or parenterally.
Hepatitis E is very similar to hepatitis A in its method of transmission (faecal–oral) and incubation (short). Neither has a carrier state, and there is no progression to chronic liver disease or carcinoma. However, hepatitis E infection does give a mortality of 10–20% in pregnant women.

1.4   All true
An embolism is the movement of solid, gaseous or immiscible material in flowing blood.
A thromboembolus is a common type of embolus. Virchow's triad suggests that changes in blood components, the vessel wall or blood flow can trigger thrombus formation.

1.5   AC
During exercise cardiac output increases sixfold (stroke volume × 2 and HR × 3). There is usually no change in PaO_2 and $PaCO_2$. An increase in systolic and a decrease in diastolic pressure is seen. Renal blood flow is reduced and there is an increase in negative intrathoracic pressure.

1.6   Classes of antibiotic
1. **D   Monobactam**
2. **B   Quinolone**
3. **A   Macrolide**
4. **C   Glycopeptide**

Vancomycin is a glycopeptide antibiotic used for the treatment of resistant infections due to MRSA, *Staph. epidermidis* and *Cl. difficile*. It inhibits bacterial cell-wall synthesis. The only other drugs that can be used to treat MRSA are teicoplanin and linezolid. Aztreonam contains a 5-monobactam ring and is resistant to β-lactamase degradation. It is active against aerobic Gram-negative organisms, and is an alternative to aminoglycosides.

1.7   ABD

During anaesthesia, a patient inhales dry gases and exhales gas saturated with water vapour. Forming this water vapour consumes heat. A condenser–humidifier 'recycles' this water vapour thereby reducing heat loss. Low-flow anaesthesia recycles water vapour in a similar fashion. By contrast, volatile (i.e. evaporating) surgical sterilising agents may cause substantial heat loss, as may the evaporation of water from bowel exposed to a dry theatre atmosphere. A 'bowel bag' reduces evaporation from exposed viscera. A laminar-flow theatre blows air over the patient thus increasing heat loss by evaporation and convection.

1.8   AD

Metabolic acidosis is characterised by a low arterial pH. The serum bicarbonate (HCO_3^-) concentration may or may not be reduced depending on whether compensatory mechanisms are functioning. Causes of metabolic acidosis include hypovolaemia, diabetic ketoacidosis, ingestion of alcohol and salicylates, septicaemia, renal failure, tissue necrosis, loss of HCO_3^- and massive blood transfusions. HCO_3^- is the main extracellular buffer, whereas proteins and phosphates represent the main intracellular buffers. Compensation occurs by an increase in alveolar ventilation (respiratory) and an increase in H^+ excretion and HCO_3^- reabsorption by the kidneys (renal). Treatment is aimed at correcting the underlying cause.

1.9   Hospital infections
1. **G** *C. albicans*
2. **E** *E. coli*
3. **A** *S. aureus* **(MRSA)**
4. **G** *C. albicans*

Steroids are immunosuppressant and predispose individuals to infections (fungal and opportunistic pathogens).
C. albicans frequently affects the oral and oesophageal mucosa causing inflammation, ulceration and dysphagia. White plaques overlie hyperaemic and ulcerated mucosa.
E. coli is the most common organism to affect the urinary tract both in patients in the community and in the hospital.
MRSA can be transmitted to patients by a single member of staff – the organisms will all be of the same strain.

1.10   All false

Patients with type I diabetes are unable to make their own insulin and therefore require an exogenous supply. In the absence of insulin, these patients metabolise their carbohydrate and lipid reserve resulting in a high blood glucose and ketone level (diabetic ketoacidosis). Initial treatment is therefore insulin and not glucose. Type II diabetics manufacture insulin, but due to insulin resistance in the tissues they are unable to control their blood glucose level. Therefore, type II diabetics usually suffer hyperglycaemia **not** hypoglycaemia or ketoacidosis. Diabetic comas may be of the hypoglycaemic (type I) or **hyper**glycaemic hyperosmolar (in non-ketotic coma in type II patients) type.

1.11   ACD

Inflammatory response is dependent on the extent of tissue injury. Inflammation is characterised by increased blood flow to the affected area, increased vascular permeability, chemotaxis of inflammatory cells and release of numerous preformed mediators such as histamine, prostaglandins, kinins and complement proteins.

1.12   E

Day-case surgery is suitable for patients undergoing operations that require a relatively short general anaesthetic or local anaesthetic, and that do not carry a risk of postoperative complications. Patients unsuitable for day surgery include: obese patients (i.e. BMI >30); elderly patients (upper age limit 65–70 years); patients with an ASA status >2 (if a general anaesthetic is required); and unfavourable/unsuitable home and personal circumstances such as those living alone, those who have no home telephone, or home is more than an hour's journey from hospital. After the anaesthetic, it is necessary for the patient to be taken home by someone else.

It is important to know the ASA scoring system. A patient with stable angina would be classified into ASA grade 2 and therefore would be deemed suitable for day-case surgery. ASA grade 3 refers to a patient with severe systemic disease, i.e. uncontrolled hypertension or heart disease with limited exercise tolerance.

1.13   Suture material
1. A   **Absorbable, braided, synthetic**
2. D   **Non-absorbable, monofilament, synthetic**
3. B   **Absorbable, monofilament, synthetic**
4. D   **Non-absorbable, monofilament, synthetic**
5. B   **Absorbable, monofilament, synthetic**
6. A   **Absorbable, braided, synthetic**
7. C   **Non-absorbable, braided, natural material**

Sutures can be classified as absorbable or non-absorbable. They can then be subdivided into: monofilament or polyfilament; and synthetic or natural.

The common absorbable braided sutures include Vicryl and Dexon.

The common absorbable monofilament sutures include PDS, Maxon and Monocryl.

The common non-absorbable monofilament sutures include prolene, nylon and steel wire. Silk is a non-absorbable braided suture.

1.14   BE

Mast cells are distributed throughout the body and can usually be found in relation to small blood vessels in the connective tissue. They are involved in type I hypersensitivity reactions and the early phases of the acute inflammatory reaction.

B lymphocytes are responsible for antibody production. In contrast, T lymphocytes are involved in cell-mediated immunity and are responsible for the presentation of antigens to the immune system, thereby playing a vital role in the up- or downregulation of the immune response. Phagocytic cells include polymorphonuclear leucocytes (particularly neutrophils), monocytes and tissue macrophages. Kupffer cells are part of the reticuloendothelial system involved in phagocytosis.

1.15   Bacterial infections
1.   F   *Strep. pneumoniae*
2.   A   *Staph. aureus*

Strep. pneumoniae is the commonest cause of primary peritonitis, followed by *Strep. pyogenes*. Primary bacterial peritonitis is most commonly seen in children and adult women. In most cases the infection is haematogenous. Paronychia is most commonly due to *Staph. aureus*, even in children.

1.16   BC

Men over the age of 50 years should have an ECG as their incidence of ischaemic heart disease is higher than in those <50 years. Smokers should have a chest X-ray as they may have concurrent cardiac problems, pneumonia or carcinoma of the lung. Consent is obtained when the patient is of sound mind, can make a balanced informed decision and can understand the information. Premedication often contains benzodiazepines, which cause drowsiness and impair concentration and cognition.

1.17   ACD

$PaCO_2$ is often lowered in severe exercise. The increase in ventilation is probably due to a neural drive to the respiratory centre, together with a voluntary drive to contracting muscles. The stroke volume increases twofold, the ventilatory rate 15-fold and the heart rate threefold; the blood pressure also rises. The relationship between heart rate and O_2 consumption is linear. There is approximately a twofold increase in oxygen consumption, therefore the mixed venous blood O_2 saturation falls to 50%.

1.18   ACD

Captopril (ACE inhibitor) and spironolactone (aldosterone antagonist) may cause hyperkalaemia. In Conn's syndrome, there is excessive production of aldosterone which causes sodium retention and potassium loss. In diabetes insipidus, there is haemodilution due to water retention caused by excessive ADH. Excessive loss of potassium-rich secretions by villous adenoma can lead to hypokalaemia.

1.19   Bacterial infections
1.   A   *S. aureus*
2.   A   *S. aureus*
3.   E   *Bacteroides* spp.

Staph. aureus is the most common cause of breast abscesses in all women (lactating and non-lactating).

Today, lung abscesses are a rare occurrence with the early use of antibiotics, but in immunocompromised individuals *Staph. aureus* is a common cause.

GI fistula infections are usually caused by *Bacteroides* spp. as they are anaerobic.

1.20   CDE
Any cause of acidosis due to lowered HCO_3^- (severe renal failure, ketoacidosis, lactic acidosis) will cause an altered distribution of potassium (hyperkalaemia). Suxamethonium chloride is a depolarising muscle relaxant, mimicking acetylcholine at the neuromuscular junction. It produces a transient rise in plasma potassium and creatinine phosphokinase concentrations.

1.21   AC
Diathermy uses the heating effect of electrical current. Although diathermy can be used in a patient with a pacemaker, the pad of the monopolar diathermy should be positioned well away from the pacemaker. Bipolar diathermy does not interfere with pacemakers and may be more suitable.

1.22   C
Metabolic alkalosis is characterised by a primary rise in the extracellular HCO_3^- concentration with a consequent fall in $[H^+]$. Causes include loss of unbuffered H^+ as in gastric aspiration, vomiting with pyloric stenosis, mineralocorticoid excess (Cushing's syndrome, Conn's syndrome) and potassium depletion. It is not usually a feature of vomiting if the pylorus is patent, as there is additional loss of HCO_3^- secretion from the upper intestine. In salicylate overdose, there is a mixed acid–base disorder of respiratory alkalosis and metabolic acidosis. A pancreatic fistula would cause a metabolic acidosis due to the loss of HCO_3^-. Acute renal failure leads to metabolic acidosis and hyperventilation.

1.23   Local anaesthetics
1.   C   1% lidocaine (lignocaine)
2.   B   0.5% bupivacaine + 1:200,000 adrenaline (epinephrine)
3.   D   Prilocaine
4.   A   1% lidocaine + 1:200,000 adrenaline
Lidocaine (lignocaine) is useful for infiltration, nerve blocks and epidurals. Bupivacaine (Marcain) is longer lasting ($t_{\frac{1}{2}}$ for lignocaine = 1.5 h, Marcain = 8 h) and is also used for nerve blocks and infiltration. However, it cannot be used intravenously (i.e. Bier's blocks) as it is very cardiotoxic.
Prilocaine is the least cardiotoxic local anaesthetic and lasts for 1.5–3 h.
The addition of adrenaline to a local anaesthetic causes local vasoconstriction, which minimises bleeding and increases the duration of anaesthesia. There is a theoretical risk of ischaemia if used near an end artery, e.g. finger/penis.

1.24   ABCD
Pneumatic calf compression is used intraoperatively to reduce the incidence of DVT. Its effect is above and beyond that of TED stockings and subcutaneous heparin. The oral contraceptive pill should be stopped 4 weeks before surgery. Prolonged surgical procedures due to increased immobility will increase the incidence of DVT. Malignant disease has a strong association with venous thrombosis and in some cases may precede presentation of the cancer.

1.25   A
If possible, hypertension needs to be corrected prior to elective surgery in all patients, as it increases the risk of myocardial complications and stroke. Hypertension is defined as 160/90 mmHg (WHO definition). However, the presence of hypertension should not delay an emergency operation as the risks of delay will outweigh the dangers of an elevated blood pressure. Nevertheless, intraoperative lowering and control of blood pressure can be performed with sodium nitroprusside or esmolol.

1.26   ABD
Day-surgery patients should not be left alone for the first 24 hours after the procedure, and they must have access to a telephone to summon assistance if required. Obesity (usually when the BMI is over 30 for day surgery) is a contraindication for day surgery because of the increased incidence of surgical and anaesthetic problems (BMI is the weight in kg divided by the height in metres squared.) Only ASA (American Society of Anesthesiologists) grade 1 and 2 patients are suitable. Patients with insulin-controlled diabetes mellitus require close glucose monitoring and therefore must be treated as inpatients. The protracted drainage after axillary clearance makes day surgery inadvisable.

1.27   Nosocomial infections
1.   B   *Streptococcus pyogenes*
2.   G   *Streptococcus viridans*
Strep. viridans is responsible for 35–50% of all cases of infectious endocarditis. Other infective causes include streptococci (*Strep. faecalis*) and *Staph. aureus* (20% of all endocarditis, 50% of acute endocarditis).

1.28   ACE
During the acute phase of injury, the body enters a catabolic phase where increased levels of catecholamines cause glycogen to be broken down in the liver and muscle to provide glucose. Insulin levels fall and the glucose levels rise. Increased sympathetic activity also causes mobilisation of fat in adipose tissue.

1.29   ACEF
The non-microbial factors influencing the incidence of postoperative infection include: dead/damaged tissue within a wound; an excessive use of diathermy; and mass ligature. Face masks contribute little to the prevention of wound infection. Excessive pressure or tension in the tissues may impair the circulation of both blood and lymph. Inadequate haemostasis results in 'dead space', haematoma or seroma formation providing a favourable nidus for bacterial growth. A well-controlled diabetes mellitus patient is no more susceptible to infection than the normal individual. Steroids and ciclosporin suppress the host's response to infection by depressing antibody function, diminishing phagocytic activity and inhibiting new capillary formation.

1.30   CE
Occupationally acquired HIV infection in health workers occurs as a result of sharps injury, with hollow needles carrying a much greater risk. The overall risk of transmission of HIV infection is about 0.36% of all needlestick injuries from HIV-positive patients. 6–12 weeks following HIV infection there is a rise in antigen titre but no detectable antibody. At 3 months, 85% of HIV-infected patients mount an antibody response and their antigen levels fall. In HIV infection the CD4 (receptors found on helper T cells and macrophages) count falls. Hepatitis B is thought to be over 1000 times more infectious than HIV.

1.31 CDE

Haematogenous infection from a primary focus elsewhere in the body is the commonest cause of osteomyelitis in neonates and children. Although this mode of infection can occur in adults, the commonest cause in this age group is following a compound fracture. *Staphylococcus* is the commonest organism in all age groups. In children, streptococci and Gram-negative organisms are found less commonly. In adults, a variety of organisms may be found but staphylococci predominate.

The treatment of osteomyelitis consists of analgesia, antibiotics and rest. If this fails, the abscess is drained through drill holes and the limb rested in a splint or plaster cast for several weeks.

1.32 Bone and joint sepsis

1. **F   Haemolytic *Streptococcus* spp.**
2. **B   *Staphylococcus aureus***
3. **A   *Mycobacterium tuberculosis***
4. **C   *Haemophilus influenzae***
5. **G   *Clostridium perfringens***

A spreading cellulitis is classically associated with a streptococcal infection. Whilst a child with sickle-cell disease is at risk of developing an osteomyelitis with *Salmonella typhi*, the most common organism is still *Staphylococcus aureus*. Even if the X-ray features do not suggest osteomyelitis the diagnosis must be considered until it can be excluded.

TB must be considered as the cause of a chronic infection in an immunosuppressed patient with sinus formation.

The prevalence of septic arthritis pathogens varies with the age of the patient, but *Staph. aureus* is still the commonest cause at all ages. In this question, the toddler was recovering from a URTI and thus *H. influenzae* is the most likely organism.

In an injury with a dirty wound and systematic features gas gangrene needs to be considered, with *Clostridium perfringens* as the causative organism.

1.33 BCE

Tourniquets should not be applied for longer than 1.5 hours and the pressure should not exceed 300 mmHg. If the tourniquet needs to be used for longer, an interval of 5 minutes should be allowed before re-applying pressure. The most common effect on peripheral nerves is neuropraxia. Mechanical effects of compression and ischaemia cause focal demyelination. Axonotmesis means disruption of the axons while the nerve sheath remains intact.

1.34   DE

Pulse oximeters monitor pulse rate, pulse volume and oxygen saturation. The oxygen saturation can be normal due to a high, inspired oxygen level. Pulse oximetry is accurate to 2%. Pulse amplitude is only an indicator of cardiac output. A high concentration of carboxyhaemoglobin can cause a pulse oximeter to give a falsely elevated reading. All colour changes are sensed. The change in path length caused by arterial pulsation allows for the subtraction of changes caused by capillary and venous blood.

1.35   Appropriate antibiotics
1. **A   Flucloxacillin**
2. **A   Flucloxacillin**
3. **C   Gentamicin**

Most breast abscesses are due to *Staph. aureus* infection. As most *Staph. aureus* organisms produce penicillinase, the use of penicillin will be ineffective. Flucloxacillin is resistant to penicillinase, and is therefore the drug of choice. Most urinary tract infections are caused by *E. coli*, and being a Gram-negative organism it is effectively treated by gentamicin. Even if the infection was due to *Pseudomonas aeruginosa* (as is common after TURP), treatment with an aminoglycoside would still be appropriate.

1.36   CDE

The Nd–YAG (neodymium–yttrium aluminium garnet) laser penetrates tissue deeply (3–5 mm). It is useful for coagulating large tissue volumes, being especially useful in the ablation of exophytic oesophageal carcinoma, controlling intestinal haemorrhage and in the treatment of low-grade bladder cancer. Safety measures are of paramount importance. There should be a designated area for laser use with a nominated user list. Adequate eye protection is required for users and patients at all times during laser procedures.

1.37   CDE

T-tubes are used to drain the common bile duct after exploration to produce a controlled fistula, so preventing possible stricturing of the bile duct. They are removed 10 days after surgery if a T-tube cholangiogram demonstrates no distal obstruction, with a free flow of contrast into the duodenum and no retained stones. The drains are made of latex rubber, which causes an intense fibrous reaction, so forming a fistula to the skin. This facilitates the external drainage of bile after removal of the tube. ERCP and sphincterotomy have reduced the incidence of intraoperative common bile duct exploration. The drain should be brought out through a separate hole to reduce the risk of wound infection.

1.38   AE

Keloid scars extend beyond the previous wound (hypertrophic scars are confined to the wound). Keloid is most common on the sternum and deltoid area. Re-excision usually leads to a recurrence unless steroids (triamcinolone) are locally injected to reduce the scar formation. Pressure dressings work well, but the use of subcuticular sutures will not reduce keloid formation.

1.39   Antibiotics
1.   A   Co-amoxiclav
2.   B   Erythromycin

Co-amoxiclav is a combination of amoxicillin and clavulinic acid, which is a β-lactamase inhibitor. It is effective against those bacteria susceptible to amoxicillin, and therefore include most strains of *Staph. aureus*, 50% of *E. coli*, some *H. influenzae* strains as well as *Bacteroides* and *Klebsiella* spp. Legionella is sensitive to erythromycin, but rifampicin can be added in severe infections.

1.40   ACE

General host factors predisposing to wound infection include hypoxia, jaundice, anaemia, increasing age, obesity, uraemia, malnutrition, diabetes mellitus, hypovolaemic shock, corticosteroids and immuno-suppressants.

1.41   CFG

Mycobacterium tuberculosis hominis is the commonest causal organism for pulmonary tuberculosis in humans, and is usually spread by air droplets. *Mycobacterium tuberculosis bovis* predominantly causes gastrointestinal tuberculosis, and is usually spread by the ingestion of infected milk. The hypersensitivity reaction is mediated by T lymphocytes, which liberate lymphokines.

The Gohn focus refers to the initial site of infection in a non-immune individual. It is usually located in the subpleural, well-aerated regions of the lung (the upper lobe and upper part of the lower lobe).

1.42   D

Actinomycetes are Gram-positive microaerophilic bacteria, present as part of the normal flora of the mouth, lower gut and female genital tract. It is therefore an endogenous infection. The commonest site of actinomycosis infection is cervicofacial, occurring in about 50% of cases. Other sites of infection include the abdomen, thorax and female genital tract. The commonest organism producing infection is *Actinomyces israelii*, though *Actinomyces propionica* is occasionally responsible. Culture of the organism is slow, taking a week or more to produce positive cultures. The discharge contains characteristic sulphur granules.

1.43   ABC

HIV is a retrovirus, and definitive diagnosis is made by Western blotting. More recently, polymerase chain reaction (PCR) techniques have been used. HIV is present in high titre in the blood of asymptomatic carriers, and in many asymptomatic HIV-positive patients. The risk of seroconversion in someone following a needlestick injury from an HIV-positive patient is about 0.03%, and from a hepatitis B-positive patient it is approximately 30%. Hence, hepatitis B is potentially more infectious following a needlestick injury than HIV. The risk of infection from an HIV individual is also dependent on the viral load of that individual.

1.44   BD

Hydatid disease is caused by the tapeworm *Echinococcus granulosus*. The intermediate host is the sheep. Dogs become infested by eating sheep offal and subsequently pass tapeworm eggs in their stool, which in turn contaminate their fur. This leads to accidental human ingestion. Therefore, humans act as an accidental intermediate host. Emergent embryos pass through the intestinal wall into the portal system and liver, and to other organs, where they develop into hydatid cysts. Hepatic lesions are often asymptomatic and discovered by chance on investigation of other problems. Diagnosis should be made on serological testing or from the typical appearances of cyst septation and daughter cysts on CT. Needle biopsy is associated with the risk of anaphylaxis and dissemination of infection.

1.45   All true

The constituents of surgical equipment vary and hence different instruments will require different sterilisation techniques. Plastics and rubber can tolerate moisture, but may melt or become deformed by the extremes of heat, as with steam sterilisation or autoclaving. Gas sterilisation is used for delicate instruments that may otherwise corrode using the chemical technique.

Dry-heat sterilisation is appropriate for equipment that can tolerate heat, but not moisture, or those that are not well penetrated by steam. Steam autoclaving is quick and effective, particularly for metal instruments and is commonly used to re-sterilise contaminated instruments if required quickly during a surgical procedure.

1.46   Adverse drug reactions
1.   C   Glyceryl trinitrate
2.   B   Cisplatin
3.   D   NSAIDs
4.   A   Atenolol
5.   A   Atenolol

Patients commencing on intravenous infusion of glyceryl trinitrate should have their blood pressure regularly monitored. In cases of acute ischaemic heart disease, the dose is titrated against pain and blood pressure.

Adverse effects of β-blockers include fatigue, sexual dysfunction, cold extremities and, rarely, vivid dreams. Their use is contraindicated in patients with airways obstruction, peripheral vascular disease and heart block.

NSAIDs block the cyclo-oxygenase pathways that lead to the formation of prostaglandin E2, which protects the gastric lining.

1.47   CE

Clostridium difficile infection is usually detected by identification of the cytotoxin. Gram staining of faeces is unhelpful in detecting the organism as it cannot distinguish *Clostridium difficile* from many of the other gut organisms.

The first step in treatment is cessation of the precipitating antibiotic(s). The two principal therapies are oral vancomycin 125 mg tds for 7–10 days or oral metronidazole 400 mg tds for 7–10 days. There is some evidence that oral vancomycin may be clinically more effective than metronidazole. Complications of *Cl. difficile* infection include electrolyte disturbances, paralytic ileus and if pancolitis develops – toxic megacolon, perforation and endotoxic shock.

1.48   Skin lesions
1. B   **Papule**
2. D   **Macule**
3. A   **Cyst**
4. E   **Hamartoma**
5. F   **Papilloma**

Definitions: a cyst is a fluid-filled sac; a macule is a flat skin lesion; a papule is a raised skin lesion; a plaque is a lesion with a large area in relation to its height and with a well-defined edge; a papilloma is an overgrowth of epithelial tissue; a hamartoma is an overgrowth of normal tissue constituents; a teratoma is an abnormal overgrowth of tissue of mesenchymal origin.

1.49   AE

Clostridium difficile infections have increased sixfold in the past few years. The ability of *Cl. difficile* to induce disease depends on the fact that the bacterium must be ingested into the colonic flora, and then become established. This usually occurs because the normal flora is disturbed. Disturbance of colonic flora is usually due to antibiotics, but chemotherapy (antineoplastic) drugs can also cause *Cl. difficile* infections. Third-generation cephalosporins (e.g. ceftazidime) are strongly associated with *Cl. difficile* infection. Diarrhoea usually starts within a few days, but up to 1–2 months may elapse before symptoms occur.

1.50   ABD

Actinomycosis is very sensitive to penicillin (antibiotic of choice). However, infection is frequently found in association with other bacteria, and therefore it is advisable to treat the patient with metronidazole as well. Pus requires appropriate drainage or excisional surgery together with antibiotics.

1.51   AD

There is good evidence that chronic hepatitis B and C infection increases the risk of developing hepatocellular carcinoma. The acute illness of hepatitis C virus infection is generally less severe than that of hepatitis A or B viruses. Patients rarely become jaundiced and there is a lower level of enzyme rise.

1.52 Commensal bacteria in different organs
1. G Sterile
2. A *Bacteroides fragilis*
3. C *Streptococcus viridans*
4. G Sterile
5. G Sterile

Cerebrospinal fluid, bile and urine should all be sterile under normal circumstances. The lower gut contains many commensal organisms, 99% of which are anaerobes (e.g. *Bacteroides* spp.). *Streptococcus viridans* is a common upper respiratory tract commensal.

1.53 AD
It is now well recognised that lower colorectal anastomoses (especially those below the peritoneal reflection) have a higher leak rate compared with higher anastomoses. There is no convincing evidence that single- or double-layered anastomoses, or the type of suture material used, provides any functional advantage. Stapled and hand-sewn anastomoses have similar clinical leak rates. Radiological leak rates are greater than clinical leak rates for both stapled and hand-sewn anastomoses. Radiological leakage in the absence of clinical manifestations is rarely of clinical importance.

1.54 D
Local anaesthetics are made 'heavy' by their preparation in 8% dextrose so that they have a more predictable spread in the cerebrospinal fluid. 0.5% bupivacaine is equivalent to 0.5 g in 100 ml, so 10 ml contains 50 mg. 1 in 200,000 adrenaline is equivalent to 1 g in 200,000 ml, so 10 ml contains 50 micrograms. The preparation here is unsuitable for intravenous injection, as bupivacaine would cause severe dysrhythmias.

1.55 AE
The risk of postsplenectomy sepsis is reduced by pneumococcal and HiB (*Haemophilus influenzae* type B) vaccination, as well as by maintenance prophylactic oral antibiotics (penicillin or amoxicillin). The vaccinations should be administered at least 2 weeks before splenectomy. The meningococcal vaccine is presently only recommended for those patients travelling to endemic areas or those who are immunocompromised.

1.56   BCDEG
Hydatid disease is caused by *Echinococcus granulosus*. This disease occurs when humans ingest the embryos of the dog tapeworm. Human infection with *Echinococcus granulosus* frequently occurs in early childhood by direct contact with infected dogs or by eating uncooked or improperly washed vegetables contaminated with canine faeces. Embryo dissemination occurs to the liver (60%), lungs (20%), kidneys (3%) and brain (1%). Complications include epilepsy (from the space-occupying effect of the cysts) and peritonitis due to rupture of the cyst.

1.57   Organisms and the infections they cause
1. **D   Pneumonia**
2. **A   Liver abscess**
3. **B   Oesophagitis**
4. **E   Osteomyelitis in a 1-year-old**

Haemophilus influenzae causes only 5% of pneumonias, typically affecting patients with COPD or pre-existing lung disease. Community-acquired pneumonias are caused by *Strep. pneumoniae* (50%), *Mycoplasma* (6%) and *H. influenzae* (5%). Nosocomial pneumonias are often caused by Gram-negative organisms (e.g. *Klebsiella* spp.). *Candida albicans* causes oesophagitis in immunosuppressed individuals, e.g. those with HIV or diabetes mellitus. Though infection with *H. influenzae* is more common in children, *Staph. aureus* is the commonest pathogen in patients of all ages with osteomyelitis.

1.58   Classification of organisms
1. **A   Fungal**
2. **A   Fungal**
3. **C   Bacterial**
4. **D   Viral**

Aspergillus is a fungus that usually causes bronchopulmonary diseases. It may be inhaled, and because it is only 3 μm in diameter it can reach the alveoli.

Nocardia is a non-sporing, aerobic, Gram-positive filamentous rod. It causes infections in patients with impaired T-lymphocyte function. *Nocardia* is often confused with fungi.

Listeria is a short Gram-positive bacillus, and is a cause of meningitis and/or septicaemia in neonates and immunocompromised patients.

Varicella zoster hides in the dorsal root ganglia post-chickenpox infection, and may emerge many years later as shingles, e.g. in times of immune deficiency.

1.59   BC

Baseline investigations for a patient with major burns include: routine haematology and biochemistry; carboxyhaemoglobin estimation; arterial blood gases; and CXR. Carbon monoxide has an increased affinity for haemoglobin and displaces oxygen from the haemoglobin molecule, shifting the oxygen–haemoglobin dissociation curve to the left. Glycosylated haemoglobin is used to assess recent blood glucose control in diabetics.

1.60   Appropriate antibiotic treatment
1.   D   Vancomycin
2.   A   Gentamicin

Clostridium difficile infection may lead to pseudomembranous colitis after antibiotic use (e.g. clindamycin). It may be treated by metronidazole or vancomycin.

Klebsiella pneumoniae is more common in hospital than in the community, especially in intensive care units. It can cause a severe illness with extensive lobar consolidation. Gentamicin ± ceftazidime or ciprofloxacin are suitable antibiotic treatments.

1.61   ABE

Interferon and interleukin-2 enhance the cytotoxic activity of natural killer cells, which play a major role in the destruction of malignant cells, virally infected cells and some normal cells without prior sensitisation.

1.62   BCE

Immunocompromise will delay wound healing and increase the risk of postoperative complications such as wound infection and breakdown. AIDS patients have a high incidence of anorectal sepsis and undergo the same treatment for anorectal sepsis as non-AIDS patients. Pyomyositis presents with pain, tenderness and swelling with overlying skin being smooth and shiny, thereby mimicking an abscess.

1.63   A

At present, there is no available vaccine against HIV. Patients do not need to be barrier-nursed. Hepatitis B is nearly 30 times more infectious than HIV. The risk of transmission of HIV is related to the depth of injury and amount of blood and viral concentration load. Hollow needles potentially contain more blood, and hence virus, so the risk of transmission is higher. HIV survives for approximately 72 hours on fomites.

1.64   Benign lesions of skin and lymphatics
1. **D   Cystic hygroma**
2. **B   Cylindroma**
3. **C   Ganglion**
4. **E   Syringoma**
5. **A   Pilomatrixoma**

A pilomatrixoma is a common, subcutaneous, often calcified, nodule of hair follicle origin. It occurs mostly on the face or scalp of young adults. A cylindroma (apocrine gland origin) typically occurs on the scalp and may be multiple. When extensive it may cover the scalp and is then known as a 'turban tumour'. A ganglion is a cystic degeneration of a synovial tendon sheath. A cystic hygroma is a lymphangioma resulting from the failure of local lymphatics to communicate with the main lymphatic system. Syringomas are small cutaneous nodules of eccrine gland origin occurring mostly on the eyelids, neck, chest and genitalia of young adults. They may be multiple.

1.65   A
The internal organs of the body are free of commensal bacteria, apart from the alimentary tract, upper respiratory tract and oropharynx, genital tract, skin, external auditory meatus and conjunctiva.

1.66   BCDE
Staphylococcus aureus produces haemolysins, fibrinolysin, hyaluronidase (may assist spread of infection), leucocidin (destroys polymorphonuclear leucocytes), coagulase, enterotoxin (heat-stable proteins causing vomiting), toxic-shock syndrome toxin (related to enterotoxins) and epidermolytic toxins (cause splitting of epidermis and blister formation).

1.67   ABCDE
In the early stages of necrotising fasciitis the skin appears normal, but if untreated subcutaneous oedema develops with gangrene of the dermal layer. The infection is typically polymicrobial (e.g. with streptococci, bacteroides, haemolytic streptococci), often developing from a simple inoculation, or occurring in a postoperative wound. It requires aggressive treatment, with resuscitation, high-dose antibiotics and radical debridement of the fascial planes affected. If the perineum is involved a colostomy is beneficial to help maintain wound cleanliness. The mortality is of the order of 30%.

1.68 CDE

Monopolar diathermy utilises an alternating current at a frequency of 400 kHz–10 MHz. Current passes down the diathermy forceps, which may be applied to surgical forceps holding tissue, causing a local heating effect (up to 1000 °C) through the patient to the patient plate electrode (which must be at least 70 cm^2 in size). Bipolar diathermy avoids the need for the patient plate, and it uses less power as the current passes down one limb of the forceps and back up the other. Bipolar diathermy may not be applied through surgical forceps and may not be used for cutting tissue down. Monopolar diathermy may be used in patients with a pacemaker, but should be used in short bursts of less than 2 s and the diathermy circuit should be away from the site of the pacemaker. It is preferable to use bipolar diathermy in these patients. Diathermy burns are usually full thickness.

1.69 ACDE

Agar plates using various media such as blood or serum are used to culture bacteria. PCR and Gram staining are also widely used techniques. Antibodies in serum may be used to identify *Helicobacter pylori* infection.

1.70 Microbiology following skin trauma

1. A *Staphylococcus aureus*
2. C *Pasteurella multocida*
3. B *Streptococcus pyogenes*
4. A *Staphylococcus aureus*
5. D *Streptococcus milleri*
6. A *Staphylococcus aureus*

Carbuncles and styes are primarily caused by *Staph. aureus*. Infected leg ulcers usually have a mixed flora, but are mostly due to *Staph. aureus*. Other organisms include coliforms, *Pseudomonas aeruginosa*, and anaerobes. *Pasteurella multocida* is frequently present in infected dog bites and cat scratches, though others may include many anaerobes. Infected human bites contain a mixture of Gram-negative organisms, other oral anaerobes, *Pasteurella* spp., *Staph. aureus* and group A streptococci. Cellulitis is most commonly caused by *Strep. pyogenes*, though other organisms such as Gram-negatives may be involved.

1.71   AB
The cell wall determines the Gram-staining reaction of the bacterium. Gram-positive bacteria have a thick peptidoglycan layer in which the mucopeptide is associated with teichoic acids. In Gram-negative bacteria the wall is more complex: the peptidoglycan layer is thinner and separated from a surrounding outer membrane by the periplasmic space. Thick blood films have been used in the past to identify malaria parasites. Culturing a tissue specimen is a better method of detecting the presence of bacteria than Gram-staining.

1.72   AD
Pseudomonas aeruginosa is a strict aerobic, Gram-negative bacillus. It is resistant to many antibiotics including ampicillin, trimethoprim and tetracycline. It is sensitive to azlocillin, aminoglycosides and ciprofloxacin. Piperacillin combined with tazobactam (Tazocin) is used to treat severe Gram-negative infections, especially in immunocompromised or neutropenic patients.

1.73   Classification of organisms
1. **B   Protozoal**
2. **C   Bacterial**
3. **B   Protozoal**
4. **A   Fungal**
5. **A   Fungal**
Immunosuppressed patients are prone to a variety of infective pathologies. These include: fungal (histoplasmosis, aspergillosis, *Nocardia asteroides* and *Cryptococcus neoformans*); protozoal (*Pneumocystis carinii* and cryptosporidiosis); bacterial (including *Mycobacterium tuberculosis* and *Listeria monocytogenes*); and viral organisms (measles virus, cytomegalovirus, Epstein–Barr virus, herpes simplex virus, and herpes zoster virus).

1.74   B
Toxoplasmosis gondii is a zoonosis. It is a protozoan that infects via the gut, lung or broken skin. Its primary host is the cat. *Toxoplasmosis* is normally transmitted by the consumption of poorly cooked infected meat, or contact with cat faeces. Often no treatment is needed, but if the eye, or an immunocompromised individual, is affected then pyrimethamine and sulfadiazine are used.

ANSWERS – CHAPTER 2: PERIOPERATIVE MANAGEMENT 2

2.1 ACE
Acute inflammation is characterised by the presence of neutrophils. Neutrophils initially marginate, adhere to endothelial cells and then actively migrate between these cells. Neutrophils migrate in response to chemical mediators such as histamine, lysosomal compounds, prostaglandins, leukotrienes (especially leukotriene B4), 5-HT and lymphokines. C5a, 6 and 7 of the complement cascade are chemo-attractant to neutrophils. In acute inflammation neutrophils survive for only 24–48 hours, after which they are replaced by monocytes. Bradykinin is a chemical mediator of pain and a vasodilator. Chronic inflammation is characterised by the presence of macrophages, giant cells, fibroblasts, epithelioid cells and lymphocytes, but few or no neutrophils. Colony-stimulating factors can stimulate the production of leucocytes and megakaryocytes and may have a role in haemopoiesis.

2.2 Selection of drains for surgical procedures
1. C   Suction
2. E   None
3. C   Suction
4. E   None

The traditional view is that cervical surgery, such as thyroid and parathyroid surgery, requires the use of a suction drain to avoid the respiratory complications of haemorrhage.

A primary inguinal hernia repair should result in minimal blood loss, so a drain is not required.

A closed, sterile system is required after hip surgery to suck out any accumulation of fluid that could harbour infection.

Following routine appendicectomy, a drain is not usually required; peritoneal lavage is usually adequate.

2.3 AD
Colloids such as Gelofusine and Haemaccel may cause anaphylaxis on rare occasions. Intestinal fluid contains large amounts of potassium and sodium and thus colloids would be an inadequate fluid replacement. Crystalloids would therefore be more suitable. Whole blood is very rarely used except, perhaps, in trauma situations. Haemaccel contains potassium and calcium, and for this reason should not be mixed with blood in a giving set as clotting will occur. Normal saline contains 154 mmol/l of sodium and 154 mmol/l of chloride.

2.4 BCD
Cardiac muscle is unable to regenerate, and thus scar tissue is formed following myocardial infarction. Peripheral nerves regenerate following injury, and growth is said to occur at a rate of 1 mm/day. Schwann cells are responsible for the myelination of peripheral nerves; these cells are involved in peripheral nerve regeneration through the production of growth factors as well as in forming growth channels for new neurites. Renal tubules (cortical) do not regenerate following injury.

2.5 Anticoagulant treatment regimens
1. **D Tinzaparin 3500 U/kg o.d.**
2. **E Tinzaparin 175 U/kg o.d.**
3. **C Unfractionated heparin intravenously to maintain an APTT ratio of 2.5–3.5**

Heparin is used in the prophylaxis and treatment of venous thrombosis and in the maintenance of anticoagulation in patients on warfarin who require surgery. The choice of treatment and prophylaxis for thrombosis lies between the use of unfractionated and low-molecular-weight heparins (LMWHs), e.g. tinzaparin.

In Scenario 1, options B and D would provide comparable thrombo-prophylaxis, but there is evidence that LMWHs are associated with less bleeding in orthopaedic surgery and thus are preferable. Furthermore, LMWHs only need a once-daily injection and routine monitoring of the coagulation screen is not required. If a patient with factor V Leiden deficiency suffers a DVT, then unfractionated intravenous heparin would be given.

Scenario 2 requires treatment of a confirmed venous thrombosis and either unfractionated or LMWH would be justified here. However, the APTT ratio target range quoted in option C should be 1.5–2.5.

The patient in Scenario 3 requires conversion to heparin to enable rapid changes to be made to his level of anticoagulation perioperatively. Although LMWHs show more predictable bioavailability than unfractionated heparins, they have a longer half-life and laboratory monitoring is less straightforward. Since the level of anticoagulation is critical in this patient, most haematologists would advocate unfractionated heparin to maintain an APTT of 2.5–3.5.

2.6 BCD
Anthropomorphic indices have been used to assess nutritional status, such as triceps skin-fold thickness and mid-arm muscle circumference. Other forms of assessment include: body mass index, biochemical tests (transferrin, retinal binding protein, thyroid binding prealbumin) and dynamometric methods (e.g. hand-grip strength testing). The serum albumin level alone is not a reliable indicator of nutritional state.

2.7   D

Body water content is 60% in the adult male and this equates to about 45 litres. Neonates comprise 75% water. The plasma volume measures about 3.5 litres and the total blood volume is around 5 litres. Approximately 400 ml of water are lost daily from the lungs. The intracellular fluid is about two-thirds of total body water, i.e. 30 litres out of a total body water content of 45 litres. Daily potassium requirements are approximately 1 mmol/kg. The normal serum potassium concentration is around 3.5–5.0 mmol/l.

2.8   Investigations for DVT
1. D   Phlebography
2. D   Phlebography
3. A   Clinical examination
4. E   Radio-iodine-labelled fibrinogen scan
5. E   Radio-iodine-labelled fibrinogen scan

Clinical examination is notoriously inaccurate for identifying DVT, with a 50% false-negative and false-positive rate.

Doppler ultrasound (Duplex) is now the most widely used method of assessment, and is extremely reliable for a thrombus at or above the popliteal fossa.

Impedance plethysmography is not widely used, but may be best used to detect major vein thrombosis.

Phlebography will usually be able to demonstrate the extent and degree of fixity of the thrombus. However, it is contraindicated in patients with severe peripheral vascular disease.

Radio-iodine-labelled fibrinogen scans do not give accurate results above the mid-thigh level. They are associated with false-positive results after lower limb incisions. The technique is contraindicated during pregnancy and may induce hepatitis. It tends to be used primarily as a research tool.

2.9   BC

Collagen provides the tensile strength, whereas elastin provides elasticity. Together they make the skin tough, flexible and deformable, but with the property of returning to its original shape once the deforming stresses are released. Type I collagen predominates during the maturation stage of wound healing. Initially, type III predominates. Collagen remodelling occurs around 14 days. Various factors can impair healing and repair: age, disorders of nutrition (e.g. zinc, vitamin C deficiency), neoplastic disorders, Cushing's syndrome and steroid therapy, diabetes mellitus and immunosuppression, vascular disturbance and denervation.

2.10   BE
A sutured, clean surgical wound heals by primary intention. Open wounds heal by secondary intention. Fibroblasts produce collagen and extracellular matrix. Myofibroblasts are the cells responsible for wound contracture. Steroids, azathioprine, diabetes mellitus, vitamin C and zinc deficiencies all delay wound healing. Hyperbaric oxygen is being used in some centres for cases of gas gangrene (as oxygen is toxic to anaerobes) but has not been proven to significantly accelerate wound healing, although it may help if there is an ischaemic element.

2.11   AB
Hypertrophy is the increase in size of a tissue due to the increase in size of the cells present. It is reversible if the stimulus is removed. An increase in cell number is defined as hyperplasia. Mitosis is the means by which cells divide and increase in number, i.e. cell division.

2.12   ABCD
Complications of TPN can be line-related and metabolic. Metabolic complications include: hyper/hypo-glycaemia, -natraemia, -kalaemia and -calcaemia. Deficiencies in folate, zinc, phosphate, magnesium, vitamins, etc. may occur. Liver function tests may become deranged, and a fatty liver and gallbladder stasis may occur.

2.13   ADF
Vitamin B_{12} is almost exclusively absorbed in the terminal ileum. Although pernicious anaemia leads to vitamin B_{12} deficiency, it specifically relates to an autoimmune condition characterised by gastric atrophy and autoantibodies to intrinsic factor (which is essential for vitamin B_{12} absorption). Iron is mainly absorbed in the duodenum and upper jejunum. Folate is absorbed in the jejunum, and therefore deficiency does not occur after ileal resection. Bile salts are normally reabsorbed in the terminal ileum as part of the enterohepatic circulation. In the absence of this re-circulation, the bile-salt pool is decreased and the solubility of cholesterol in the bile diminished. This can in turn lead to the formation of gallstones. Increased faecal loss of bile salts will result in watery diarrhoea.

2.14 BCD

Asplenic patients are at an increased risk of overwhelming sepsis caused by capsulated organisms such as *Streptococcus pneumoniae*, *Neisseria meningitidis* and *Haemophilus influenza*. At present in the UK, vaccination is recommended against *Haemophilus* and *Pneumococcus* spp. It reduces the risk of infection and ideally should be given 2 weeks before surgery. Prophylactic oral antibiotics are effective at preventing postsplenectomy sepsis, which carries a 50% mortality. The antibiotic of choice is penicillin, but erythromycin is indicated in cases of allergy.

2.15 Sites of drug action in the kidney
1. C Ascending loop of Henle
2. A Distal convoluted tubule
3. E Collecting ducts
4. A Distal convoluted tubule

Furosemide (frusemide) is a loop diuretic and inhibits sodium–potassium chloride co-transport in the thick ascending limb of Henle's loop and produces potassium loss in addition to sodium loss. Increased elimination of salt or water reduces oedema and decreases cardiac preload.

Amiloride is a non-competitive antagonist of aldosterone, producing an effect in the distal convoluted tubule. Its effect on sodium transport at this site is responsible for its therapeutic action. Amiloride is commonly used in combination with furosemide because of its potassium-sparing action.

ADH acts on the collecting ducts making them more permeable to water. Consequently, water passively leaves the collecting ducts down its osmotic gradient from the tubules into the highly concentrated papillary interstitium. This process results in the formation of a small volume of highly concentrated urine.

Aldosterone is secreted by the adrenal cortex and has approximately 1000 times more mineralocorticoid activity than hydrocortisone. Aldosterone acts on the distal convoluted tubule binding to the intracellular mineralocorticoid receptor that controls sodium–potassium exchange. The effect of aldosterone is to increase the plasma sodium concentration and to produce a urinary loss of potassium ions.

2.16 BCDE

Feeding by the enteral route is nutritionally, immunologically and metabolically superior to feeding using the parenteral route. Enteral nutrition provides a degree of protection against stress ulceration. The presence of nutrients in the upper small bowel stimulates the release of gut peptide hormones – it is by this mechanism that enteral nutrition promotes biliary flow and prevents cholestasis. A low nasogastric aspirate (<250–300 ml/24 h) is the most appropriate prompt to initiate feeding.

2.17   ABD

Postoperative hypoxaemia in its episodic form can occur up to 3 days postoperatively. Although it is more common following narcotic infusions than with bolus doses, it does not occur with regional anaesthesia. Upper abdominal incisions are painful and patients often fail to make full respiratory incursions if analgesia is inadequate.

2.18   C

Lifelong aspirin is advocated for the long-term prevention of further myocardial events and subsequent manifestations of atherosclerosis. Coronary artery stenting is a useful technique for recurrent coronary artery disease. Warfarin is not required following CABG unless a mechanical valve has been inserted.

2.19   ABE

Macrophages are part of the mononuclear phagocytic system and are derived from bone marrow haemopoietic cells. Macrophages are well-known phagocytic cells. The function of macrophages includes antimicrobial defence against intracellular organisms such as *Mycobacteria*, *Listeria* and *Histoplasma* spp.

Macrophages also play a vital role in several aspects of the immune response. They take up antigen and degrade it to short polypeptides that can be expressed on their surface. Furthermore, the macrophages play a role in delayed-type hypersensitivity reactions; and also have antitumour activity. In addition, they produce various colony-stimulating factors, which promote the growth and development of different white blood cells, and a number of factors that act on other cells (monokines), such as interleukin-1 (IL-1) which stimulates T-helper cells. Indirectly, macrophages also promote the production of more erythrocytes, since they have a greater affinity for the iron-transport compound transferrin. Once transferrin has been converted to ferritin by phagocytes, this storage form of iron is delivered to the bone marrow where it speeds up the production of haemoglobin, which in turn shortens the maturation time of new red blood cells.

Macrophages are involved in granulomatous and chronic inflammation, whereby macrophages and monocytes differentiate into epithelioid cells. Giant cells are formed by fusion of macrophages in response to exogenous insoluble material (e.g. talc and silica) and in reaction to insoluble material, e.g. keratin, fat, cholesterol and certain organisms such as those causing tuberculosis and syphilis.

2.20 BCDE

The normal CVP range is 3–8 cm H_2O. A low or negative reading confirms a low circulating blood volume. The response of the CVP to a fluid challenge of colloid gives much information regarding the state of the circulation. A dehydrated patient's CVP will rise in response to a challenge but fall to the original value as the circulation vasodilates. A sustained rise indicates a well-filled patient, but an elevation of greater than 4 cm H_2O indicates overfilling or a failing myocardium.

A bolus of any intravenous fluid may produce a rise in the CVP reading but it will not necessarily be sustained. If the patient is dehydrated there will be a drop in the reading after the initial rise. A sustained CVP rise of >4 cm H_2O *may* indicate that the patient is overfilled, but this value should clearly be looked at with the clinical picture in mind. There is a well-recognised incidence of allergic reaction to the gelatins, but this is rare.

2.21 Nutrition

1. **A Nasogastric feeding**
2. **B Postoperative jejunostomy feeding**

If possible, nutrition should always be administered enterally as numerous studies have shown enteral nutrition to have many beneficial effects (decreased peptic ulceration, decreased bacterial translocation, reduced liver dysfunction and reduced feeding-line complications). However, in certain instances enteral feeding would be inappropriate, e.g. in short bowel syndrome or a high small bowel fistula.

A feeding jejunostomy is a popular route for feeding after oesophagectomy or total gastrectomy. The use of special feeds containing glutamine, for example, is gaining in popularity but is not yet widely accepted.

2.22 ABD

Steroids are associated with oseoporosis and also with avascular necrosis of bone, e.g. of the femoral head. Mineralocorticoid side-effects include hypertension, hypernatraemia, hypokalaemia and water retention. Glucocorticoid side-effects include diabetes, mental disturbances (usually depression or serious paranoid state), Cushing's syndrome and obesity. Topical steroid use on eyes may lead to cataract formation. Hepatotoxicity and bone marrow suppression is seen with azathioprine use.

2.23   A

On administration, 5% dextrose is isotonic but becomes hypotonic as the dextrose is metabolised. Although it is evenly distributed through all the fluid compartments, only a small amount stays within the intravascular space because it passes easily into the interstitial space. It contains 278 mmol/l dextrose and has a negligible calorific content (30 kcal (~125.7 J)/l). Type I respiratory failure may be caused by the infusion of 5% dextrose.

2.24   ABCD

GFR varies during life. Adult levels are reached at 2 years of age and decline linearly from 40 years of age due to glomerular sclerosis. In research laboratories, GFR can be measured by inulin clearance. Inulin is a polymer of fructose that is not secreted, metabolised or reabsorbed by the kidney. This means that the amount of inulin excreted in urine (per minute) equals the amount of inulin filtered at the glomerulus (per minute). In clinical practice, GFR is estimated by creatinine clearance. A 50% increase in GFR occurs during pregnancy. GFR increases after a protein-rich meal.

2.25   CDF

Metabolic acidosis is characterised by a low plasma pH and low bicarbonate ion concentration. It can be caused by the addition of acid or the removal of alkali from the body, or by failure of the kidneys to excrete acid. Vomiting causes a loss of acid and so will result in a metabolic alkalosis. Hyperaldosteronism (Conn's disease) will cause alkalosis, hypokalaemia and hypertension. Diabetic ketoacidosis and renal failure will both cause a metabolic acidosis, as will septic shock (lactic acidosis).

2.26   ABE

Respiratory acidosis occurs when the $PaCO_2$ is raised and the pH lowered. It is caused by hypoventilation. The causes can be divided into airway obstruction, intrinsic lung disease, neuromuscular problems, chest wall problems and central respiratory-drive depression. Pulmonary embolus classically causes a respiratory alkalosis due to hyperventilation. Respiratory depression and failure may occur in a patient with a severe, massive pulmonary embolus, so causing a respiratory acidosis.

2.27   BDEFG

Excess steroids lead to hypernatraemia and hypokalaemia due to their mineralocorticoid effects on the distal convoluted tubule, namely sodium and water retention and potassium loss. Pyrexia leads to water loss and hence hypernatraemia. Irrigation during TURP may lead to excessive water absorption (the TUR syndrome). Small bowel obstruction, diarrhoea and vomiting can all cause hyponatraemia.

2.28   AB

Absorption of irrigating fluids can lead to the so-called TURP syndrome, causing metabolic acidosis, hyponatraemia, hypertension (due to water overload) and confusion (due to cerebral oedema), as well as a clotting abnormality due to the release of thromboplastins from the prostate. Hyperglycaemia may occur if dextrose irrigation is used. Glycine in the irrigation fluid can cause temporary blindness. Other symptoms include vomiting, headache, fatigue, weakness, muscle twitching and coma.

2.29   BC

Wounds of the skin, subcutaneous tissues, muscle, fascia and tendon only ever regain 80–90% of their preinjury strength. The development of wound strength depends on the type of collagen produced. Type III collagen is produced during the early phase of wound healing, which is weaker than the later-appearing type I collagen (maturation stage). The process of skin healing includes a lag phase lasting 1–2 weeks after injury, followed by a proliferative phase lasting 2–12 weeks and finally a scar maturation phase lasting months to years.

2.30   BCE

Hyponatraemia after surgery is usually due to inappropriate fluid therapy with hypotonic intravenous fluids (e.g. 5% dextrose) and increased ADH secretion (leads to water retention). Patients who have had upper abdominal incisions are more prone to developing respiratory complications as a result of increased pain. The most common respiratory complication following general anaesthesia is atelectasis. This usually presents with pyrexia and tachypnoea and should be treated with physiotherapy and oxygen. Septic shock usually produces a clinical picture of warm, dilated peripheries, but in advanced states it may cause peripheral vasoconstriction – cold, clammy extremities.

2.31   BC
The laboratory findings in haemolytic anaemia include the biochemical markers of increased red cell breakdown: unconjugated hyper-bilirubinaemia; increased excretion of urobilinogen in the urine; and stercobilinogen in the faeces. Haptoglobins normally eliminate free haemoglobin in the plasma – in the presence of haemolysis they characteristically become saturated and are absorbed by reticulo-endothelial cells. Hyperbilirubinaemia may lead to pigment gallstones. Increased red cell turnover leads to marrow hyperplasia and increased production of reticulocytes, hence leading to an increased mean cell volume.

2.32   AE
Excessive crystalloid administration results in: increased filtration pressure; reduced colloid osmotic pressure; and increased capillary permeability. The end result is interstitial and intra-alveolar oedema, promoting the development of ARDS. Initial volume expansion is more quickly achieved with colloid than with crystalloid. Neither colloid nor crystalloid administration prevents a fall in the haematocrit level following blood loss. Stored blood has a low pH and infusion may exacerbate an existing acidosis. Stored blood is also high in potassium and low in clotting factors and functioning platelets. Blood is the fluid of choice to replace continuing haemorrhage and hypotension. Bleeding sites need to be urgently identified and controlled.

2.33   ABC
Third-space loss is the internal temporary loss of extracellular fluid into a space that does not participate in the normal transport of nutrients or waste products. In moderately major operations, e.g. a cholecystectomy, such a loss would be approximately 3 ml/kg per h. In more extensive operations such as aortic aneurysm repair, third-space fluid loss could initially be 10–20 ml/kg per h. Dextrose–saline is a hypotonic solution, so when the dextrose is metabolised it increases the free-water content and so leads to hyponatraemia. Balanced salt solutions should be used to replace third-space losses. Transcellular losses that might be measured include ascites, pleural effusions and intraintestinal losses.

2.34   D
Carbon dioxide is the standard gas used for insufflation. While pressures up to 15 mmHg can be used, they are not usually recommended. A pressure of 12 mmHg is preferable. Even at a pressure of 12 mmHg venous return to the heart is decreased. The Veress needle is a major cause of visceral and vascular injury in laparoscopic surgery despite its spring-loaded shield. Shoulder-tip pain is a common occurrence following laparoscopic procedures and may be reduced at the end of the procedure by allowing the gas out of the peritoneal cavity. However, retained CO_2 is not the only cause of shoulder-tip pain, peritoneal fluid (e.g. blood or bile) and injury to the liver or spleen are other recognised causes.

2.35   CE
A median sternotomy involves detaching the sternal origin of the muscular diaphragm. If possible, the pleura should not be opened. However, if the pleura are inadvertently opened, the pleural space should be drained postoperatively. Most retrosternal goitres can be removed via the neck, but a partial sternal split may be needed.

2.36   BDE
Cytology does not give architectural histology. Gram staining is not part of FNAC. A C2 cytological result means that the tissue sample is benign. FNAC can be used to diagnose thyroid lumps but cannot distinguish between follicular adenoma and follicular carcinoma.

2.37   ABC
Cytotoxic T cells recognise foreign transplant antigens and have a major role in graft rejection. IgE is involved in the allergic response of atopic dermatitis. IgA is involved in the protection of mucosal surfaces.

2.38   ABD
Microcytic anaemia is characteristic of iron deficiency and is usually associated with chronic bleeding from the gut or with menorrhagia. Microcytic anaemia may occur in α- or β-thalassaemia and in sideroblastic anaemia (defect in haem synthesis). Hereditary haemochromatosis is a disorder of iron absorption characterised by iron overload and has no direct haematological manifestations. The anaemia of chronic renal failure is normocytic.

2.39 BCD

Fresh-frozen plasma (FFP) contains all the non-cellular components of blood, including all clotting factors, immunoglobulin, albumin and other plasma proteins. Although FFP contains some fibrinogen, in certain situations (such as severe hypofibrinogenaemia associated with disseminated intravascular coagulation) it is usual to supplement FFP with cryoprecipitate which has a higher fibrinogen concentration. FFP is supplied as 150–200-ml units separated from a single whole-blood donation; or, in some centres, as a 300-ml unit obtained from a single-donor plasmapheresis. Units are stored at –30 °C for up to 1 year. FFP should be thawed in a waterbath in the transfusion laboratory and administered within 4 hours, usually at a dose of 12–15 ml/kg. Repeated transfusion should be prescribed according to the results of a post-transfusion coagulation screen. Donor FFP may contain anti-A or anti-B antibodies, which can sometimes cause dramatic haemolysis of recipient red cells. FFP is therefore usually issued as ABO-compatible.

2.40 Wounds
1. C   Clean-contaminated
2. C   Clean-contaminated
3. D   Contaminated
4. B   Clean
5. D   Contaminated
6. B   Clean
7. E   Dirty

Wounds can be divided into four categories:

Clean: incision through non-inflamed tissue; no entry into GU, GI or respiratory tracts

Clean-contaminated: entry into a hollow viscus other than the colon

Contaminated: breaching of a hollow viscus with spillage of contents, e.g. opening the colon, open fractures, animal or human bites.

Dirty: gross pus, perforated viscus producing faecal peritonitis or traumatic wounds >4 h old.

2.41 DE

Haemophilia A is a sex-linked inherited disorder characterised by a complete or partial deficiency of factor VIII. Heterozygous female carriers have a factor VIII level of approximately 50%, although some individuals have sufficiently low levels to cause clinical symptoms. Severe disease (factor VIII <1%) is characterised by painful joint and muscle bleeds that eventually lead to a chronic arthropathy. Rarer manifestations include pseudotumour formation following muscle bleeds, nerve entrapment, compartment syndromes, haematuria and post-traumatic intracranial bleeds. Significant mortality arises from replacement therapy associated with HIV, hepatitis B and hepatitis C infection. Haemophilia B is a sex-linked disorder arising from deficiency of factor IX. The clinical pattern is similar to haemophilia A.

2.42 ABCF

The daily folic acid requirement is 50 μg, but increased amounts are needed during pregnancy. The storage capacity for folic acid is sufficient for about 80–100 days and it is mainly stored in the liver. Any malnutritional state such as anorexia will predispose to folic acid deficiency, e.g. alcoholism. Other causes include coeliac disease, tropical sprue, Crohn's disease and drugs such as phenytoin, trimethoprim and methotrexate.

2.43 ABD

Postoperative DVT is confirmed in 30% of patients when no prophylactic anticoagulant measures are taken. Factor V Leiden is a mutation that causes resistance to activated protein C and is found in 60% of idiopathic DVTs. Other inherited causes of an increased risk of DVT include antithrombin III deficiency and protein S and C deficiencies.

2.44 ABD

The spleen is the second commonest organ to be damaged following blunt abdominal trauma. Such an injury must always be suspected if there is pain or tenderness in the lower left chest or hypochrondrium, lower rib fractures or pain over the left shoulder-tip (Kehr's sign). Splenic conservation is routinely practised in all centres as there are problems with postsplenectomy sepsis. However, a splenectomy would be indicated if there is evidence of haemodynamic instability or generalised peritonitis. Splenic rupture most frequently occurs 2 weeks after injury.

2.45   BDE

Laboratory features of iron deficiency anaemia include: decreased serum iron concentration; a raised TIBC; and absent iron in both the marrow and erythroblasts. Tissue oxygen delivery is dependent on haemoglobin and therefore will be affected. Anaemia does not cause a shift in the oxygen-dissociation curve. The presence of a posterior cricoid web and iron deficiency is a recognised association (Plummer–Vinson–Paterson–Kelly syndrome). Treatment with aspirin can cause gastritis, and associated haemoglobin loss over a prolonged period can deplete iron stores.

2.46   BDE

Fibrin dissolution can be reduced by tranexamic acid, which acts by inhibiting plasminogen activation and fibrinolysis. It is useful in cases where it is difficult to stop haemorrhage directly, as in prostatectomy. Epsilon-aminocaproic acid also inhibits the fibrinolytic system. Protein C is an important natural inhibitor of blood clotting. Factor XII acts upon prekallikrein to form kallikrein, which activates the fibrinolytic system through the intrinsic pathway. tPA (tissue plasminogen activator) is produced by endothelial cells; it binds to fibrin, converting fibrin-bound plasminogen to plasmin, which in turn degrades to fibrin.

2.47   AC

Vitamin B_{12} is involved in the red cell maturation process and haemopoiesis, but not in haemoglobin synthesis directly. In deficient states, megaloblastic erythropoiesis results. Vitamin B_{12} cannot be absorbed except in the presence of intrinsic factor, a glycoprotein secreted by the stomach. The intrinsic vitamin B_{12} complex is selectively absorbed in the terminal ileum. Stores of vitamin B_{12} are very great in the liver. A vitamin B_{12} deficiency takes approximately 5 years to develop.

2.48   A

Aspirin and clopidogrel are both antiplatelet agents and have no effect on blood cross-matching. Warfarin increases the INR by inhibiting the production of vitamin K-dependent factors II, VII, IX and X, but it does not affect cross-matching and compatibility testing *per se*. Haemaccel too does not affect blood cross-matching, which is one of the advantages of using this fluid in resuscitation.

2.49   CE

Human albumin solution is available in 20-g units, either as 400 ml of a 5% solution or 100 ml of a 20% solution. The 20% solution is hyperoncotic and will therefore expand the plasma volume by more than the volume infused. The 5% solution has a sodium content of 130–150 mmol/l and may precipitate hypernatraemia. Human albumin is manufactured from large pools of donations and is subjected to virus-inactivation procedures, hence the viral safety is excellent. The freeze-dried product has a long shelf-life at room temperature. Clinical indications include the treatment of hypoproteinaemic oedema with nephrotic syndrome and ascites in liver failure. There is no evidence that a 5% human albumin solution is superior to colloids in acute volume replacement.

2.50   BE

Autologous transfusion of preoperatively donated blood is a useful technique that minimises the hazards of infection transmission and alloantibody stimulation. It is particularly useful in patients who already have multiple alloantibodies and who are difficult to cross-match. The procedure still carries a small risk of a transfusion reaction, either through bacterial contamination of the donor units or by human error in transfusing the wrong blood. Patients who are unable to tolerate large venesections (e.g. children and those with pre-existing anaemia, cardiac or respiratory disease) or those with HIV or hepatitis B or C are unsuitable. Donations must be made at not less than weekly intervals and not within 4 days of surgery. The finite shelf-life of stored blood therefore limits the maximum collection to 4–5 units.

2.51   AF

Coagulation is initiated *in vivo* by the exposure of circulating factor VII to tissue factor, which in turn activates factor X (extrinsic pathway). Activated factor X subsequently sustains and amplifies the pathway by activating more factor VII and by activating factors XII, XI, IX, VIII and V (intrinsic pathway). Both pathways generate more activated factor X which, in sufficient concentration, converts prothrombin to thrombin – this in turn converts fibrinogen to fibrin (common pathway) so producing a fibrin clot. The process is completed by factor XIII which stabilises the fibrin clot.

Clotting factors are predominantly synthesised in the liver – factor II, VII, IX and X synthesis being vitamin K-dependent.

The coagulation cascade is inhibited *in vivo* by antithrombin III and the protein S and C pathways, hence deficiency of these proteins predisposes to thrombosis. Deficiency of the extrinsic, intrinsic and common pathway factors predisposes to haemorrhage, with the exception of factor XII deficiency which is asymptomatic.

intravascular coagulation (DIC) is characterised by the simultaneous activation of the coagulation and fibrinolytic pathways, which results in the consumption and depletion of platelets and clotting factors. Clinical presentation is usually with haemorrhage, but thrombosis may occur and tissue ischaemia may be apparent if the coagulation pathways are dominant. Common causes of DIC include sepsis, malignancy (especially adenocarcinoma), trauma and obstetric emergencies. Laboratory features include prolongation of all clotting times and a progressively falling platelet count and fibrinogen concentration. Increasing fibrin-degradation products (FDP) indicate activation of the fibrinolytic system, and, in the context of the other laboratory abnormalities, support a diagnosis of DIC. An isolated raised FDP level is seen in other conditions, including liver disease, and may cause diagnostic confusion. Treatment involves intensive blood-product support with correction of the underlying cause.

2.53   CE
The intravenous giving set should be removed but the cannula retained as intravenous access is required. The patient should be given large quantities of intravenous fluids to promote a urine output of >1.5 ml/kg per h. Furosemide (frusemide) should be given to promote diuresis, and a central line should be inserted if the patient remains oliguric. 100 ml of 20% mannitol are recommended for 'renal protection'. Hyperkalaemia and DIC may both occur and require specific treatment.

2.54   BCDE
A raised mean cell volume occurs with macrocytosis associated with the dietary deficiency or malabsorption of vitamin B_{12} and folate, liver disease (especially associated with alcohol abuse), hypothyroidism, myelo-dysplasia and after exposure to some drugs (cytotoxic). Vitamin B_{12} is found exclusively in animal products and deficiency is a hazard of veganism. Conditions such as haemolytic anaemia or recovery from acute haemorrhage lead to an increased erythropoietic drive and hence the appearance of reticulocytes in the circulation. This may manifest as a raised mean cell volume because reticulocytes have a higher cell volume than mature red cells. Iron deficiency is associated with microcytosis.

2.55 BDE

The activated partial thromboplastin time (APTT) measures the integrity of the intrinsic and common coagulation pathways. Hence, it is sensitive to a deficiency of factors VIII, IX, XI, XII and to a lesser extent factors V, X and prothrombin. The APTT is prolonged in patients on warfarin, except in the very early stages, due to impaired synthesis of the vitamin K-dependent factors II, VII, IX and X. Intravenous heparin potentiates the activity of the endogenous anticoagulant antithrombin III and prolongs the APTT by inhibiting the intrinsic and common pathway factors. Low-molecular-weight heparin selectively inhibits factor Xa and at therapeutic doses has little or no effect on the APTT. Thromboprophylaxis with subcutaneous heparin does not usually prolong the APTT. Lupus anticoagulant is an example of a coagulation factor inhibitor that has affinity to factors in the intrinsic pathway. The presence of a lupus anticoagulant impairs the function of these factors and so prolongs the APTT.

2.56 AB

Petechial haemorrhages are usually associated with vascular or platelet disorders. Coagulation disorders are typically associated with haemarthrosis and muscle haematomas. Scurvy is usually associated with swollen spongy gums with spontaneous bruising, haemorrhage and perifollicular haemorrhages. However, vitamin C deficiency may cause petechial haemorrhages.

2.57 All false

Aspirin and warfarin reduce the risk of arterial emboli in patients with atrial fibrillation. The international normalised ratio (INR) is a measure of prothrombin time (PT) and warfarin dosage should be adjusted to maintain the INR at 1.5–2.5. Warfarin should be stopped before surgery as it predisposes to major haemorrhage, outweighing the risk of emboli. The risk of bleeding is small once the INR is less than 1.5. To prepare this patient for surgery, warfarin should be stopped 3 days before scheduled surgery to allow the INR to fall to <1.5. Generally, aspirin does not need to be stopped before surgery. Warfarin could be recommenced after the operation once bleeding has stopped. For an elective operation such as this, stopping the warfarin several days before the surgery and administering heparin or a low-molecular-weight heparin is the accepted course of management. The use of vitamin K and FFP in this instance is wasteful of limited expensive resources.

2.58   D

Although it is popularly believed that all patients with a preoperative haemoglobin of <10 g/dl should be transfused, clinical studies show that cardiac output does not increase sharply until the haemoglobin falls well below 7 g/dl. Young patients tolerate haemodilution well, especially women. For an acute perioperative blood loss of less than 20% of total blood volume, resuscitation with a suitable crystalloid is usually sufficient unless there is a contraindication. In the elderly, pre-existing cardiorespiratory disease is much more likely and more aggressive transfusion is usually required, although rapid transfusion is unwise because of the risk of volume overload. Total blood volume is approximately 70 ml/kg in adults and 80 ml/kg in children.

2.59   ABDE

The other features of acute haemolytic transfusion reaction include pyrexia, flushing, lumbar pain, DIC, haemoglobinaemia and haemoglobinuria. Hypotension, not hypertension, may also occur. Immediate haemolytic transfusion reactions are usually due to ABO incompatibility. Delayed haemolytic transfusion reactions may occur in patients alloimmunised by previous transfusions or pregnancies. The haemolysis is usually extravascular and the patient may develop anaemia and jaundice a week after transfusion (most are clinically silent).

2.60   BDE

Thrombocytopenia is a common haematological abnormality, and usually arises from increased peripheral destruction of platelets in disorders such as immune thrombocytopenia, disseminated intravascular coagulation, hypersplenism or following heparin therapy. Thrombocytopenia may also occur in infiltrative bone marrow disorders such as carcinomatosis. Artefactual thrombocytopenia may result from platelet clumping *in vitro* following difficult venesection. Spontaneous bleeding in an afebrile patient with otherwise normal haemostasis is unlikely at platelet counts above 10×10^9/l. Thrombocytosis may indicate an acute-phase response in sepsis, inflammatory disorders or malignancy. It is common for the platelet count to rise transiently after splenectomy.

2.61   BCDE

Coagulation is initiated *in vivo* by the interaction between tissue factor (TF) in the tissues and factor VII in the plasma. Anatomical separation of TF from the plasma prevents activation of the pathway, unless vascular integrity is breached. Alternatively, coagulation can be initiated if TF is pathologically expressed on vascular cells, as in malignancy, disseminated intravascular coagulation and inflammation. If TF and factor VII interact, the resultant complex activates factor X and so completes the extrinsic pathway. In turn, factor X activates small quantities of thrombin that back-activates factors V, VIII, IX and X (intrinsic and common pathways) in the presence of anionic phospholipids on the surface of activated platelets. This provides amplification of the pathway by generating larger quantities of thrombin. Eventually, sufficient thrombin is formed to cleave fibrinogen to fibrin to form a thrombus. Coagulation is limited *in vivo* by the activation of the anticoagulants antithrombin III, protein S and protein C by thrombin.

2.62   BDE

Although acute haemolytic transfusions are almost exclusively caused by ABO incompatibility, haemolysis may also occur due to anti-Rh D, Rh E, Rh C and anti-Kell antibodies. In these cases, haemolysis occurs within the liver and spleen. The usual presentation is with fever, nausea and shivering usually about an hour after transfusion. Alternatively, in parous women or previous recipients of transfusions, there may be undetectable pretransfusion antibodies that increase dramatically after re-exposure as a secondary antibody response. This may manifest as a delayed haemolytic transfusion reaction presenting 5–10 days after transfusion with fever, a falling haemoglobin level, jaundice and haemoglobinuria. Fever and rigors occur in about 1–2% of red cell and platelet transfusions and may indicate a non-haemolytic febrile transfusion reaction. This is most common in parous women and those previously transfused. It represents a recipient antibody response to donor white cell antigens. Allergic reactions ranging from mild urticaria to anaphylaxis are usually due to an antibody response to donor plasma proteins.

2.63   All true

Graft-versus-host disease (GVHD) is a near-universally fatal condition caused by T lymphocytes in donor blood, and is characterised by fever, skin rash and gastrointestinal and liver dysfunction starting 4–30 days after transfusion. GVHD is prevented by using gamma-irradiated blood products. Lymphocyte contaminants in red cell products have immunosuppressant activity even in immunocompetent recipients. There is some evidence that recurrence of malignancy and sepsis is more common in heavily transfused patients undergoing surgery for malignant disease. Iron overload is inevitable in patients on long-term transfusion programmes. This may manifest as hepatic cirrhosis, endocrine insufficiency and cardiomyopathy. Post-transfusion purpura is a potentially fatal disorder, which is due to the production of antibodies against foreign platelet antibodies after transfusion. Thrombocytopenia in the recipient occurs when these antibodies crossreact with the recipient's own platelets. In the United Kingdom, blood products are not screened for the human T-cell leukaemia viruses (HTLV-I and -II) and a small number of patients acquire the lifelong risk of T-cell leukaemia from transfusions each year.

2.64   ABCD

Massive blood transfusion is defined as replacement of the whole-blood volume within 24 hours. Since red cell donations contain few platelets and low concentrations of coagulation factors, dilutional thrombocytopenia and coagulopathy can occur. Other sequelae include: hypocalcaemia; hyperkalaemia; and metabolic alkalosis. Correction of these biochemical and haematological abnormalities should be on an 'as needed' basis. Hypothermia is a recognised hazard and a blood warmer should be used routinely. Adult respiratory distress syndrome is a well-recognised complication.

2.65   B

Cardiopulmonary bypass is often associated with thrombocytopenia and platelet dysfunction. It is usually combined with induced hypothermia to reduce tissue metabolic demand. Plasma coagulation factor levels drop due to haemodilution. Heparin is routinely used to prevent extracorporeal clotting in the oxygenerator. Protamine sulphate is used at the end of a bypass to neutralise the remaining circulating heparin.

2.66   ADE

The prothrombin time measures the integrity of the extrinsic and common pathways of coagulation and is therefore sensitive to a deficiency or inhibition of factors II, V, VII and X. It is particularly sensitive to the global impairment of coagulation factor synthesis seen in severe liver disease or to vitamin K deficiency (impaired synthesis of factors II, VII, IX and X). Coagulation factor deficiencies, which affect only the intrinsic pathway, such as haemophilia A (factor VIII deficiency), will not prolong the prothrombin time. The prothrombin time is usually expressed as an international normalised ratio (INR) when monitoring oral anticoagulant dose. This allows standardisation of reagents between different laboratories.

2.67   All true

Inherited deficiencies or defects in components of the coagulation cascade with anticoagulant activity predispose to spontaneous and perioperative venous thrombosis. These include: antithrombin III, protein S and protein C deficiencies; and the factor V Leiden mutation. Acquired risk rises with increasing age, malignancy, a previous history of thrombosis, immobilisation, obesity, the combined oral contraceptive pill, hormone replacement therapy and pregnancy. Thrombosis also occurs more frequently in patients with sickle-cell disease, inflammatory bowel disease and myeloproliferative disorders.

2.68   A

Warfarin is an orally active anticoagulant that rapidly depletes hepatic vitamin K by impairing its recycling. It acts by preventing the synthesis of the vitamin K-dependent factors II, VII, IX and X, therefore it requires at least 48 hours to become effective. Although warfarin treatment will prolong both the APTT and the PT, the PT is a more reliable index of anticoagulant activity. It is usual practice to express the PT as an international normalised ratio (INR) when measuring anticoagulation. Complications of treatment include bleeding and, rarely, skin necrosis. Warfarin has numerous interactions with other drugs, commonly antibiotics (either reducing or enhancing its bioavailability).

2.69   A

Aspirin is an irreversible inhibitor of platelet cyclo-oxygenase and therefore reduces platelet thromboxane A2 (which usually promotes platelet aggregation and local vasoconstriction). Its main use is in the prevention of arterial thrombosis, which is more critically dependent on platelet activation and aggregation than venous thrombosis. Because patients who have received aspirin continue to show impaired platelet function until the platelet pool has been replaced from the marrow, aspirin should therefore be discontinued at least 7 days before surgery for its full antithrombotic effects to be eliminated. Aspirin is orally active and carries with it the risk of upper gastrointestinal haemorrhage, but very seldom bleeding at other sites.

2.70   BCE

Low-molecular-weight heparins (LMWHs) are prepared by enzymatic degradation of unfractionated heparin, so reducing their mean molecular weight from 15 to 4–7 kDa LMWHs therefore have a longer half-life than unfractionated heparin and better bioavailability after subcutaneous injection. Only a once-daily administration is required. LMWHs act predominantly by inhibiting factor Xa; and, unlike unfractionated heparin, they have low antithrombin activity. Consequently, a patient may be adequately anticoagulated with an LMWH without prolongation of the APTT. Excretion is almost exclusively renal and so dose reduction is required in patients with renal failure.

2.71   BDE

von Willebrand's disease is the commonest inherited bleeding disorder in white populations and is usually autosomal dominant in inheritance. Affected individuals have reduced or dysfunctional von Willebrand factor (vWF), a protein normally present in platelets and endothelium. vWF stabilises factor VIII in the circulation and mediates platelet adhesion at the site of vascular injury. The associated laboratory abnormalities therefore include a prolonged APTT (due to reduced factor VIII), a normal PT and a prolonged bleeding time (platelet-adhesion defect). Clinically, affected individuals usually show a mild bleeding tendency with epistaxis, easy bruising, menorrhagia and gingival bleeding. Although factor VIII levels are characteristically reduced, levels are rarely sufficiently low to cause haemarthroses, the hallmark of haemophilia A. Preoperative management usually involves treatment with desmopressin (which liberates platelet stores of vWF) or factor replacement with either intermediate-purity factor VIII or a specific vWF concentrate.

2.72 AB

Bleeding time is a global test of small-vessel haemostasis. It may be altered in thrombocytopenia, disorders of platelet function and collagen disorders affecting the vessel wall. However, the correlation with surgical bleeding is poor. Aspirin irreversibly inactivates platelets by inhibiting cyclo-oxygenase and therefore prolongs the bleeding time. Fibrinogen is manufactured in the liver and its synthesis is increased as part of the acute-phase response. A reduced fibrinogen concentration may indicate a consumptive coagulopathy. The thrombin time (TT) is a measure of the conversion of fibrinogen to fibrin and is therefore prolonged in hypofibrinogenaemia. Inhibitors of fibrin polymerisation – such as heparin, fibrin degradation products and severe hypoalbuminaemia – also prolong the TT. Heparin may cause significant prolongation of the TT at concentrations well below that needed to prolong the APTT.

2.73 BD

Following splenectomy there is an early thrombocytosis, usually peaking between 7 and 10 days. There are increased circulating Howell–Jolly bodies (DNA fragments of nuclear origin, normally present in <2% of circulating RBCs) and an increased proportion of target cells, sideroblasts (RBCs containing granules of free iron) and RBCs containing Heinz bodies (degraded haemoglobin, usually found in ageing RBCs). An early leucocytosis (usually neutrophils) is seen within hours and may last for several weeks. There is also increased platelet adhesiveness and platelet dysfunction.

2.74 ACE

Human albumin solution is a purified derivative of pooled, whole-blood donations and is subject to heat-inactivation of viruses. 20-g units are supplied as a freeze-dried product, which is stable at room temperature either as 400 ml of 5% solution or 100 ml of 20% solution. The 20% solution is hyperosmolar and may expand the plasma volume by more than the volume infused. The most common clinical uses are in the treatment of hypoproteinaemic oedema in nephrotic syndrome and ascites in chronic liver disease. Human albumin solutions should not be used as acute volume replacement because there is no evidence that they offer advantages over alternative fluids. The 5% solution has a sodium content of 130–150 mmol/l and may precipitate hypernatraemia in susceptible individuals.

2.75   BDE

Acute haemolytic transfusion reactions are the result of administration of ABO incompatible blood: group A, B or AB to a group-O recipient; group A or AB to a group-B recipient; or group B or AB to a group-A recipient. Human error outside the transfusion laboratory is the commonest cause. Clinically, the reaction can be recognised by the very rapid onset of agitation, flushing, pain at the venepuncture site, abdomen, flank or chest, a fever, hypotension, haemoglobinuria or haemoglobinaemia. This may be clinically indistinguishable from the effects of transfusing blood contaminated with Gram-negative organisms. Management should be the immediate cessation of transfusion, supportive measures and confirmation of the diagnosis with serological and haematological investigations.

2.76   Analgesia
1. **C   Dexamethasone**
2. **G   Opioid patient-controlled analgesia**
3. **D   Tricyclic antidepressants**
4. **E   Non-steroidal anti-inflammatory agent**

The three-step regimen for analgesia is useful: non-opioids for mild pain (e.g. paracetamol); mild opioids for moderate pain (e.g. co-dydramol); strong opioids for severe pain (e.g. diamorphine). Some types of pain are not sensitive to opioids and are best managed with alternative analgesia.

Pain from stretching of the liver capsule by metastases responds well to steroid therapy, which reduces liver swelling and capsular stretch.

Young patients will find an opioid PCA (patient-controlled analgesia) easy to understand and use. The on-demand intravenous analgesia acts rapidly and provides a continuous level of analgesia when compared to intermittent pethidine, for example. Haemophiliacs should avoid intramuscular injections.

Pain due to infiltration of nerves responds well to drugs that alter neurotransmission. Non-steroidal agents and steroid therapy run a risk of causing gastrointestinal ulceration.

The colicky pain associated with renal stones responds particularly well to the NSAID diclofenac.

2.77   BE

L5 cord lesions cause an ipsilateral loss of fine touch and a contralateral loss of pain and temperature sensation below the lesion. There is an ipsilateral upper neurone lesion with brisk reflexes, a Babinski sign, but no muscle wasting.

ANSWERS – CHAPTER 3: TRAUMA

3.1   All false
Severe burns may give rise to acute respiratory distress syndrome (ARDS). Also, full-thickness burns to the thorax can reduce skin compliance and impair chest wall movement. Pulse and BP alone are not reliable indicators of fluid resuscitation as they do not provide an accurate index of tissue perfusion and oxygenation. Full-thickness burns are usually anaesthetic, whereas partial-thickness burns are characteristically painful. According to ATLS guidelines for adults, partial- or full-thickness burns of over 20% body surface area should be referred to a burns centre. This threshold is reduced to 10% in children. The American Burn Association guidelines have an even lower threshold for referral (second-degree burns >10% total body surface area, third-degree burns >5% total body surface area).

3.2   E
Full-thickness burns can have a variety of colours, including cherry-red, white or black, but they typically result in anaesthesia due to destruction of the neural elements in the skin. Fluid resuscitation is not restricted to full-thickness burns. Lesser degree burns can still result in significant third-space loss due to capillary leakage and oedema. Inhalational injuries increase mortality and it is recommended that they be treated in a specialist burns unit.

3.3   Peripheral nerves of the upper limb
1. G   Deep branch of the ulnar nerve
2. E   Anterior interosseous nerve
3. C   Ulnar nerve at the elbow

The ulnar nerve divides into its deep (motor) and superficial (sensory) branches as it leaves the canal of Guyon. The deep branch is prone to compression where it passes round the pisiform bone in the palm.

The anterior interosseous branch of the median nerve (which supplies the flexor pollicis longus and flexor digitorum profundus to the index and middle fingers) may be compressed (usually by muscle hypertrophy from repeated forced pronation) where it passes through pronator teres, giving rise to muscle weakness but no motor signs.

One of the commonest nerve compressions is of the ulnar nerve at the cubital tunnel. Although the nerve is a mixed nerve, sensory signs and symptoms predominate in the early stages as the smaller diameter of the sensory fibres renders them more prone to neuropraxia.

3.4   BCD

Hyperkalaemia occurs as a result of tissue damage leading to potassium moving out of cells. Partial-thickness burns characteristically cause pain and blistering. It is only in full-thickness burns that there is a loss of sensation.

3.5   Upper limb fractures
1. A   Neck of the humerus
2. G   Olecranon fracture
3. F   Acromioclavicular joint disruption
4. D   Colles' fracture

A surgical neck of humerus fracture is treated with a collar and cuff, and gravity aids the reduction of the fracture.

Olecranon fractures are usually internally fixated with a tension band wire. This is to restore congruity in the joint line as this is an intra-articular fracture. It also restores the distal attachment of triceps, thereby restoring active extension.

The Colles' fracture typically results from a fall onto the outstretched hand and can be diagnosed from the 'dinner fork' deformity of the wrist caused by dorsal angulation at the fracture site in the wrist. The median nerve can be compromised. A load-bearing film is usually necessary to confirm the diagnosis of a disrupted acromioclavicular joint; treatment is with a broad arm sling.

3.6   ABCDF_ Nof

Compartment syndrome is associated with (but not exclusive to) closed fractures, particularly of the femur, elbow, forearm and proximal third of the tibia. It occurs when pressure within an osteofascial compartment increases, compressing the arteries passing through it. This can lead to ischaemia and necrosis of tissues supplied by those arteries. One well-known end-result is Volkmann's ischaemic contracture. Compartment syndrome may present with pain, pallor, paraesthesia, paralysis and pulselessness. The presence of a pulse does not exclude the diagnosis.

3.7   C

Haemorrhagic shock can be divided into four classes of severity, which are summarised in the following table:

	Class I	Class II	Class III	Class IV
Blood loss (ml)	<750	750–1500	1500–2000	>2000
Blood loss (% vol)	<15%	15–30%	30–40%	>40%
Pulse rate	<100	>100	>120	>140
Blood pressure	Normal	Normal	Decreased	Decreased
Pulse pressure	Normal	Decreased	Decreased	Decreased
Respiratory rate	14–20	20–30	30–35	>35
Urine output (ml/h)	>30	20–30	5–15	Negligible
Mental state	Slight anxiety	Mild anxiety	Anxious/ confused	Confused/ lethargic

The patient in this question is in Class III shock. The systolic blood pressure will be markedly reduced, the pulse pressure will be narrowed, and urine output will be significantly reduced. His respiratory rate will be elevated and he will be anxious and even disorientated. A decrease in blood pressure is a relatively late event in haemorrhagic shock and only occurs once 30% of the circulating blood volume has been lost.

3.8   ABDEG

Circulating fat globules larger than 10 mm in diameter and histological traces of fat emboli in the lungs occur in most adults after closed fractures of long bones. These fat emboli can impact not only in the lung microvasculature, but also in the brain. Fortunately, only a small number of patients develop the fat embolism syndrome. The source is thought to be the bone marrow. Early warning signs are a slight rise in temperature and pulse rate. Petechiae should be sought on the front and back of the chest, axilla and conjunctival folds. Fat droplets may be found not only in sputum, but also in urine, blood and CSF. Restlessness, drowsiness and even chest pain may occur. Some studies suggest that steroids can both prevent and treat the fat embolism syndrome.

3.9   Lower limb injuries
1.   C   **Saphenous nerve**
2.   A   **Common peroneal nerve**
Due to his lateral position on the operating table, the first patient has suffered a neuropraxia of his saphenous nerve, which supplies sensation to the medial side of his leg and foot.
The sural nerve arises from branches of the tibial and common peroneal nerves. It passes posterior to the lateral malleolus and supplies the lateral side of the foot and the little toe.
The second patient has sustained an injury to the common peroneal nerve which supplies the peroneal muscles (eversion of the ankle) and dorsiflexors of the ankle.

3.10   Brachial plexus injuries
1.   D   **Axillary nerve**
2.   B   **Lower brachial plexus**
3.   E   **Radial nerve in the spiral groove**
4.   F   **Long thoracic nerve**
The axillary nerve passes though the quadrilateral space, where it is particularly vulnerable to damage by downward displacement of the femoral head or after fracture of the surgical neck of the humerus. This may result in paralysis of the deltoid and teres minor muscles and loss of sensation over the lower part of the deltoid.
The lower brachial plexus (C8–T1) is susceptible to injury by forcible abduction, as in grabbing to save oneself from a fall. This is called a Klumpke's palsy. The first thoracic nerve is usually torn, resulting in a clawed appearance of the hand.
The radial nerve as it lies in the spiral groove is susceptible to injury at the time of fractures or during callus formation. Prolonged pressure on the back of the arm, for instance from the edge of the operating table, may result in a temporary wrist drop.
The long thoracic nerve of Bell crosses the axilla and is susceptible to damage during axillary dissection. This results in an inability of the serratus anterior muscle to rotate the scapula during abduction of the arm above 90°, such that the inferior pole of the scapula wings outwards. The other nerve commonly injured or sacrificed in axillary surgery is the sensory intercostobrachial nerve.

3.11   Peripheral nerve injury
1.   B   Common peroneal nerve
2.   D   Superficial peroneal nerve

An anterior compartment syndrome may compress the deep peroneal nerve and give rise to loss of sensation in the first web space between the first and second toes.

The common peroneal nerve is often damaged at the level of the fibular neck by severe traction when the knee is forced into varus (e.g. lateral ligament injuries and fractures around the knee) or from pressure from a splint or plaster cast. It is commonly associated with fractures of the head of the fibula, especially caused by impact from a car bumper. The patient has foot drop and loss of sensation over the front and outer half of the leg and dorsum of the foot.

The superficial peroneal nerve innervates the peroneal muscles, and emerges through the deep fascia 5–10 cm above the ankle to supply the skin over the dorsum of the foot and medial four toes.

3.12   BCD

Application of the PASG can raise systolic pressure through increasing peripheral resistance and myocardial afterload. However, the efficacy of PASG remains unproven. The PASG is indicated for splinting pelvic fractures with continuing haemorrhage and hypotension, and for intra-abdominal trauma with severe hypovolaemia in patients who are *en route* to theatre or to another facility. PASG is contraindicated in pulmonary oedema, suspected diaphragmatic rupture or when there is uncontrolled haemorrhage outside the confines of the garment (chest, arm, head or neck). The use of the PASG must not delay or reduce volume replacement.

3.13   ACDE

During the catabolic phase of the metabolic response to trauma, increased levels of ADH lead to water retention. Increased aldosterone levels lead to sodium retention. There is negative potassium balance in the first few days, although this rarely amounts to more than the average daily intake. Therefore during the first couple of days post-trauma, water and salt requirements are likely to be less than normal and potassium supplements are not required. Gluconeogenesis in the liver is stimulated by cortisol, amino acids from the catabolism of muscle acting as the substrate, leading to a negative nitrogen balance, which may persist for up to 2 weeks in patients with severe burns. Amongst the haematological responses are a thrombocytosis and neutrophilia.

3.14   Chest injury management
1.   A   **Oral analgesia**
2.   B   **Oral analgesia and admission**
3.   C   **Chest drain**

Rib fractures may be extremely painful. The importance of treating rib fractures lies in the management of the underlying lung injury and the prevention of pulmonary complications such as pneumonia and collapse. Atelectasis will occur if the lung is not fully aerated. This would occur if there is poor chest expansion due to pain. Young patients can tolerate a rib fracture more easily than elderly patients. With good physiotherapy and analgesia, young patients may be managed conservatively at home.

However, elderly patients (especially those living alone or who have co-morbid conditions) will tolerate rib fractures less well and necessitate admission with regular analgesia, physiotherapy and prophylactic antibiotics.

In a polytrauma patient, it is wise to insert a chest drain for the treatment of the pneumothorax, and also to prevent a recurrent or tension pneumothorax from developing when the patient is ventilated.

3.15   DE

Open chest wounds are most frequently caused by penetrating chest injuries, usually by firearms. A defect more than two-thirds the diameter of the trachea will lead to air preferentially entering via the defect rather than via the bronchus. The initial management is to close the defect with an occlusive dressing sealed on three of its four sides, to act as a valve and allow air to escape out but not to enter via the defect (this prevents a tension pneumothorax being formed). A chest drain should be inserted on the side of the lesion, some distance from the defect. Surgical repair is usually required.

3.16   BCE

Catecholamines are secreted by the adrenal medulla, and a decrease in atrial pressure stimulates ADH secretion by the Henry–Gauer reflex. Decreased PaO_2 stimulates chemoreceptors, and with increased ventilation (tidal ventilation) and reduced cardiac output there is an increase in V/Q mismatch. The oxygen–haemoglobin dissociation curve shifts to the left.

3.17   Sensation of lower limb
1.   C   Lateral cutaneous nerve of the thigh
2.   I   Tibial nerve
3.   F   Branch of the infrapatellar nerve
4.   H   Saphenous nerve

The woman in the first scenario has a lateral femoral cutaneous nerve palsy. The lateral femoral cutaneous nerve is a branch of the lumbar plexus, L2, L3. As it passes from the lateral border of the psoas major across the iliac fossa it lies at first behind the fascia iliaca and then passes behind, or pierces, the inguinal ligament, where it lies free in a fibrous tunnel a centimetre from the medial aspect of the anterior superior iliac spine. This nerve is sometimes compressed as it passes through the inguinal ligament or where it pierces the fascia lata. It causes pain on the lateral side of the thigh (meralgia paraesthetica).

Posterior lag of the knee would indicate cruciate ligament laxity, and together with medial collateral ligament laxity is due to tibial nerve damage. The tibial nerve gives off articular branches which supply both the medial collateral ligament and cruciate ligaments.

Pain and numbness on the medial side of the leg following knee arthroscopy is due to damage of the infrapatellar nerve.

The superficial peroneal nerve is susceptible to damage from surgery to short saphenous vein perforators in the lateral compartment of the leg. It passes downwards over the peronei and divides above the ankle into medial and lateral branches which supply the skin of the dorsum of the foot. The medial branch further divides to supply the medial side of the dorsum of the foot and sides of the second cleft. The lateral branch divides to supply the third and fourth clefts. Note that the first cleft is supplied by the deep peroneal nerve.

The saphenous nerve is the longest peripheral nerve in the body. It runs beside the long saphenous vein and may be damaged if the vein is stripped too far below the knee. It supplies sensation to the lateral side of the foot and leg.

3.18   ABD

Spontaneous breathing is a prerequisite for nasotracheal intubation. A laryngoscope is not used; the tube is advanced as the operator listens to breathing sounds through the tube. No tube should be passed into the nose when there is clinical evidence of either a facial or base-of-skull fracture, as the tube could inadvertently pass through into the brain. In trauma, oxygen must be given through a mask with a reservoir bag at 12–15 litres/min, nasal prongs are insufficient. Either needle or open cricothyroidotomy is indicated when endotracheal intubation has failed. The airway must be managed with the in-line neck immobilisation until it has been cleared radiologically. The neck must not be extended to open the airway.

3.19   Spinal injuries
1. F   A C1 Jefferson fracture
2. C   Cord transection at the C5 level
3. E   C2 odontoid dens dislocation
4. B   Neurogenic shock
5. A   Cauda equina syndrome
6. D   Hangman's fracture
7. B   Neurogenic shock
8. C   Cord transection at the C5 level
9. C   Cord transection at the C5 level

A Jefferson fracture is caused by axial compression, typically from a head injury, and results in a blow-out fracture of the C1 ring.

A hangman's fracture involves the posterior elements of C2 and is usually caused by distraction.

Neurogenic shock is caused by the loss of sympathetic outflow after a cord injury. Careful use of vasopressors may be indicated.

A fracture in the thoracolumbar region may result in injury to the nerve roots that comprise the cauda equina, as the spinal cord terminates at this level. With such cauda equina injuries, there will be bladder and bowel signs and patchy lower limb sensory and motor losses along the affected roots (as opposed to sensory or motor levels seen in spinal cord injuries).

A cord injury at the C5 level will result in flaccid areflexia, diaphragmatic breathing and an ability to flex but not extend at the elbow. The patient will grimace to pain above but not below the clavicle, as this represents the axial line between dermatomes C4 and T1. Priapism may be present in males.

3.20   All true

Fracture of the frontal skull can cause anosmia due to damage to the cribriform plate (olfactory nerve) and visual defects by damage to the orbit and optic chiasm. Discharge from the nose or ear may indicate leakage of CSF. Other indications of a basal skull fracture are: bruising over the mastoid bone (retroauricular ecchymoses, Battle's sign); periorbital ecchymosis ('racoon eyes'); and cranial nerve VII palsy.

3.21   Cerebral pathology
1.   A   CT head
2.   A   CT head

Any patient who has a falling Glasgow Coma Scale should have a CT scan. In instances where there is suspected raised intracranial pressure it would be unwise to do a lumbar puncture for fear of coning.

In the first case scenario, one would need to exclude an extradural haematoma. For the second patient, one would suspect a subarachnoid haemorrhage. Both these can be investigated with CT scanning.

3.22   ABCD

Extradural haematoma is associated with fracture and is usually the result of damage to the anterior part of the middle meningeal artery. The dura has strong attachments to the cranium along the suture lines; as a result these attachments can limit the extent of the haematoma. Subdural haematomas tend to follow a contre-coup injury, whereas extradural haematoma typically occurs with a direct local impact (coup).

3.23   A

Tracheal stenosis following tracheostomy may occur at three possible sites: level of the stoma; level of the cuff; and at the tip tube. The incidence is approximately 10%. The standard approach is a 2-cm transverse incision 2 cm above the sternal notch. The thyroid isthmus may need to be tied as it lies over the 2nd and 3rd tracheal rings. This has no effect on the thyroid status of the patient. In adults, the tracheostomy is placed between the 2nd and 4th tracheal rings, and in children at the 2nd and 3rd tracheal rings. The cough reflex is lost in someone with a tracheostomy and the patient is therefore unable to clear secretions from the tracheobronchial tree, so frequent suction is necessary.

3.24   CDE

Children have a relatively larger head which tends to flex the head on the neck, making airway obstruction more likely. The relatively larger tongue tends to flop back and obstruct the airway in the obtunded child and gives less room in the mouth when intubating. The larynx is positioned more cephalic (glottis at C3 in infants compared with C6 in adults) and the angle of the jaw is larger in children (140° in infants, 120° in adults), both making intubation more difficult. In addition, the trachea is shorter and the cricoid ring is the narrowest part of the airway (compared with the glottis in the adult).

3.25   Peripheral nerve anatomy
1.   **B   Lingual nerve**
2.   **A   Facial nerve**
3.   **F   Oculomotor nerve**
4.   **H   Cervical sympathetic trunk**
5.   **C   Ophthalmic nerve**

Misapplication of dental forceps during extraction of a lower 7 or 8 tooth can crush or sever the lingual nerve as it passes in a groove in the alveolar bone of the mandible under the gum. Such lesions cause ipsilateral loss of proprioception from the muscles of the tongue, predisposing to laceration between the occlusal surfaces of the teeth. The lingual nerve also subserves general sensation to the mucous membrane over the anterior two-thirds of the tongue (taste is from the chorda tympani nerve – VII).

Facial paralysis often goes unnoticed by patients with Bell's palsy, but other ipsilateral symptoms including dry eye (loss of lacrimal secretion) leading to corneal ulceration, impaired vision, some loss of taste (from the anterior two-thirds of the tongue), inability to close the mouth and the collection of food in the vestibule (paralysis of the buccinator muscle) are of concern. This particular lesion is located in the nerve at or before the origin of the superior petrosal branch.

IIIrd nerve lesions give rise to ipsilateral ptosis (paralysis of the striated component of the levator palpebrae superioris muscle), and pupillary dilatation (paralysis of the constrictor pupillae muscle). There is also an ipsilateral depressed lateral (down and out) strabismus (paralysis of all extraocular muscles, except the superior oblique and lateral rectus).

In Horner's syndrome, signs include ptosis (paralysis of the smooth muscle component of the levator palpebrae superioris muscle), and pupillary constriction (paralysis of the dilator pupillae muscle).

In herpes zoster infection of the ophthalmic division of cranial nerve V, a rash appears over the forehead from the vertex to the upper eyelid extending over the ala of the nose (the external nasal branch of the nasociliary nerve). If the cornea is involved (ciliary branch), blindness may result from scarring.

3.26   BCD
Post-traumatic stress disorder (PTSD) arises as a delayed and/or protracted response to a stressful event or situation of an exceptionally threatening or catastrophic nature, which is likely to cause pervasive distress in almost anyone. The symptoms include episodes of reliving the trauma via intrusive memories ('flashbacks') occurring against a background of a sense of 'numbness' and emotional blunting, detachment from other people and avoidance of activities and situations reminiscent of the trauma. Anxiety and depression are commonly associated, and excessive alcohol or drug abuse may be a complicating factor. PTSD symptoms, by definition, last at least a month. Acute stress disorders, by definition, begin within a month of the trauma and last less than a month, but PTSD symptoms may begin at any time.

3.27   AD
Below the L1 vertebra (transpyloric plane), the anterior and posterior nerve roots pass almost vertically downwards through the subarachnoid space and form the cauda equina. This consists only of anterior and posterior nerve roots. The subcostal plane lies at L3. A positive Babinski sign represents an upper motor neurone defect.

3.28   Operative procedures in the resuscitation room
1.   A   Pericardiocentesis
2.   C   Needle thoracocentesis
3.   J   Passage of a nasogastric tube
4.   H   Intraosseous infusion
A cardiac tamponade must be aspirated by pericardiocentesis with a large needle through a subxiphoid approach.
A tension pneumothorax is a clinical diagnosis, and is treated initially by needle aspiration through the second intercostal space in the mid-clavicular line. Formal chest drainage is performed later, towards the end of the primary survey.
Before diagnostic peritoneal lavage can be performed, both a urinary catheter and a nasogastric tube must be in place.
After two attempts at peripheral cannulation in the child, intraosseous infusion is recommended. Central lines should be avoided. In the adult, a venous cutdown is the procedure of choice after peripheral cannulation fails. It is easier to cannulate peripherally with venous cutdown than centrally if the patient's veins are collapsed.
In all cases of trauma, the first procedure is to secure the airway. In penetrating chest injury, up to 30% of pulseless patients can be saved by emergency thoracotomy if performed immediately by a qualified operator when the patient still has some electrical cardiac activity.

3.29   EF

Chronic subdural haematomas are most commonly found in the older age groups. Chronic alcohol ingestion is also an associated factor due to the frequent incidence of falls. Chronic subdural haematomas are collections of altered blood and are most frequently triggered by minor trauma. The symptoms include progressive headache, failing intellect, hemiparesis and a fluctuating conscious level. Acute subdural haematoma is more commonly associated with anosmia and rhinorrhoea as there is usually a concomitant skull fracture.

3.30   Trauma
1. **E   Ruptured diaphragm**
2. **C   Basal skull fracture**
3. **A   Flail chest**
4. **G   Jefferson's fracture**
5. **D   Fractured 1st rib**
6. **B   Fracture of C3**

Trauma resuscitation follows the ABC principles of ATLS training. In multiple trauma, the initial assessment will include three X-rays (cervical spine, chest and pelvis), which are likely to yield the most important clinical information during the resuscitation stage. If there is no neck tenderness and no focal neurology, a cervical spine X-ray may not be indicated. A full secondary survey is necessary to identify other less serious injuries, and also to detect deterioration or the development of new pathology. Battle's sign may not become obvious until several hours after injury. A hangman's fracture passes through the pedicles of C2.

3.31   B

A spontaneous pneumothorax causes reduced breath sounds on the affected side with hyper-resonance (if large enough). There is a tracheal shift to the affected side. A tension pneumothorax pushes the trachea to the opposite side. Spontaneous pneumothoraces typically resolve at 1% per day. Both lungs are affected equally. They have a male to female preponderance of 6:1. Only pneumothoraces with a >20% radiographic volume loss require aspiration.

3.32   BE

Rising intracranial pressure presents with headache, drowsiness, vomiting, seizures and there is often history of trauma. Signs include listlessness, irritability, drowsiness, falling pulse, rising blood pressure, coma, irregular breathing (respiratory depression from compression of the medulla) and later papilloedema. Lumbar puncture is contraindicated in raised intracranial pressure.

3.33   ABC
Systemic features of the crush syndrome include hyperkalaemia, hypocalcaemia, myoglobinaemia, anuric renal failure and coagulopathy. This occurs as a result of ischaemia and subsequent muscle necrosis. Myoglobin and other breakdown products are released following muscle necrosis, thereby causing acute tubular necrosis. Haemoconcentration, oliguria and uraemia are well documented.

3.34   A
A CT scan is most useful for diagnosing a solid-organ injury such as to the spleen or liver. The spleen is the most commonly injured solid organ in blunt trauma (the liver in penetrating trauma). Retroperitoneal organs such as the pancreas are rarely injured (10% of cases). The sole absolute contraindication of diagnostic peritoneal lavage is an indication for laparotomy.

3.35   CE
Damage to the long thoracic nerve causes winging of the scapula owing to weakness of the serratus anterior. Spinal accessory nerve damage will cause weakness in shrugging the shoulders. The axillary nerve contains fibres of C5 and C6 to predominantly supply the deltoid muscle. It conveys some sensory fibres to the lateral aspect of the forearm. The radial nerve supplies the extensor carpi radialis and ulnaris, plus extensor digitorum, so its injury results in wrist drop. Froment's (pincer) sign is associated with an ulnar nerve injury, where the adductor pollicis is weak and so the flexor pollicis longus accommodates. When a sheet of paper is placed between the thumb and index finger of a patient with a weak adductor pollicis, he/she will flex their thumb at the interphalangeal joint to grip the sheet. Sciatic nerve injuries result in foot drop, thus the high-stepping gait.

3.36   Anatomy of the cerebral vasculature
1.   E   Vertebral artery
2.   B   Posterior inferior cerebellar artery
3.   A   Posterior cerebral artery
4.   G   Striate arteries
The medial medullary syndrome results from an infarct in the ventromedial medulla oblongata after occlusion of the medullary branch of the vertebral artery. This results in destruction of the pyramid (contralateral hemiparesis), medial lemniscus (contralateral loss of all posterior column sensations) and rootlet of XII (ipsilateral lower motor neurone). With such alternating hemiplegias, the ipsilateral lower motor neurone component is the localising element.

The lateral medullary syndrome results from an infarct in the lateral medulla oblongata after occlusion of the medullary branches of the posterior inferior cerebellar artery. There is destruction of the: lateral spinothalamic tract (spinal lemniscus – contralateral loss of pain and temperature); nucleus ambiguus (paralysis of the muscles of the soft palate, pharynx, and larynx – difficulty in speaking and swallowing); and spinal tract and nucleus of V (ipsilateral loss of pain and temperature of the distribution of V).

The posterior cerebral artery supplies the visual cortex. Occlusion of the artery thus causes the above signs and symptoms. Macular sparing is attributed to a dual blood supply to the occipital pole from both the posterior and middle cerebral arteries.

Striate artery occlusion is the commonest cause of a stroke, affecting the posterior limb of the internal capsule, where both the descending corticospinal/corticobulbar projections, the ascending spinothalamic and the trigeminal sensory tracts to the thalamus are located.

3.37   CE

Brain death is defined as the irreversible loss of consciousness and breathing. All brainstem reflexes are absent. It is confirmed by: fixed, unresponsive pupils; absent corneal, gag, cough and vestibulo-ocular reflexes; and no spontaneous respiratory effort. The GCS would be 3.

3.38   BCDE

A fall of more than 15 feet (4.6 m) is associated with a significant probability of sustaining a major trauma, as is an extrication time of >20 minutes or a vehicular impact speed >30 mph (~19 kph) (>25 mph (~16 kph) with no restraints). In addition, a pedestrian impact with a car travelling >20 mph (~13 kph) is associated with a significant risk of injury.

3.39   Anatomy of the brachial plexus and nerves of upper arm

1. **A   C5, C6, C7 roots of brachial plexus**
2. **B   C8, T1 roots of brachial plexus**
3. **C   Long thoracic nerve**
4. **E   Axillary nerve**
5. **F   Radial nerve**

Erb's palsy (upper brachial plexus injury) may be found after difficult deliveries. It is much more common than Klumpke's paralysis (the corresponding lower brachial plexus injury).

Pure lower brachial plexus injuries are rare. The presence of Horner's syndrome suggests a C8 and T1 root avulsion and helps to differentiate this injury from an ulnar nerve lesion. It is essential to establish how proximal the injury is in these cases as preganglionic avulsions are irreparable, whereas postganglionic avulsions may be amenable to repair.

Injuries of the long thoracic nerve (of Bell) may occur following axillary dissection.

Damage to the axillary nerve may occur after shoulder dislocation. In addition to loss of deltoid contraction, there may be loss of sensation in the regimental badge area, although this is not universal. Recovery usually occurs within 3 months, but on occasions the nerve is completely divided and requires repair or shoulder stabilisation.

'Saturday night palsy' of the radial nerve occurs after drinking binges. The usual mechanism is direct pressure on the nerve in the spiral groove of the humerus as the arm hangs over the back of a chair when the patient has passed out. Recovery is usual, and the condition is treated with a wrist splint.

3.40   Operative procedures in the resuscitation room

1. **E   Venous cutdown**
2. **K   Endotracheal intubation**
3. **D   Emergency thoracotomy**
4. **B   Chest tube drainage**

In the adult, a venous cutdown is the procedure of choice after peripheral cannulation fails. It is easier to cannulate peripherally with venous cutdown than centrally if the patient's veins are collapsed.

In all cases of trauma, the first procedure is to secure the airway. In penetrating chest injury, up to 30% of pulseless patients can be saved by emergency thoracotomy if performed *immediately* by a qualified operator when there is still some electrical cardiac activity.

3.41 ACE

Tachycardia in response to haemorrhage may be absent in: the elderly; patients on β-blockers and calcium antagonists; in those with hypothermia; and in patients who have a pacemaker. Infants will develop a tachycardia and the rate will be much higher than in adults. Athletes have a higher cardiac output and stroke volume but a lower resting pulse than the average population. The usual responses to hypovolaemia may not be manifest in athletes until a significant blood loss has occurred. Oxygen has no affect on this response.

3.42 Shock
1. **C Neurogenic shock**
2. **F Hypovolaemic shock >40% volume loss**
3. **B Septic shock**

Neurogenic shock is due to the loss of sympathetic tone, and combines the symptoms characteristic of hypovolaemic shock with a profound bradycardia.

Generally in hypovolaemic shock:

<15% loss leads to slight anxiety, no change in pulse, BP or respiratory rate, urine output is maintained.

15–30% loss leads to mild anxiety. The BP is maintained, the pulse is generally >100 and the pulse pressure is reduced, urine output is maintained at 20–30 ml/h.

30–40% loss leads to an anxious patient. The BP is decreased with a pulse >120 bpm. Urine output is 5–15 ml/h.

>40% loss causes confusion. The pulse is generally >140, the BP and pulse pressure fall. There is no urine output. Fit athletic individuals may initially compensate for massive blood loss causing hypovolaemia and maintaining their pulse and BP, then rapidly decompensate.

Septic shock should be considered in cases of delayed presentation. This is similar in presentation to hypovolaemic shock, but is characterised by a wide pulse pressure. Patients who are hypothermic from exposure may initially appear to be apyrexial.

3.43 BCE

Internal fixation will not lead to faster healing but will give rapid stability to the bone. If large opposite forces are present then splinting is unlikely to be successful and fixation is needed. In the multiply injured patient, stabilisation of fractures with internal fixation has been shown to reduce the incidence of complications and improve outcome. Internal fixation should be avoided in compound fractures because of the risk of infection.

3.44   Burns in children
1. F   18%
2. F   18%
3. A   1%
4. F   18%
5. C   7%
6. D   9%
7. E   14%

The relative body surface areas in children are different from adults. The head and neck make up a larger proportion of an infant's total body area than a child's – 18% and 14%, respectively. The legs make up a smaller proportion at 14% each. Other regions include the: genitals, 1%; anterior trunk (chest and abdomen), 18%; posterior trunk (upper and lower), 18%; and each arm, 9%.

3.45   ACE

A surgical airway is indicated where the trachea cannot be intubated and when there is an immediate need for an airway. In emergency situations, insertion of a needle through the cricothyroid membrane is a useful technique for providing oxygen on a short-term basis. A surgical cricothyroidotomy is performed by making a skin incision through the cricothyroid membrane and inserting a small endotracheal/tracheostomy tube (5–7 mm).

3.46   CE

In the immediate aftermath of a traumatic insult to the body, a complex series of responses are set in motion. Underperfusion of the tissues leads to a decrease in metabolic rate and body temperature, and an increase in anaerobic metabolism with the formation of lactic acid and a secondary metabolic acidosis. Increased levels of catecholamines stimulate lipolysis and glycogenolysis, which lead to hyperglycaemia in the presence of decreased insulin levels, this hyperglycaemia is exacerbated by the conversion of lactic acid in the liver to glucose.

3.47   DE

This procedure is limited to children 6 years of age or younger, in whom venous access is impossible due to circulatory collapse or for whom percutaneous peripheral venous cannulation has failed on two attempts. The puncture site is on the anteromedial surface of the proximal tibia 1–3 cm below the tubercle. The Seldinger technique is one of needle puncture followed by the insertion of a guide-wire, over which a larger cannula can be inserted. This is used for the placement of central lines, Swanz–Ganz catheters or femoral lines.

3.48   ACD
Cervical cord injury is characterised by flaccid areflexia, diaphragmatic breathing and the ability to flex but not extend the elbow. Priapism is an uncommon but characteristic sign. Full immobilisation of the neck is required at all times.

3.49   Neurotransmitters in the body
1. **C   Adrenaline (epinephrine)**
2. **E   GABA**
3. **A   Substance P**
4. **D   Noradrenaline (norepinephrine)**
Catecholamines are produced by the chromaffin cells of the adrenal medulla and sympathetic nervous tissue. Adrenaline is produced mainly in the adrenal medulla and noradrenaline in the sympathetic tissue.
Adrenaline vasoconstricts the gut and skin and vasodilates skeletal muscle, whereas noradrenaline is a very potent general vasoconstrictor.
GABA is an inhibitory neurotransmitter.
Substance P is a paracrine neurotransmitter that contracts smooth muscle, and is involved in neurogenic inflammation.

3.50   ACDE
ADH, catecholamines and corticosteroids are elevated following trauma. This has the effect of conserving sodium, water and producing a hyperglycaemia.

3.51   Upper limb injuries
1. **A   Axillary nerve**
2. **B   Median nerve**
3. **C   Ulnar nerve**
The axillary nerve passes through the quadrangular space and winds around the surgical neck of the humerus with the posterior circumflex humeral artery and vein. It supplies the teres minor and deltoid muscles and an area of skin around the mid-lateral arm-badge area. The median nerve and brachial artery are classically at risk in supracondylar humeral fractures, as they cross anterior to the fracture site. This form of injury is more common in children. The ulnar nerve passes behind the medial humeral epicondyle and can be stretched in elbow dislocations.

3.52   AC

Cerebrospinal fluid is predominantly produced by the choroid plexuses in the ventricles, which are connected via the foramen of Monroe. CSF is produced at a rate of 0.3–0.5 ml/h. The arachnoid granulations (villi) are involved in the reabsorption of CSF into the venous sinuses and so into the systemic circulation.

3.53   BD

Cerebral perfusion pressure is calculated by the mean arterial blood pressure minus the intracranial pressure. It is tightly regulated so that perfusion pressure, and hence cerebral blood flow, fluctuates very little despite many postural changes. The autoregulatory stimuli are PO_2 and pH (PCO_2 exerts its effect via dissociation into HCO_3^- and H^+ ions and hence a fall in pH). Mannitol is used to reduce intracranial oedema, and hence intracranial pressure, in cases of head injury. This has the effect of increasing cerebral blood flow, but it has no effect in normal subjects.

3.54   BDE

Immediately after a fracture, a haematoma forms at the site. A vascular pannus is associated with rheumatoid disease. Two specialised cell types are involved in fracture healing: osteoblasts lay down seams of uncalcified new bone; osteoclasts reabsorb bone and play a key role in remodelling. Immediately after a fracture, haemorrhage results in the formation of a blood clot, which is invaded by macrophages and replaced by granulation tissue. The inflammatory process extends to involve the periosteum on either side of the fracture. Bony necrosis is seen after 24–48 hours. A provisional callus of woven bone is laid down; this is then slowly reabsorbed and replaced with lamellar bone.

3.55   Lower limb trauma
1. B   Posterior compartment syndrome
2. A   Anterior compartment syndrome

Pain on stretching the suspected compartment by passive force indicates a compartment syndrome. The first patient is likely to have a posterior compartment syndrome as the muscles of the posterior compartment are stretched by ankle dorsiflexion.

The second patient is also likely to have a compartment syndrome. The deep peroneal nerve which supplies the 1st web space runs in the extensor or anterior compartment of the leg.

3.56   ADG

The classical symptom triad of cardiac tamponade (Beck's triad) includes muffled heart sounds, distended neck veins and hypotension, and is seen in the majority of patients. Pulsus paradoxus is defined as a fall in systolic blood pressure of over 10 mmHg on inspiration. This only occurs in 1 in 10 cases of tamponade. In cardiac tamponade, the cardiac outline on CXR is classically globular. Charcot's triad refers to fever, jaundice and abdominal pain, and is suggestive of cholangitis. In severe haemorrhage, the CVP may not be elevated even in cardiac tamponade.

3.57   CDE

Split-skin grafts contain epidermis and varying amounts of dermis, and rely totally on the vascularity of the recipient site for survival. Thinner split grafts are more likely to 'take' than thicker ones because there is less tissue to be supported by imbibition. Lesser degrees of recipient-site bacterial contamination, such as tissues containing $<10^5$ organisms/mm^3, will usually allow a graft to 'take'.

3.58   Injury patterns following RTA trauma
1. **B   Side-impact RTA**
2. **A   Frontal-impact RTA**
3. **B   Side-impact RTA**
4. **A   Frontal-impact RTA**
5. **D   Pedestrian in an RTA**

Different mechanisms of injury give rise to different related-injury patterns, though there is much overlap between each.

Frontal impact is more likely to produce cervical spine fractures, anterior flail chest, myocardial contusion, pneumothorax, aortic transection, liver/spleen rupture and posterior dislocation of the femur on the acetabulum.

Side impact is more likely to produce cervical spine fractures, lateral flail chest, pneumothorax, pelvic compression fractures and liver/spleen rupture.

Rear impact is more likely to produce cervical spine injury.

Pedestrians in RTAs are likely to suffer head injury, thoracic and abdominal injuries, and fractures of the lower limbs (e.g. tibial plateau fractures).

3.59   CE

A chronic subdural haematoma (CSH) is produced by rupture of veins passing from the cerebral hemispheres to the venous sinuses as a result of displacement of the brain inside the skull. It is bilateral in 50% of cases. CSH may occur after only slight force and there may be no preceding loss of consciousness. In many cases the patient will be unable to recall any history of head trauma. Features may not be apparent for weeks or months, and can range from undramatic (mental slowness) to significant symptoms (weakness, seizures, gait disturbance). Papilloedema is rare.

3.60   B

The only absolute contraindication to DPL is any existing indication for laparotomy. DPL under these circumstances would not alter management decisions and would only delay transfer to theatre and the subsequent correction of potentially life-threatening injuries. Relative contra-indications include advanced pregnancy, advanced cirrhosis, previous abdominal operations, morbid obesity and established pre-existing coagulopathy.

3.61   BEF

Good-quality lateral cervical spine films will identify approximately 85% of significant cervical spine injuries in adults. In combination with AP and peg views, this sensitivity can exceed 90%. An acceptable quality lateral cervical spine X-ray should include the upper border of T1 (to exclude a cervicothoracic dislocation). If the upper border of T1 is not visualised despite applying traction to the arms, then a swimmer's view, or even a C7–T1 junction CT scan, can be attempted. Flexion and extension views are not recommended in an acute setting. Significant cervical spine injury may exist even in the absence of radiological abnormalities on standard views, particularly in children. Spinal cord injury without radiological abnormality is commoner in children than in adults.

3.62   E

A collapsed L5–S1 disc presses on the S1 spinal nerve (the L5 nerve passes above the prolapsed disc in the intervertebral foramen and thus escapes damage). At the level of prolapse, the spinal canal contains the cauda equina and not cord *per se*. The S1 dermatome lies over the lateral malleolus. Exaggerated reflexes are diagnostic of an upper motor neurone lesion. The S2 dermatome occupies the posterior aspect of the calf.

3.63   Anatomy of intracranial haemorrhage/thrombosis
1. E   **Internal carotid artery**
2. C   **Middle meningeal artery**
3. F   **Cerebral vein**
4. H   **Cerebral artery**
5. A   **Cavernous venous sinus**

Expanding, internal carotid artery aneurysms in the cavernous sinus can erode into the sphenoidal air sinus medially and also compress the lateral wall of the cavernous sinus damaging CN III, IV, Va and Vb. CN VI is most commonly involved as it passes through the venous sinus in the adventitia of the artery. Rupture of the aneurysm into the cavernous sinus creates a carotid–cavernous sinus fistula (causing eyeball pulsation); blood may dissect through the eroded passage medially into the sphenoid air sinus from whence it drains through the sphenoethmoidal recess into the nasal cavity, relieving the pressure in the sinus. In this case, only VI is affected, giving diplopia and a medial strabismus. Diplopia is worse on looking to the left as abduction is paralysed in the affected eye.

Scenario 2 is a typical history of a developing extradural haematoma from a middle meningeal artery bleed after skull fracture at the pterion. The lucid interval is extended because the bleed is contained between the meningeal and endosteal layers of the dura mater, which are dissected apart as the bleed progresses.

Scenario 3 is a typical history of a subdural haematoma after tearing a cerebral vein as it lies in the subdural space above the arachnoid mater at the point of entry into the superior sagittal sinus. The tear occurs by shearing at the vein/sinus interface when a forward accelerating movement of the head is suddenly arrested. Movement of the skull and associated dural sinuses are halted, but the forward movement of the brain and cerebral veins continues. The lucid interval is protracted because of the low and often negative pressures in the system.

Scenario 4 is a typical history of a massive subarachnoid haemorrhage. This is usually from a rupture of a cerebral artery aneurysm arising from the circle of Willis – a Berry aneurysm. The lucid period is short and commonly absent altogether. Intracranial pressure quickly builds and, unless relieved, death rapidly ensues.

Cavernous sinus thrombosis may result from the spread of infection from areas drained by the venous tributaries of the sinus; in scenario 5, ophthalmic veins draining the chronically infected ethmoidal air sinuses. There is oedema of all drainage areas and resulting exophthalmos. Complete ophthalmoplegia may ensue as CN III, IV and VI become involved. Damage to CN Va (and Vb) causes severe pain over cutaneous distributions.

3.64   ABE
The liver is the most frequently injured solid organ in penetrating abdominal injuries. Penetrating hepatic trauma in the unstable patient requires emergency treatment, but can, occasionally, be managed conservatively in stable patients. Although it usually presents with hypotension and shock, it can sometimes present late with symptoms such as haemobilia. It is rarely fatal if treated aggressively (less than 10%). At operation, excessive bleeding is usually controlled by pressure, direct suture or packing swabs around the liver – but not into the hepatic defect. Pringle's manoeuvre consists of compression of the porta hepatis (and thus the portal vein and hepatic artery) to reduce the haemorrhage.

3.65   AEF
The duration of post-traumatic amnesia (not retrograde amnesia) correlates well with primary brain injury. Blood alcohol levels correlate very poorly with the degree of depression of conscious level in a patient with a head injury. The depression of conscious level must be assumed to be due to the head injury.
Adequate analgesia improves the cerebral perfusion pressure. Codeine phosphate does not interfere with pupillary reflexes. Haemodynamic stabilisation takes priority over evacuation of intracranial haematomas. In diffuse axonal injury, the distal segment of a disrupted axon undergoes wallerian degeneration.

3.66   Cerebral injury
1. E   Basal skull fracture
2. B   Subarachnoid haemorrhage
3. A   Subdural haematoma
4. D   Extradural haematoma
Basal skull fracture is suggested by a number of signs, including bleeding or CSF leaking from the nose or ears. Battle's sign (bruising around the mastoid) and 'racoon eyes' (periorbital ecchymoses) usually occur later. Subarachnoid haemorrhage is characterised by a sudden, dramatically severe onset of headache. Subdural haematomas often occur following the rupture of bridging veins in the elderly and are easy to miss because of the fluctuating levels of consciousness. A lucid phase is classical in an extradural haematoma. Treatment is usually emergency drainage.

3.67   CD

Extradural haematomas are usually biconvex in appearance, whereas subdural ones are crescenteric. In contrast to subdural haematomas, extradural haematomas do not usually cross suture lines as the dura is normally very adherent to the cranium. Both subdural and extradural haematomas can cross the midline. Decreased attenuation of a haematoma is usually a feature of a chronic (over 21-days-old) subdural haematoma.

3.68   ACEG

Traumatic rupture of the thoracic aorta usually follows rapid deceleration and is usually fatal. The commonest site of injury is just distal to the origin of the left subclavian artery. The ascending or distal descending aorta are much less commonly involved. Arch aortography is still the 'gold standard' and the diagnostic modality of choice. Transoesophageal echo and CT scan are alternative imaging modalities.

3.69   Radial nerve injury
1.   C   Axillary compression
2.   B   Fracture at the level of the mid-humerus
3.   A   Compression at the level of the elbow

In low radial nerve lesions – i.e. those due to fractures or dislocations at the elbow – the posterior interosseus nerve may be injured and the patient is unable to perform finger extension with weakness of thumb abduction (weak abductor pollicis longus) and extension. In high lesions, e.g. with fractures of the humerus or prolonged tourniquet pressure, there is weakness of the radial extensors of the wrist and numbness over the anatomical snuff-box. Triceps function is preserved in these lesions as the nerve to the triceps branches off in the axilla. The radial nerve may be compressed in the axilla by a crutch palsy.

3.70   AD

Blood loss is a leading cause of death in severely injured patients, and hypotension must be assumed to be hypovolaemic in origin until proven otherwise. A shorter neck makes for a more difficult intubation. Tourniquets produce anaerobic metabolism and increase blood loss if incorrectly applied. They may also result in limb ischaemia. A high-riding prostate may indicate significant urethral injury and is a contraindication to urethral catheterisation. A urethrogram is used to assess urethral integrity. Neck wounds penetrating through the platysma require formal surgical exploration.

3.71   CE

Traumatic diaphragmatic rupture following blunt trauma occurs in the left hemidiaphragm in around 70% of cases. The initial CXR changes are usually non-specific. In fact, the X-ray will be normal in half the cases. DPL is unreliable for the detection of isolated diaphragmatic injury.

3.72   Head injury
1. D   **Diffuse axonal injury**
2. C   **Base-of-skull fracture**
3. A   **Extradural haematoma**
4. E   **Concussion**
5. A   **Extradural haematoma**
6. C   **Base-of-skull fracture**
7. B   **Subdural haematoma**

Diffuse axonal injury (DAI) is characterised by prolonged coma often lasting weeks. One-third of the patients will usually die from increased intracranial pressure secondary to cerebral oedema. DAI results from widespread microscopic damage and therefore no mass lesion is seen on a CT scan of the head.

Base-of-skull fractures are often not apparent on skull X-rays, but may reveal themselves indirectly as air-fluid levels in the sphenoid sinus. Clinically there may be rhinorrhoea, otorrhoea, bilateral periorbital haematoma (racoon eyes) and ecchymosis over the mastoid process (Battle's sign).

Acute extradural haemorrhage almost always occurs from a tear in a dural artery or vein, usually always associated with a linear fracture in the temporal or parietal regions of the skull. Typically, there is a period of loss of consciousness, followed by a lucid interval. Following this, there is a secondary depression of consciousness and subsequent development of a contralateral hemiparesis and ipsilateral pupillary dilatation.

Subdural haematomas result from the rupture of subdural bridging veins. A skull fracture may or may not be present. However, the underlying brain injury is often severe.

3.73   ACE

Composite grafts include skin, subcutaneous tissue and other tissue elements such as cartilage. They are free grafts and rely on imbibition and diffusion. Therefore, they are size-limited. Human epithelial cells can be cultured to provide sheets for grafting. This is useful for large burns. Free flaps generally rely on a blood supply from an artery of least 1 mm in diameter, with microvascular anastomosis being able to restore the blood supply. Advancement flaps depend on the laxity of their skin to provide excess tissue when separated from their underlying structures. They are useful when there is excessive skin with a good blood supply, such as in the ageing face.

3.74   BD

Major burns are associated with splanchnic vasoconstriction on both the arteriolar and venular sides of the circulation. Curling's ulcers are stress ulcers related to major burns. They have a propensity to massive bleeding and have a poor prognosis.

3.75   Theme: Tubes used in trauma
1. **C   Urethral catheter**
2. **D   Nasogastric tube**
3. **F   Cuffed endotracheal tube**
4. **B   Short, wide-bore intravenous cannula**
5. **A   Long, wide-bore central line**
6. **F   Cuffed endotracheal tube**

Hourly measurement of urinary output is a fairly reliable indicator of organ perfusion in shocked patients. Blood pressure alone is of limited value. An arterial line is useful to determine oxygen saturation and blood gases, in addition to providing a continuous measurement of peripheral blood pressure. A definitive airway is one that has a cuffed endotracheal tube. No tube should be passed into the nose in the presence of either facial or base-of-skull fractures.

Fluids are best given quickly through large-bore, short cannulas. A central line gives a good indication of right atrial pressure, but is not a good indicator of overall perfusion. A cuffed endotracheal tube gives definitive airway protection against gastric aspiration.

3.76   CEF
Injuries to the urethra, bladder, lumbosacral nerve roots, genitalia, rectum and pelvic contents often accompany pelvic fractures. About 90% of bleeding from pelvic trauma is from the fracture site or pelvic veins. Major bleeding is rarely arterial in origin. The prevailing philosophy is to tamponade the low-pressure retroperitoneal bleeding by splinting the pelvis and transfusing. If this fails, pelvic vascular embolisation is advocated. Open surgical approaches for haemostasis are a last resort and are associated with a high mortality. The overall mortality of open pelvic fractures approaches 50% and reflects associated abdominal, rectal, thoracic and head injuries. Cystography requires at least two views to exclude a bladder rupture. With a pelvic bleed, over 4 litres of blood can collect in the retroperitoneum.

3.77   BCD
Clinical indicators suggestive of acute inhalational injury include a history of confinement in a burning environment or history of explosion, facial burns, carbonaceous sputum, oesophageal carbon deposits, hoarseness, wheezing or singeing of the eyebrows, eyelashes or nasal hair.

3.78   BCD
Acute traumatic diaphragmatic rupture is more common on the left side, reflecting the degree of protection offered to the right diaphragm by the liver. Abdominal viscera (such as the spleen, stomach, omentum and small bowel) can migrate into the chest, especially on the left side, causing mediastinal displacement and cardiorespiratory compromise. Once in the chest, migrated viscera are at risk of obstruction or strangulation. Treatment is surgical and involves reduction and repair of abdominal viscera, closure of the diaphragmatic defect and drainage of the pleural cavity.

3.79   AD
The femoral nerve supplies the quadratus femoris muscle, the contracting fibres of which elicit the knee jerk. The nerve supplies the L2–4 dermatomes over the anterior skin of the thigh. The genitofemoral nerve mediates the cremasteric reflex. The saphenous nerve (L4), a branch of the femoral nerve, innervates the skin over the medial malleolus. The lateral cutaneous nerve of the thigh, and the genitofemoral nerve, both branches of the lumbar plexus, also supply the L2 dermatome.

3.80   Patterns of injury
1. C   **Explosion**
2. E   **Restrained front-seat passenger in rear-end car shunt**
3. E   **Restrained front-seat passenger in rear-end car shunt**
4. A   **Fall from height**
5. B   **Rear car-seat passenger**

A fall from height, whereby the victim lands on both feet, causes the force to be transmitted from the heels through the legs and up through the axial skeleton. Thus, fractures may occur at any site from the heels to the base of the skull.

A restrained driver involved in a head-on collision will slide forwards at impact, striking the knees on the dashboard. This may result in patellar fractures, femoral shaft fractures and posterior hip dislocations with or without acetabular fractures. The steering wheel can also impact the anterior chest wall resulting in sternal fractures and myocardial contusion as well as duodenal and pancreatic injuries.

The restrained passenger involved in a (less forceful) rear-end shunt will experience hyperextension of the neck, causing a neck sprain or whiplash type injury.

A rear car-seat or aeroplane passenger with a loop seatbelt applied above the anterior superior iliac spine, rather than between it and the femur, gives rise to anterior lumbar compression (Chance) fractures or visceral damage (e.g. duodenum, pancreas).

An explosion can cause a rupture of the tympanic membrane resulting in deafness. There are also likely to be lacerations secondary to flying debris.

3.81   ACD

Hyperbaric oxygen refers to an oxygen tension of significantly greater than one atmosphere. An anaesthetic breathing circuit can only achieve approximately one atmosphere, so a pressurised chamber is required for the administration of hyperbaric oxygen. Typically, treatment involves several sessions of an hour or more. Among other effects, hyperbaric oxygen therapy is thought to improve oxygen delivery to cells and to reduce smoke-induced pulmonary oedema. Uses include the treatment of gas gangrene, necrotising fasciitis and carbon monoxide poisoning (though there has been conflicting evidence as to its efficacy). Exposure to more than two atmospheres tension of oxygen may cause acute oxygen toxicity, which can manifest as convulsions.

3.82   BCD
Although less than 10% of trauma admissions have sustained cardiac or major vascular injury, thoracic trauma is responsible for 25% of trauma deaths. Most injuries (around 85%) can be managed without surgery. Tracheal rupture is an immediate threat to the airway and most people die before reaching hospital. A small number will reach hospital in a stable condition and undergo successful surgical repair.

3.83   Radiological signs in trauma
1.   C   Apical capping
2.   D   Talar shift
3.   E   Loss of psoas shadow
4.   B   Posterior fat-pad sign
An anterior fat-pad sign on an elbow X-ray is non-specific, it can occur in any condition that produces an effusion (e.g. septic arthritis or rheumatoid arthritis). A posterior fat-pad sign is specific for a traumatic fracture. An apical capping represents extrapleural blood that tracks upwards and appears as a density at the left apex of the lung. Signs of aortic injury in descending order of frequency are: a widened mediastinum, tracheal deviation to the right, elevation of the right main bronchus and depression of the left main bronchus, loss of contour of the aortic knuckle, left apical capping, left haemothorax, obscured descending aorta, left mediastinal stripe and widened right paratracheal area. The widened mediastinum is the most sensitive sign, but is only 8% specific. It is defined as being >8 cm or >25% of the width at that level on a supine CXR or >6 cm on an erect PA (more accurate) CXR.
Loss of the psoas shadow may be seen in the presence of a major retroperitoneal haemorrhage.

3.84   ABC
During the management of a multi-traumatised patient, primary and secondary surveys should be repeated frequently to ascertain deterioration in patient status. They guide any changes to treatment. Blood at the penile meatus, perineal bruising or a high-riding prostate indicate urethral damage. They are thus contraindications to urethral catheterisation without a preceding urethrogram to assess urethral integrity. Cribriform plate fractures may lead to intracranial passage of a per-nasally inserted gastric tube. In such circumstances gastric tubes should be placed *per orum*. Skull X-rays are not usually valuable in making decisions for the initial management of major trauma situations or in the absence of penetrating cranial injuries. Blood pressure is not a reliable measure of actual tissue perfusion.

3.85   BD

High-velocity bullets have enormous kinetic energy and displace tissue, producing cavitational effects that can result in tissue necrosis distant from the bullet track. Gunshot wounds to the abdomen are associated with significant visceral injury in about 95% of cases, so laparotomy is mandatory. If an exit wound is absent, AXRs may help determine the missile trajectory by tracing the sites of entry to residual bullet fragments. Gunshot wounds are contaminated and broad-spectrum antibiotics should be routinely administered for at least 24 hours. The kinetic energy of an object is proportional to its mass and square of its velocity (kinetic energy = $\frac{1}{2} mv^2$). Thus, velocity is a more important factor.

3.86   ACD

Pulmonary ventilation–perfusion mismatch results from lung contusion, haematomas and alveolar collapse. Reduced ventilation results in hypercarbia. Hypovolaemia from blood loss and changes in intrathoracic pressure relationships (from tension or open pneumothoraces) clearly compromise oxygen exchange.

3.87   ABEF

According to ATLS, the primary survey includes:
A   Airway maintenance with cervical spine control
B   Breathing and ventilation
C   Circulation and haemorrhage control
D   Disability: neurological status
E   Exposure/environmental control – prevent hypothermia

The purpose of the primary survey is to identify and manage life-threatening injuries. Abdominal, musculoskeletal and detailed neurological assessment form part of the secondary survey.

3.88 Orthopaedic procedures
1. A Intramedullary nail
2. E Amputation
3. A Intramedullary nail

Patients with multisystem trauma and multiple fractures are best stabilised by having their fractures internally fixed within 48 hours. This allows for more rapid improvement, a reduction in the incidence of ARDS and earlier mobilisation.

In Scenario 1, the patient's other injuries (chest and head) took precedence and, now that he is stabilised, the fracture should be internally fixated.

In severe lower limb trauma, a careful evaluation is needed. Reconstruction is determined by the nature and severity of the injuries. In Scenario 2, there is gross soft tissue (muscle and nerve) and bony damage that precludes any possibility of limb salvage.

3.89 BCE

Haemorrhage is defined as an acute loss of circulating blood. The normal adult blood volume is approximately 5% of body weight (a 70-kg man has a 5-litre circulating blood volume), and in children it is approximately 8–9% of their body weight. The blood volume of obese patients is estimated by their ideal body weight, as their true weight gives an overestimation of blood volume. Tachycardia is the earliest measurable sign of haemorrhage.

3.90 ABEF

The secondary survey is a head-to-toe assessment. It includes assessment of vital signs, all body systems (head, neck, chest, abdomen, extremities, neurological) and GCS scoring. Chest and pelvic X-rays are performed during the primary survey as they may reveal a life-threatening injury requiring prompt intervention that may have otherwise remained undetected. Special investigations and procedures such as DPL, USS, further X-rays and CT are conducted during the secondary survey. Furthermore, the secondary survey includes 'a tube and finger' in every orifice.

3.91 AE

The Glasgow Coma Scale is a tool for measuring and following a patient's level of consciousness. It is scored according to the table, with the total score ranging from 3 to 15. Vital signs do not impact on the score. An unconscious patient with no eye opening and no verbal or motor response to stimuli scores 3, as does a deceased person. A score of 8 or less indicates coma. A neurologically normal and alert patient scores 15. A deteriorating Glasgow Coma Scale is of great clinical significance and indicates progressive cerebral insult.

		Score
Eye opening	Spontaneous	4
	To voice	3
	To pain	2
	None	1
Verbal response	Oriented	5
	Confused	4
	Inappropriate	3
	Incomprehensible	2
	None	1
Motor response	Obeys commands	6
	Localises to pain	5
	Withdraws from pain	4
	Flexes to pain (decort.)	3
	Extension to pain (decereb.)	2
	None	1

3.92 ACE

Catheter aspiration of the normal uninjured peritoneal cavity may yield up to 5 ml of clear fluid. Lavage fluid exiting via a chest drain is an indicator of diaphragmatic injury and requires laparotomy. Accepted criteria for laparotomy on laboratory analysis of peritoneal lavage fluid (unspun) are >100,000 RBCs/mm^3 or >500 WBCs/mm^3. The presence of bile draining from the catheter is also a positive result.

3.93   B

Intravenous methylprednisolone, 30 mg/kg initially, then 5.4 mg/kg per hour for 23 hours, has been shown to improve neurological recovery. Other treatments such as naloxone and mannitol have not. Unstable thoracic spine fractures can safely be treated by maintaining the spine in the neutral position ('postural reduction'). Although many centres operate early to allow early mobilisation, there is no evidence that this improves neurological recovery. Fractures of the pedicles of C2 are unstable fractures in which the cord is put at risk by distraction. They should initially be treated by in-line immobilisation. The initial neurological examination is a poor predictor of prognosis as spinal shock can mimic complete cord injury.

3.94   Knee injuries
1.   A   **Cruciate rupture**
2.   E   **Patella fracture**
3.   D   **Collateral ligament injury**

Cruciate ligament rupture characteristically produces swelling within 1–2 hours of the injury. In contrast, meniscal tears tend to produce a swelling the following day, which is less dramatic. Blood aspiration suggests severe intra-articular damage.

The presence of fat globules usually signifies a fracture.

Collateral ligament injuries cause pain and discomfort with straining of the knee in valgus and varus positions.

3.95   BCDE

The odontoid peg is the ascension of the atlas fused to the ascension of the axis. The peg has an articular facet at its front and forms part of a joint with the anterior arch of the atlas. It is a non-weight-bearing joint. The alar ligaments, together with the apical ligaments, are attached from the sloping upper edge of the odontoid peg to the margins of the foramen magnum. The inner ligaments limit rotation of the head and are very strong. The weak apical ligament lies in front of the upper longitudinal bone of the cruciform ligament, and joins the apex of the deltoid peg to the anterior margin of the foramen magnum. It is the fibrous remnant of the notochord.

3.96   DE

Abduction of the thumb is weakened, but not lost, after paralysis of the abductor pollicis longus muscle (radial nerve), because the abductor pollicis brevis muscle remains functional (median nerve). Extension of the forearm is unaffected, since branches to the triceps muscle leave the radial nerve before it enters the spiral groove. Despite paralysis of the supinator muscle, supination is unaffected because the biceps muscle remains functional (musculocutaneous nerve). Loss of sensation over the first dorsal web and the brachioradialis tendon reflex (mainly C6 through a branch coming off the radial nerve after leaving the spiral groove) are features of radial nerve damage at this site.

3.97   ACD

Major burns are associated with numerous complications, as are other forms of major trauma. Muscle loss/injury due to electrical burns may lead to myoglobinuria. Potassium levels tend to rise due to cellular damage and sodium levels can be raised or lowered due to excessive or inadequate fluid resuscitation.

3.98   Chest trauma
1. **F   Flail chest**
2. **E   Massive haemothorax**
3. **D   Tension pneumothorax**
4. **C   Cardiac tamponade**
5. **A   Traumatic rupture of the thoracic aorta**
6. **A   Traumatic rupture of the thoracic aorta**

CXR findings of a traumatic rupture of the thoracic aorta (aortic dissection) include: a widened mediastinum; pleural capping; oesophageal and tracheal deviation to the right; depression of the left main bronchus; and obliteration of the window between the pulmonary artery and aorta.

Massive haemothorax presents as shock associated with the unilateral absence of breath sounds and dullness to percussion.

Findings of a tension pneumothorax include: tracheal displacement to the opposite side; respiratory distress; cyanosis; tachycardia; hypotension; distended neck veins; unilateral absent breath sounds; and hyperresonance.

Cardiac tamponade is associated with muffled heart sounds, pulsus paradoxus and dilated neck veins.

There is restricted chest wall movement with rib crepitus in cases of flail chest.

3.99 BCD

The branches of the posterior cord are the upper and lower subscapular, thoracodorsal and axillary nerves. It terminates as the radial nerve. Through the axillary nerve, the posterior cord supplies the deltoid muscle. The musculocutaneous nerve leaves the lateral cord to supply the coracobrachialis muscle. The suprascapular nerve supplies infra- and supraspinatous muscles and is derived from the upper trunk.

3.100 C

Signs of S1 nerve root compression include: reduced sensation in the S1 dermatome (sole of the foot); weakness of plantar flexion of the ankle; and absent or reduced ankle jerk.

3.101 Adult burns

1. D 9%
2. F 18%
3. A 1%
4. F 18%
5. D 9%
6. B 4.5%
7. F 18%

The 'rule of nines' gives a practical guide to the rapid calculation of the extent of body burns. The adult body is divided into anatomical regions each comprising 9% of the total body surface. The head and neck comprise 9% of the total body surface, the anterior trunk (chest and abdomen) 18%, the posterior chest (upper and lower) 18%, each arm 9%, and each leg 18%. The genitals comprise 1% of the total body surface area.

3.102 BD

Ulnar nerve damage results in sensory loss over the hypothenar eminence, the whole of the little finger and the medial side of the ring finger. There is denervation of the flexor carpi ulnaris muscle, the ulnar half of the flexor digitorum profundus muscle, the muscles of the hypothenar eminence, the two ulnar lumbricals, all the interosseous muscles and the adductor pollicis muscle. Thus, both flexion of the little finger and abduction of the fingers are lost. Adduction of the wrist is still possible through the action of the extensor carpi ulnaris muscle. Claw hand, a feature of ulnar nerve damage at the wrist, is usually not present with high lesions at the elbow or above, because the distal interphalangeal joints cannot be flexed if the ulnar half of the flexor digitorum profundus muscle is paralysed.

3.103   BCD
In Erb's palsy (traction injury of the upper roots and trunk – C5/6), there is paralysis of the abductors and lateral rotators of the shoulder, the elbow flexors and the supinator muscles. The arm hangs by the side medially rotated, extended at the elbow, and pronated. There is also loss of cutaneous sensation over the lateral aspect of the arm and forearm.

3.104   Shock
1. E   Septic shock
2. B   Neurogenic shock
3. D   Haemorrhagic shock
4. A   Cardiogenic shock
Spinal shock relates to the areflexic flaccid paralysis of the limbs and anaesthesia below the level of cord injury. Over a period of weeks, spasticity develops.
Neurogenic shock is the state of cardiovascular collapse due to sympathetic denervation after a cord injury.
Septic shock may occur after a perforated viscus some hours after injury.

3.105   Spinal trauma
1. H   Cervical cord injury
2. E   Left posterior column
The findings in Scenario 125 suggest a cervical cord injury as there is flaccid areflexia, flaccid anal sphincter and priapism. Injury above T1 stops intercostal involvement in respiration, and injury below C5 allows the phrenic nerve to function (supplying the diaphragm).
The posterior columns carry proprioceptive impulses (two-point discrimination and vibration nerve) and fine touch from the same side of the body. The spinothalamic tract supplies pain, temperature and crude touch.

ANSWERS – CHAPTER 4: INTENSIVE CARE

4.1 ACDE
The causes of a PEA arrest include hypovolaemia, hypoxia, hypothermia, hyper/hypokalaemia, tension pneumothorax, cardiac tamponade, drug toxicity, electrolyte abnormalities, thromboembolism and mechanical obstruction. The treatment is basic life support, adrenaline (1 mg per 3 minutes) and treatment of the underlying cause. Electric shock usually causes a ventricular fibrillatory arrest or occasionally an asystolic arrest.

4.2 Lung segments
1. D Medial (right)
2. A Apical
3. C Lateral basal (left)
4. D Medial (right)
5. A Apical
6. D Medial (right)

Inhaled foreign objects which enter the bronchial tree most frequently lodge in the medial right lung segment, as the right main bronchus is not only wider but also more vertical than the left main bronchus. Pneumonia tends to affect the basal lung segments as they are less well ventilated. Tuberculosis may colonise areas of calcification in the apical lobes of the lung, and re-emerge years later as active disease, e.g. during periods of immunosuppression.

4.3 BCE
Enteral nutrition is more effective than parenteral nutrition and has an advantage in maintaining intestinal mucosal integrity, so preventing the translocation of gut organisms which can result in sepsis in critically ill patients. Nutritional support should not be delayed in obese individuals as protein for wound healing is needed, rather than calories which can be provided from fat stores.

4.4 ACD
Myocardial blood flow is approximately 250 ml/min at rest (which represents 5% of the cardiac output) and is dependent on arterial pressure. The right coronary artery supplies one-third of the blood to the left ventricular muscle. Myocardial blood flow is only seen in diastole. Pain and vasopressin (ADH) may reduce myocardial blood flow. Coronary vessels have both α- and β-adrenergic receptors. Coronary vessels generally have more α-receptors and therefore vasoconstrict slightly with sympathetic stimulation.

4.5   Cardiovascular physiology
1. **B   Isometric ventricular contraction**
2. **C   Ventricular ejection**
3. **D   Isometric ventricular relaxation**
4. **B   Isometric ventricular contraction**
The cardiac cycle is divided as follows:
Phase 1 – Atrial contraction (atrial systole)
Phase 2 – Isometric ventricular contraction lasts from the closure of the AV valves until ventricular pressure exceeds the aortic and pulmonary pressures and the aortic and pulmonary valves open
Phase 3 – Ventricular ejection lasts until the aortic and pulmonary valves close
Phase 4 – Isometric ventricular relaxation lasts until the AV valves open
Phase 5 – Passive ventricular filling

4.6   ABDE
IPPV creates a positive intrathoracic pressure (versus normal negative) and a compression tamponade, thereby reducing venous return, cardiac output and thus blood pressure. With a reduction in cardiac output there is reduction in liver, kidney and intestinal blood flow. The alveoli may be subjected to high inflation pressures and result in subsequent PCO_2 barotrauma and pneumothorax. IPPV causes an increase in intracranial pressure, along with PEEP and obstruction of central venous drainage.

4.7   A
Cardiac index = cardiac output/body surface area. (It allows comparison of cardiac function corrected for size of the individual.)
Cardiac output = stroke volume × heart rate.
Systemic vascular resistance = [(mean arterial pressure – CVP)/cardiac output] × 80.

4.8   ACDE
Respiratory failure can be divided into type 1 and type 2. Type 1 is where the PaO_2 is low and the PCO_2 is normal or low, and type 2 is where the PO_2 is low and the $PaCO_2$ is high. In practical terms this occurs when the PO_2 is <8 kPa and the $PaCO_2$ >7 kPa. Certainly, an inability to clear secretions would will lead to respiratory insufficiency. This often occurs after abdominal surgery (especially upper) when pain prevents deep inspiration and coughing with subsequent basal atelectasis and retention of secretions. The symptoms of respiratory insufficiency include confusion, agitation and drowsiness. In pancreatitis, inflammatory mediators are released into the circulation and this can produce respiratory impairment through acute lung injury, which may progress to fulminant ARDS.

4.9   ABE

The left coronary artery arises from the left posterior aortic sinus behind the pulmonary trunk. After a short course it divides into two main arteries: the circumflex and the left anterior descending, otherwise known as the anterior interventricular artery. 60% of hearts have the right coronary artery supplying the SA node; in 40% of hearts, the SA nodal artery arises from the left coronary artery. The left coronary artery supplies the vast majority of the left ventricle and left atrium. Part of the right ventricle is supplied by the left coronary artery through a conus branch.

4.10   CD

Heart rate is determined by the electrical discharge of the SA node and is normally 60–80/min. The SA node spontaneously fires at 140/min and resting vagal tone reduces this to approximately 70/min. Baroreceptors in the carotid and aortic sinuses produce a reflex response to hypertension by inhibiting the SA node and decreasing the heart rate. Inspiration increases heart rate and decreases blood pressure via stretch receptors in the lung and the respiratory centre in the medulla.

4.11   Structures in the transthoracic plane (of Louis)
1. G   Vagus nerve
2. D   T4 vertebra
3. F   Left pulmonary artery
4. H   2nd costal cartilage

The left recurrent laryngeal nerve is given off by the vagus as it descends between the concavity of the aortic arch and left pulmonary artery. The left recurrent laryngeal nerve loops round the ligamentum arteriosum and ascends into the neck in a groove between the trachea and oesophagus.

The prevertebral fascia fuses with the T4 vertebra.

The ligamentum arteriosum is a remnant of the fibrosed ductus arteriosum, which interconnects the left pulmonary artery with the concavity of the aortic arch in the fetus.

The sternocostal joint has an intra-articular ligament (connecting the 2nd costal cartilage to the fibrocartilage of the manubriosternal joint) and two synovial cavities (an upper compartment for articulation with the manubrium, and a lower compartment for articulation with the body of the sternum).

4.12   ADE
Central venous pressure is the pressure in the right atrium. It is dependent on the tone of the peripheral veins. CVP rises in right-sided heart failure. However, it does not regulate stroke volume *per se*, which is controlled by baroreceptors in the aortic arch and carotid arteries. Atrial natriuretic peptide, a substance secreted by the atrium, produces a net sodium loss.

4.13   DF
The haemodynamic features of septic shock are, in the most part, due to the effects of endotoxins from Gram-negative bacteria. Endotoxin has a direct myocardial depressant effect. The classical picture is of septic-shock tachycardia, hypotension and peripheral vasodilatation. Typically, the white cell count is raised.

4.14   All false
Feeding by the enteral route is the preferred means of nutritional support. However, it is not always suitable. It would be inappropriate, for instance, in those with short gut and bowel obstruction; absorption of the nutrients would not take place in such patients. A common side-effect of enteral feeding is diarrhoea, occurring in 20% of cases.

4.15   BE
Functional residual capacity (FRC) is the volume of gas in the lung after a normal expiration. It can be calculated from the total lung capacity minus the vital capacity. FRC can be measured by the helium dilution technique or body plethysmography. FRC is often increased in diseases where there is increased airway resistance, e.g. emphysema, chronic bronchitis and asthma. A reduced FRC is seen in patients with reduced lung compliance, e.g. with diffuse interstitial fibrosis.

4.16   C
Following any trauma or sepsis there is a negative nitrogen balance. Metabolic rate increases and protein from muscle stores is mobilised for repair and energy, which results in increased urea production and a net nitrogen loss. This may be prolonged for many weeks if sepsis or multiorgan failure occurs.

4.17   All true
JVP is a measure of pressure in the right atrium and usually reflects intravascular volume reasonably well. However, there are a few instances where a falsely elevated JVP may occur, as in conditions that cause or lead to right-sided cardiac failure or pulmonary hypertension.

4.18   ABC

Atrial fibrillation (AF) may be treated by intravenous or oral digoxin. Digoxin does not convert the patient to sinus rhythm but merely controls the rate. Verapamil and amiodarone can both potentially convert AF into sinus rhythm. Amiodarone should be administered via a central line if infusion is prescribed (5 mg/kg over 20–120 minutes with ECG monitoring, max 1.2 g over 24 hours). Isoprenaline primarily increases heart rate and is used in severe bradycardia and heart block. Phentolamine is a short-acting blocker used to control hypertensive crises due to phaeo-chromocytoma.

4.19   Respiratory physiology

1. A   Compliance
2. I   West's zones
3. B   Functional residual capacity
4. F FEV_1
5. H   Shunt
6. G   Dead space
7. J   Starling resistor
8. D   Vital capacity

The definitions are self-explanatory. It is essential to have a thorough understanding of respiratory physiology and its terminology.

4.20   Structures in the transthoracic plane (of Louis)

1. J   Thoracic duct
2. A   Trachea
3. C   Mediastinal parietal pleura
4. B   Superior vena cava

The thoracic duct forms on the left side and continues upwards, ascending on the bodies of the thoracic vertebrae. The trachea divides slightly to the right of the midline. The carina is a keel-shaped cartilage at the bifurcation. The mediastinal pleura on each side meet in the midline in front of the aortic arch. The azygos vein arches over the hilum of the right lung, indenting the upper lobe before joining the superior vena cava. The thoracic duct drains into the confluence of the left brachiocephalic vein and internal jugular vein.

4.21   DE

The scalenus anterior is attached to the scalene tubercle. The scalenus medius is attached to the area behind the posterior groove. The subclavian artery passes anterior to the 1st thoracic nerve root.

4.22   ABCE

Hyperventilation causes a respiratory alkalosis. Rebreathing into a bag causes expired CO_2 to be stored in this reservoir and reabsorbed. Due to the physiological shifts, a change in the negatively charged protein buffers leads to a fall in free unbound calcium thereby causing tetany.

4.23   ABCD

The pressure in the veins situated above the level of the right atrium is below that of the atmosphere; therefore when a wound involves the wall of such a vein, air may be sucked into it and pass into the circulation. It may also happen where positive pressure is used in venous or arterial catheterisation and in venous infusion of fluids. *Cl. perfringens* causes gas gangrene; hydrogen peroxide is used to irrigate wounds during debridement, and formation of gas emboli has been described.

4.24   AB

The risk factors for postoperative renal failure include sepsis, jaundice and hypotension. Jaundice is a well-known risk factor for developing renal failure, which may lead to the hepatorenal syndrome. Sepsis is one of the most common causes of acute renal failure in surgery. Benign prostatic hypertrophy leads to acute urinary retention, but does not lead to postoperative renal failure unless it is left unrecognised.

4.25   BCD

ARDS is the most extreme manifestation of acute lung injury. It produces diffuse alveolar shadows on CXR. Early radiographic signs are non-specific. The final common pathway of ARDS involves neutrophil activation, release of inflammatory mediators and free radicals causing increased alveolar permeability. ARDS should be managed in the ITU/HDU environment as rapid deterioration can occur requiring advanced circulatory support.

4.26   BCDE

Each half of the diaphragm is supplied by its own phrenic nerve (C3, C4, C5) which is both motor and sensory. The intercostal nerves send some proprioceptive fibres to the periphery of the diaphragm. The oesophageal opening is opposite the T10 vertebra behind the seventh costal cartilage. It lies in the fibres of the left crus, but a sling of fibres from the right crus loops around it. The greater, lesser and least splanchnic nerves pierce each crus.

4.27   AC

Acute renal failure results in a metabolic acidosis. Thus, the blood pH and plasma bicarbonate level drop. To compensate, respiratory rate increases and carbon dioxide levels are lowered. The biochemical features of ARF include a hyperkalaemia, hyponatraemia and elevated urea and creatinine. Phosphate is elevated and calcium lowered.

4.28   AB

Nitric oxide is a molecule with broad and diverse effects. It was first described in 1980 as a product of endothelial cells that causes vasorelaxation. This product was called endothelium-derived relaxing factor (EDRF) and was eventually shown to be nitric oxide. Nitric oxide is known to be produced by many cell types and to exert a wide range of biological effects. The physiological actions of nitric oxide include relaxation of gastrointestinal smooth muscle and bronchial smooth muscle, maintenance of vascular integrity, inhibition of smooth muscle migration and proliferation. Endothelial nitric oxide also plays a critical role in haemostasis, making an important contribution to the normal inhibition of platelet function. Inhibition of platelet adhesion is a property of nitric oxide. Nitric oxide is also an important determinant of cell blood flow and is thought to be involved in immune and inflammatory responses via its production in macrophages, lymphocytes and neutrophils. Nitric oxide is synthesised by a family of enzymes known as nitric oxide synthetases.

4.29   BCD

Fluid resuscitation is essential to ensure the patient is adequately filled with a blood pressure sufficient for renal perfusion (prerenal failure). All nephrotoxic drugs should be stopped. The initial management is supportive; dialysis is used for chronic renal failure. In the emergency setting haemofiltration is used when there is fluid overload, hyperkalaemia (>6.0 mmol) or metabolic acidosis (pH <7.2 and deteriorating base excess) resistant to treatment.

4.30   ACDE

FRC represents the volume of the lungs at the end of a normal tidal breath. It is reduced intraoperatively because of the increased activity of muscles of respiration and elevation of the diaphragm. Pain and splinting of the diaphragm occur postoperatively in abdominal surgery. With age there is loss of elastic tissue and hence the FRC rises.

4.31 BDE

An intercostal drain should be inserted in the 5th intercostal space in the mid-axillary line and so should not penetrate pectoralis major. The visceral pleura overlies the lung and should not be entered, although this may occur inadvertently.

4.32 ABD

The right ventricle is the most anterior chamber of the heart and most likely to be injured in penetrating trauma to the chest. Being anterior it is best visualised by standard transthoracic echo. It is supplied by the right coronary artery and receives blood from the bronchial veins (remember the dual circulation of the lungs).

4.33 BCD

Dissection of the ascending aorta (DeBakey types I and III) may disrupt the ostia of the coronary arteries and so cause cardiac ischaemia and infarction. Distortion of the aortic valve may occur leading to valvular incompetence. Rupture into the pericardium can cause tamponade, but this is rare.

4.34 BCDE

Atrial fibrillation is associated with, but does not cause, mitral valve disease. However, atrial fibrillation may lead to thrombus formation in an enlarged atrium and so lead to embolic pneumonia causing stroke, digital gangrene and intestinal infarction. Dyspnoea may be secondary to left ventricular failure as a result of an excessively rapid heart rate, rate-dependent ischaemia or infarction.

4.35 CE

Dopamine at low doses has an effect on pure dopaminergic receptors, only at higher doses does it have a truly inotropic effect via β-receptors. Calcium and digoxin are both inotropes. Furosemide (frusemide) and GTN may have an indirect inotropic effect if used to off-load a failing ventricle, but they themselves are not inotropic. Isoprenaline is a chromotropic agent and is occasionally used in bradycardic states.

4.36 ACD

At rest, there is tonic vagal tone on the heart. This is lost after cardiac denervation, and, as a result, the heart rate increases. Adenosine induces heart block, and if given in sufficient doses can cause transient asystole. Salbutamol and adrenaline have β-effects on the heart and cause a tachycardia. Metronidazole has no effect on the heart rate.

4.37   ABCE

ARDS can broadly be divided into direct and indirect insults to the lung. Direct insults include lung contusion, aspiration and pneumonia. Indirect insults include massive blood transfusion, pancreatitis and fat embolus. Renal failure may be associated with ARDS especially in the presence of multiorgan failure. It is, however, not a cause of ARDS. Other causes include acid aspiration, traumas, severe pneumonia and massive blood transfusion.

4.38   Ventilation

1.   B   CPAP
2.   H   Reversed I:E ratio
3.   D   High-frequency jet insufflation
4.   F   Volume-controlled ventilation
5.   H   Reversed I:E ratio
6.   A   PEEP
7.   C   Intermittent mandatory ventilation

In general, ventilators control either the volume or pressure of gas delivered to the patient. When ventilating a patient who has a low arterial oxygen pressure, oxygenation can be improved by a combination of increasing the FiO_2, adding positive end-expiratory pressure (PEEP), or by reversing the inspiratory:expiratory (I:E) ratio. The latter is most useful when the lungs are poorly compliant (stiff), but may be detrimental to CO_2 transfer. If the patient's major problem is hypercapnia, increasing the minute volume (by increasing rate and/or tidal volume) will lower the end tidal CO_2 (a reflection of alveolar and arterial CO_2).

4.39   B

Emergency tracheostomy is a formal operation and should be carried out under controlled circumstances under general anaesthetic. However, percutaneous tracheostomy is performed under local anaesthetic in some centres. It is useful in enabling adequate toilet of the lungs and reduction in dead space may aid weaning from ventilation. Anatomical dead space of the respiratory tract refers to all areas not involved in gas exchange, e.g. the oropharynx.

4.40   AE

The absolute indications for intubation and ventilation are GCS <8 (definition of coma) as protective airway reflexes may be lost, a tiring or exhausted patient with a high and rising $PaCO_2$ (>6.5 kPa), or a PaO_2 of <8 kPa on >60% oxygen.

4.41   BCE

By adequately inflating the lungs, artificial ventilation will help to prevent the collapse of small airways. However, overforceful ventilation pressures may cause a pneumothorax and subsequent surgical emphysema. The use of positive end-expiratory pressure to reduce alveolar closing may lead to a positive intrathoracic pressure, which in turn may reduce venous return to the heart so reducing cardiac output. Artificial ventilation can be used to induce hypocarbia and so reduce intracranial pressure. Acute gastric distension may occur with ventilation, which usually responds well to the insertion of a nasogastric tube.

4.42   AC

To obtain an inspired oxygen concentration of 100% there must be a closed circuit, which can be achieved with an endotracheal tube or with a tightly fitting face-mask as used in CPAP. The normal face-mask and nasal specula are variable-performance devices and do not deliver a constant FiO_2. Their maximum inspiratory flow is 15 litres/minute.

Fixed-performance devices such as Venturi masks deliver a fixed FiO_2 according to the type of mask (maximum 60%). With a mask and reservoir, an airtight seal is unlikely and an FiO_2 of 1.0 is not attainable in practice.

4.43   BDF

The phrenic nerve is sensory and motor to the diaphragm. The main motor root is C5 and injury to the phrenic nerve causes paralysis of the corresponding hemidiaphragm. This leads to paradoxical movement of the diaphragm, rising on inspiration.

4.44   ADE

The vertical dimension of the chest increases on inspiration. The ribs move upwards and outwards. However, the first rib does not move during respiration. The serratus anterior (supplied by the long thoracic nerve) is involved in respiration.

4.45   Renal failure
1. **C   Acute tubular necrosis**
2. **H   Pulmonary oedema**
3. **F   Prerenal renal failure**

A story of prolonged hypotension followed by a period of oliguria/anuria which eventually makes a complete recovery is typical of acute tubular necrosis (ATN). Cortical necrosis may produce a similar picture but does not usually recover.

Any patient who has received large volumes of fluid and becomes hypoxic must be considered to have pulmonary oedema until proven otherwise. It is particularly likely to occur in those with compromised cardiovascular or renal function, especially elderly people.

The patient in scenario 3, although oliguric initially, did not develop and progress to acute renal failure. Once renal perfusion was restored she was able to produce urine normally. This suggests that the cause of the renal impairment was poor perfusion, secondary to hypovolaemia. This is a prerenal cause of renal failure and, if inadequately treated, will progress to acute tubular necrosis (see above), an intrinsic cause of renal failure.

4.46   BCD

The most pronounced metabolic response to trauma begins to fall approximately 24 hours after the surgery. Catabolism that accompanies trauma increases urea production and excretion. ADH levels rise as part of the endocrine response to stress. Increased serum cortisol leads to sodium and water retention.

4.47   AB

Pain often causes an elevation of systemic arterial pressure via sympathetic nervous system stimulation. This is often related to the wound or occasionally urinary retention. The volatile anaesthetic agents do not cause hypertension and epidurals most frequently cause postoperative hypotension due to sympathetic blockade and loss of vasomotor tone.

4.48   ABDE

Theatre temperature is usually maintained between 22 and 24 °C but may need to be higher for neonatal surgery. Humidification and covering exposed surfaces will minimise heat loss. Anaesthesia obtunds the normal mechanisms of heat production, so the patient is vulnerable to hypothermia from conductive, convective and evaporative heat loss. Hypothermia also delays recovery from anaesthesia and postoperative shivering increases oxygen demands.

4.49   EF

Hyperkalaemia produces peaked T waves, slows conduction time and inhibits the myocardium so leading to ventricular standstill. Acidosis causes a shift of potassium from the intracellular to extracellular compartment. The pancreatic juices are rich in potassium and the presence of a high-output fistula may lead to hypokalaemia.

4.50   ABCD

Arteriovenous fistulas can develop when an adjacent vein is punctured or damaged during line placement. The arterial line itself can cause damage to the vessel wall with subsequent development of an aneurysm. This in turn can produce microemboli, so causing infarction and gangrene. A less common cause of gangrene is when an end artery is cannulated with no collateral supply, e.g. radial artery cannulation with no ulnar collateral supply to the hand. This is rare, but should be avoided by performing an Allen's test prior to cannulation.

4.51   BCE

Respiratory failure is a $PaCO_2$ of <8 kPa or $PaCO_2$ 7kPa. Type I respiratory failure is otherwise considered as hypoxaemic respiratory failure. Here the patient is able to eliminate their CO_2. In contrast, CO_2 accumulates in type II respiratory failure (ventilation failure). Satisfactory oxygen saturation does not signify adequate oxygen delivery to the tissues. Bicarbonate may be high despite acidosis in a metabolically compensated respiratory acidosis, e.g. COPD; a patient with type II respiratory failure who has been given too much oxygen now retains CO_2 because of the loss of hypoxic drive.

4.52   DE

Angiotensin II stimulates aldosterone synthesis and secretion through the activity of a specific receptor found in the zona glomerulosa. Angiotensin II is one of the most potent endogenous vasoconstrictor agents and inhibits renin release through a negative feedback loop. Renin stimulates the formation of angiotensin I from angiotensinogen. Angiotensin I is converted to angiotensin II in the lung by angiotensin converting enzyme (ACE).

4.53   ABDE

Nephrotoxicity arises through several mechanisms: general and local vascular effects (diuretics, β-blockers, ACE inhibitors) or by direct tubular effects (proximal: aminoglycosides, radiocontrast, mannitol; distal: NSAIDs, ACE inhibitors, ciclosporin), tubular obstruction (sulphonamides, aciclovir), acute interstitial nephritis (β-lactams, vancomycin, ciprofloxacin, furosemide (frusemide), thiazides) and acute glomerulonephritis (penicillamine). Furosemide is itself a nephrotoxic drug, but it may also be beneficial in renal failure. It reduces oxygen consumption and requirement in the medullary tubules of the kidney by inhibiting solute reabsorption and clearing tubular debris.

NSAIDs cause nephrotoxicity through several mechanisms: vasoconstriction within the renal circulation, reduction of medullary blood flow and oxygen delivery, alteration of potassium balance and inhibition of compensatory mechanisms protecting renal tubular blood flow in the volume-depleted kidney. In addition, NSAIDs may cause an interstitial nephritis.

4.54   Anatomy of the heart
1.   F   Anterior cusp of the mitral valve
2.   K   Oblique pericardial sinus
3.   C   Membranous interventricular septum
4.   H   Interatrial septum

The anterior cusp of the mitral valve is large, with a massive papillary muscle giving rise to multiple chordae tendinae attached along the edge of the cusp. The muscle prevents herniation of the cusp into the left atrium during systole when the cusp has to withstand the pressure of blood flowing over it towards the aortic opening.

The oblique sinus separates the left atrium from the oesophagus posteriorly.

The atrioventricular bundle of His traverses the membranous part of the interventricular septum before dividing into the left and right bundle branches which travel towards the ventricular apices in the muscular interventricular septum.

The atrioventricular node lies in the interatrial septum to the left of the opening of the coronary sinus.

4.55   ABDF

Vasoconstriction is widespread and occurs on both the venous and arterial sides of the circulation. The result is increased peripheral resistance to blood flow. Changes in vascular pressures lead to an influx of extracellular water into the circulation, a phenomenon known as transcapillary refilling. This leads to haemodilution. Tachycardia occurs as a fall in blood pressure and is sensed by baroreceptors in the carotid arteries and aortic arch.

4.56   AE

In acute respiratory failure the PaO_2 falls and the $PaCO_2$ rises with a consequent drop in pH. In chronic respiratory failure, the serum bicarbonate concentration increases to correct the acidaemia. The rise of bicarbonate concentration in the CSF renders the respiratory centre in the brainstem insensitive to hypercarbia but not hypoxia. Thus, a hypoxic respiratory drive is the predominant mechanism and is the only stimulus to increase ventilation rate.

4.57   BCD

Acute renal failure (ARF) occurs in about 30% of critically ill patients. Loss of renal function leads to a 60% increase in mortality and morbidity. The common causes of ARF include postoperative hypovolaemia, CCF, radiocontrast and drugs (aminoglycosides, NSAIDs). Only 20% of ARF is drug induced. In 60% of cases, ARF is potentially avoidable, as it is the result of fluid or drug mismanagement. The histological appearance of the kidney bears little relevance to the level of renal dysfunction. Severe functional renal deficit can occur with minimal histological appearances. The proximal tubule is the segment that is most susceptible to injury and reflects the relative hypoxia in the outer medulla and inner cortex.

4.58   AB

The CVP reflects pressure in the right atrium and thus is elevated in right-sided heart failure. The Valsalva manoeuvre raises central venous pressure by impeding venous return to the heart. CVP is low in all types of shock except for cardiogenic shock. CVP does not directly reflect cardiac output and, at best, is an indicator of intravascular fluid volume.

4.59   ACE

The oxygen–haemoglobin dissociation curve is sigmoid-shaped and reaches a plateau at 70–100 mmHg (PO_2). A left shift is produced by a high pH, alkalosis, a fall in PCO_2, a fall in temperature and a fall in 2,3-DPG concentration. As a result of a left shift, less oxygen is released (a higher % saturation for a given PO_2, leading to a fall in oxygen delivery). Anaemia produces no shift of the curve but alters the percentage oxygen saturation of the blood.

4.60   CE

Shock is the inadequate perfusion and delivery of tissues with oxygen and other nutrients. Of all the shock states, cardiogenic shock is unique, in that cardiac output is reduced and the systemic arteriolar vessels constrict, increasing the SVR in an attempt to maintain the blood pressure. In all other forms of shock there is a primary vasodilatation of inappropriate vascular beds causing maldistribution of blood flow. This inappropriate vasodilatation causes a fall in SVR and blood pressure. Cardiac output (CO) increases passively as a result of reduced afterload on the heart, and actively as a result of increased sympathetic drive.

4.61   ACEF

Changes in cellular metabolism associated with shock include accumulation of lactic acid and reduced ATP production due to anaerobic metabolism. Changes in membrane function result in the passage of sodium into cells and the passage of potassium out of cells. Lysosomal fragmentation occurs as a result of autodigestion. Fatty acid mobilisation results in increased ketone production.

4.62   AB

The principles of management of severe anaphylactic shock include: airway maintenance and oxygen; intravenous fluids to provide circulatory support; and subcutaneous or intramuscular adrenaline (epinephrine). Intravenous adrenaline may, in rare circumstances, be given but at a much lower dose and only with ECG monitoring. Nebulised bronchodilators can help counteract the bronchospasm. Other drugs that might be helpful include aminophylline and hydrocortisone. β-Blockers are contraindicated as they lower blood pressure and may cause bronchoconstriction.

4.63   Vascular resistance
1. **C   Decreased peripheral vascular resistance**
2. **C   Decreased peripheral vascular resistance**
3. **A   Increased peripheral vascular resistance**
4. **D   No change in peripheral vascular resistance**

Due to endotoxin production in septic shock, there is a reduction in peripheral vascular resistance thus leading to vasodilatation. Calcium-channel blockers decrease peripheral and not pulmonary vascular resistance. Amputations have no known effect on the peripheral vascular resistance.

4.64   Surface/radiological anatomy of the thorax
1.   C   Right sternoclavicular joint
2.   F   4th rib
3.   A   5th intercostal space

The brachiocephalic artery bifurcates behind the right sternoclavicular joint, behind the commencement of the right brachiocephalic vein (confluence of the right subclavian and right internal jugular veins).

The horizontal fissure of the right lung passes along the line of the right 4th rib from the right mid-clavicular line to the 4th costal cartilage of the right sternal margin.

The oblique fissure of both lungs runs from the 2nd thoracic vertebra posteriorly to the 6th costal cartilage anteriorly.

The left ventricle lies behind the left 5th intercostal space from the left sternal margin to the left mid-clavicular line.

4.65   ACDE

Pulmonary thromboembolism may produce the classical ECG pattern of $S_1Q_3T_3$, and reduced arterial PCO_2 tension due to hyperventilation. Mismatched ventilation–perfusion defects on lung scan may be found. On CXR a pleural effusion, pulmonary atelectasis, pulmonary infarct area of oligaemia and a raised hemidiaphragm may be observed. It is important to note that approximately 30% of CXR are normal in PE. Obstruction in the pulmonary circulation on angiography (which provides the definitive diagnosis) may be observed.

4.66   B

ARDS is initially due to pulmonary oedema of non-cardiac origin. Complement activation is the final common pathway independent of the causal factors. Aggregated neutrophils release superoxide radicals as a by-product of phagocytosis, which may promote protein destruction (e.g. of collagen and elastin). There is increased shunting and associated pulmonary ventilation–perfusion mismatch. It is associated with diffuse pulmonary infiltrates on X-ray.

4.67   ACE

Physiological and histological features of ARDS include: increased capillary permeability; interstitial and alveolar oedema; fibrin exudation; hyaline membrane formation; and diffuse late interstitial and alveolar fibrosis.

4.68   Pathological chest conditions
1. **C   Aspergilloma**
2. **D   Malignant mesothelioma**
3. **A   Pulmonary cysts**
4. **E   Idiopathic mediastinal fibrosis**
5. **B   Bronchogenic cysts**

Bronchogenic cysts are congenital cysts of bronchial origin. They are usually closely related to the trachea, hilum of the lung or oesophagus. They usually present as an asymptomatic mass on CXR.

Pulmonary cysts differ from bronchogenic cysts in that they are embedded in the pulmonary parenchyma. They are connected to the airways, and their walls do not contain cartilage.

An aspergilloma is the result of *Aspergillus fumigatus* infection, which can cause an asthma-like condition or invasive lung infections.

Malignant mesothelioma is asbestos-related and has a poor prognosis. It affects both parietal and visceral pleura.

Idiopathic mediastinal fibrosis is due to diffuse collagenous fibrous replacement of the normal mediastinal connective tissue. It is thought to have an autoimmune aetiology.

4.69   C

MODS is the dysfunction of more than one organ, requiring intervention to maintain homeostasis. The overall prognosis of established MODS is very poor, despite aggressive treatment, and is partly dependent on the number of organ system failures. To optimise chances of recovery, the underlying problem should be corrected and supportive therapy (including nutrition) instituted. There is presently no evidence to show that antiendotoxin antibodies improve survival rates. Pulmonary artery catheters have not been shown to improve outcome.

4.70   C

A CT at this level is at the level of T4. At this level, the arch of the aorta is terminating, the azygos vein enters the SVC, left recurrent laryngeal nerve loops round the ligamentum venosum and the bifurcation of the pulmonary trunk can be seen. The thoracic duct crosses the midline at T5.

4.71　BE

Bleeding from the middle meningeal artery following head injury usually leads to an extradural haematoma. This is usually a tear of the anterior branch of the middle meningeal artery, with an underlying linear skull fracture. The characteristic picture is of a head injury with a brief episode of unconsciousness followed by a lucid interval. The patient then develops a progressive hemiparesis, stupor and rapid transtentorial coning with an ipsilateral dilated pupil. This is followed by bilateral fixed dilated pupils, tetraplegia and death.

4.72　ADE

The left lung has two lobes, in contrast to the right which has three lobes. The left lung has two bronchial openings and ten bronchopulmonary segments. Two pulmonary veins arise from the left lung, one above and one below the oblique fissure. The arterial supply is from the bronchial arteries which arise from the aorta.

4.73　Trauma and shock
1.　D　Hypovolaemic shock
2.　B　Septic shock

Any patient who is brought hypotensive into the A&E department should be considered to be suffering from hypovolaemic shock until proven otherwise. Neurogenic shock occurs following damage to the spinal cord with resultant loss of sympathetic tone. It characteristically produces a picture of low BP without tachycardia or peripheral vasoconstriction; a narrowed pulse pressure is not a usual feature. The earliest sign of hypovolaemic shock is a tachycardia. In young patients there may not be a fall in blood pressure until there is nearly a 2-litre blood loss.

Septic shock is usually due to circulating endotoxins producing warm dilated peripheries. However, in advanced cases there may be vasoconstriction. Liver function may also be affected.

4.74　AC

The foramen spinosum transmits the middle meningeal vessels and meningeal branch of the mandibular nerve. The foramen rotundum contains the maxillary nerve. The foramen ovale transmits the mandibular nerve, lesser petrosal nerve and accessory meningeal artery. The foramen lacerum transmits the internal carotid and greater petrosal nerve, which leaves as a nerve of the pterygoid canal.

4.75   ABCE
The right main bronchus is shorter (approximately 2.5 cm long), wider and runs more vertically than the left main bronchus. The right main bronchus gives off the upper lobe branch (before entering the lung) and passes inferior to the pulmonary artery before entering the hilum of the lung (approximately T5). It is important to remember the azygos vein, which arches over the right main bronchus from the posterior aspect as it passes to the SVC, and the pulmonary artery which lies inferior and then anterior to it. The left main bronchus is about 5 cm long and, unlike the right, does not give off any branches before entering the hilum of the left lung at the level of T6.

4.76   CE
The recurrent laryngeal nerve supplies all the intrinsic muscles of the larynx except the cricothyroid and is sensory inferior to the vocal folds. In the neck, the recurrent laryngeal nerves on both sides follow the same course ascending in the tracheo-oesophageal groove. As the nerve passes the lateral lobe of the thyroid it is closely related to the inferior thyroid artery. The superior laryngeal nerve supplies the vocal cord mucosa.

4.77   All true
The external jugular vein drains most of the scalp and side of the face. It begins near the angle of the mandible and is formed from the union of retromandibular and postauricular veins, receiving branches from the posterior external and transverse cervical veins. The external jugular vein has no valves and lies anterior to the scalenus anterior and pierces the deep fascia of the neck, usually posterior to the clavicular head of the sternocleidomastoid muscle before draining into the subclavian vein.

4.78   ABE
The left main bronchus passes downwards and outwards below the aortic arch, anterior to the descending aorta and oesophagus. The pulmonary artery loops over it, the vagus nerve lies just posterior, the phrenic nerve in front and the hemiazygos vein is posterior to the aorta.

4.79   All true
The sinoatrial node artery passes backwards between the right auricle and aorta, and forms a vascular ring around the termination of the superior vena cava. Arteriolar anastomoses between the terminations of the right and left coronary arteries exist, but are too few and small in calibre to compensate significantly in acute coronary artery occlusion.

4.80   Anatomy of the lungs and airways
1. **D   Left pulmonary artery**
2. **F   Trachea**
3. **E   Left pulmonary vein**
4. **G   Lobes of the lungs**
5. **A   Left main bronchus**

The left pulmonary artery is separated from the arch of the aorta by the left vagus, the recurrent laryngeal nerve and the ligamentum arteriosum.

The left brachiocephalic vein passes in front of the trachea in the midline. The left upper pulmonary vein is the most anterior structure in the left hilum.

There are 10 bronchopulmonary segments in each lung, despite the left medial basal segment being small: 3 in the upper, 2 in the middle and 5 in the lower lobes.

The left main bronchus is longer than the right and crosses in front of the oesophagus, providing a potential obstruction to food during deglutition.

In the superior mediastinum, the trachea lies directly anterior to the oesophagus.

4.81   ABCD

The right atrium forms the right border of the heart, lies anterior to the left atrium and thus the posterior wall is the interatrial septum. The sinoatrial node lies near the opening of the superior vena cava, lateral to the sulcus limitans, and the coronary sinus opens into the atrium above both the opening of the inferior vena cava and the septal cusp of the tricuspid valve.

4.82   BCDE

The left crus is attached to the L1/2 vertebrae, and both crura are pierced by the sympathetic splanchnic nerves. Inferior phrenic arteries (the first branches of the abdominal aorta) supply the diaphragm. Both suprarenal glands lie against the diaphragm retroperitoneally. Both kidneys lie on the lateral arcuate ligaments and thus a pneumothorax is a possible complication of nephrectomy.

4.83   BE

The vagus nerve lies just posterior to the right main bronchus and the azygos vein is at first posterior and then arches over the bronchus. The phrenic nerve is anterior to the bronchus. The right recurrent laryngeal nerve hooks around the right subclavian artery superior to the right main bronchus.

4.84   All true
The thyroid gland is supplied by the inferior thyroid artery, a branch of the thyrocervical trunk. The internal thoracic artery supplies: the breast, through anterior intercostal vessels, usually in the 2nd and 3rd intercostal spaces; the rectus abdominis muscle, through the superior epigastric branch; and the diaphragm, through the musculophrenic artery. The vertebral arteries supply the brainstem through the posterior inferior cerebellar arteries.

4.85   ABDE
The phrenic nerve lies anterior and the vagus posterior to the left hilum. The left main bronchus lies inferior and posterior to the pulmonary artery and does not divide before entering the lung. The hilum is separated from the aortic arch and descending thoracic aorta by the vagus nerve.

4.86   ABE
Neurological complications are not uncommon following cardio-pulmonary bypass and usually manifest clinically as mild neuro-psychological deficits, e.g. poor short-term memory, lack of concentration and mood changes. These deficits are usually reversible and thought to result from cerebral microemboli or hypoperfusion. Less than 1% of patients suffer a severe stroke. Cardiopulmonary bypass causes platelet depletion and also reduces platelet activity. Acute pancreatitis occurs in 25% of open-heart procedures and may be severe in 5% of cases.

4.87   Cardiorespiratory physiology
1.   B   Metabolic acidosis
2.   C   Low MCV
3.   D   Shift of the O_2 dissociation curve to the right
The 45-year-old man in Scenario 1 is in hypovolaemic shock. Due to decreased tissue perfusion there is a build up of lactate resulting in a metabolic acidosis.
Chronic blood loss leads to a hypochromic microcytic anaemia.
A right shift of the O_2 dissociation curve is caused by a decrease in pH, hypercapnia, raised temperature and release of 2,3-DPG. In chronic bronchitis, the CO_2 concentration in the blood is increased, producing a lowered pH and causing a shift of the O_2 dissociation curve to the right.

4.88   BEF

Cardiac output is decreased upon standing from a lying position as venous return to the heart is suddenly reduced. Above a certain heart rate the stroke volume falls, so reducing cardiac output. Cardiac output is increased only in the short term when first arriving at high altitude. After this initial rise, cardiac output gradually returns to normal but the haematocrit level increases to improve the blood's oxygen-carrying capacity. Other causes of increased cardiac output include AV shunts, hyperthyroidism, severe anaemia and Paget's disease.

4.89   BE

Perioperative myocardial ischaemia occurs most commonly in those with a history of a previous infarction, in the intraoperative period and on day 3 postoperatively. The more recent the MI, the greater the risk of re-infarction. Close intraoperative monitoring has been shown to reduce the risk of infarction in the higher risk patient.

The risk in patients without a cardiac history is less than 1 in 70,000.

4.90   ADE

The FRC is the residual volume plus the expiratory reserve volume and represents less than 50% of the vital capacity. FRC decreases when supine and increases on standing. It also varies with height and body build. Expiratory reserve can be measured directly by spirometry, but residual volume is measured by the helium dilution technique.

4.91   BDE

The spirometer is able to measure the forced vital capacity (not the total lung capacity), the FEV_1 (forced expiratory volume in 1 s) and thus the FEV_1:FVC ratio.

Residual volume is measured by helium dilution. The peak expiratory flow rate measures the amount of air expired in 1 s and extrapolates it to the volume that would be expired in 1 m (and thus can be calculated by measuring the FEV_1).

4.92   C
Pulse oximetry measures the oxygen saturation of arterial blood (not partial pressure of oxygen). This relationship is sigmoid and not linear. Pulse oximetry does not reflect whether delivery to the tissues is adequate as this is dependent also on cardiac output and haemoglobin concentration. The adequacy of ventilation is better reflected by the PCO_2. Carbon monoxide leads to the presence of carboxyhaemoglobin, which decreases the oxygen available to the tissues. Pulse oximeter readings in excess of 95% reflect the adequacy of arterial oxygen saturation in the peripheries, nothing more. Readings can be unreliable when there is poor peripheral perfusion (e.g. in vasoconstriction, hypothermia, severe anaemia, excess ambient light and patient movement).

4.93   CE
The central tendon is pierced by the inferior vena cava and right phrenic nerve (caval opening) at the level of T8 and the 6th costal cartilage. The vagal trunks, oesophagus and left gastric vessels pass through the oesophageal opening in the muscle of the right crura (T10). The greater splanchnic nerves pierce the crura. The aorta, azygos and hemiazygos veins as well as the thoracic duct pass posterior to the diaphragm through the aortic aperture.

4.94   BDE
The apex of the arch, which gives attachment to the pretracheal fascia, lies posteroinferior to the left brachiocephalic vein. The lower border of the arch lies in the transthoracic plane and on the left is directly related to the left pulmonary artery (the superior vena cava lies over the right pulmonary artery). The arch is symmetrically covered by the pleura from both sides, which meet in the midline behind the manubriosternal joint.

4.95   ABCD
The autonomic fibres in the phrenic nerve are sympathetic and pass from the superior (C1–4) and middle (C5/6) sympathetic cervical ganglia as grey rami into the C3–5 roots of the phrenic nerve, and innervate blood vessels in the diaphragm. The nerve lies on the fibrous pericardium and is sensory to the mediastinal and diaphragmatic pleura, and also to the diaphragmatic peritoneum. The phrenic nerve enters the chest by descending from the medial lower border of the scalenus anterior muscle between the subclavian vein anteriorly and artery posteriorly.

4.96   AC

Impressions on the mediastinal surface of the right lung include the trachea, vagus, superior vena cava, right atrium and subclavian artery. The oesophagus grooves the left lung above the arch of the aorta and below the hilum.

4.97   The denervated heart
1. **A   Lack of parasympathetic stimulation**
2. **B   Release of catecholamines**
3. **D   Transplant rejection**

The transplanted or denervated heart has no vagal/parasympathetic innervation and thus has a higher basal heart rate. The transplanted heart relies on circulating catecholamines to produce inotropic and chronotropic effects.

4.98   Blood gases
1 **B   Metabolic alkalosis**
2 **C   Respiratory acidosis**
3 **A   Metabolic acidosis**
4 **F   Normal acid–base balance**

The patient in Scenario 1 has an alkalosis, as indicated by a pH of 7.6. This is metabolic in origin as the bicarbonate level is high. The PCO_2 is normal. The patient in Scenario 2 has respiratory acidosis, as indicated by a pH of 7.3 and PCO_2 of 8.2 kPa. The bicarbonate level is normal and therefore there is no compensation.

A low pH, low HCO_3^-, low PCO_2 and low PCO_2 represent a picture of metabolic acidosis.

The patient in Scenario 3 has normal acid–base balance.

4.99   ABE

The trachea commences at the lower border of the cricoid cartilage, is palpable in the jugular notch, bifurcates in the transthoracic plane and is innervated by the recurrent laryngeal nerves. The left main bronchus bifurcates inside the left lung and is not as vertical as the right main bronchus.

ANSWERS – CHAPTER 5: NEOPLASIA: TECHNIQUES AND OUTCOME OF SURGERY

5.1   ACDF

α-Fetoprotein is secreted in high amounts by hepatocellular carcinomas and teratomas. It also occurs in some lung, gastric and pancreaticobiliary tumours. Medullary thyroid carcinoma is known to secrete calcitonin and is a reasonably good tumour marker. However, there are no known markers for parathyroid tumours. Acid phosphatase, but not alkaline phosphatase, is a tumour marker for prostate carcinoma. However, prostatic specific antigen is a superior tumour marker for prostate carcinoma. Placental alkaline phosphatase is associated with some tumours but its lack of specificity means that it is not a clinically useful marker.

5.2   BG

Male sex, increased tumour thickness, the presence of ulceration, older age and mucosal involvement are predictors of poor outcome in melanoma. The prognosis also depends upon the lymph node involvement and growth pattern. The 5-year survival rate is 90% for stage I, 50% for stage II, 30% for stage III and <1% for stage IV disease. While the so-called 'Celtic type' race appear more susceptible to the development of melanoma, non-White populations with melanoma have a worse overall outcome.

5.3   Audit
1. **D   Strategic**
2. **C   Criterion**

Audit is the systematic critical analysis of the quality of medical care, including the procedures used for diagnosis and treatment, the use of resources, resulting outcome and quality of life for the patient.

Audit may be subdivided into medical audit (assessment of patient treatment by doctors) and clinical audit (assessment of patient treatment by all healthcare professionals).

5.4   ABEF

Preconditions for a good screening test include:
- The disease must be an important health problem.
- There should be an accepted treatment.
- Facilities for diagnosis and treatment must be available.
- There should be a latent stage.
- The screening test should have both high sensitivity and specificity.
- The test should be acceptable to the population.
- The natural history of the disease should be adequately understood.
- There should be an agreed policy on whom to treat.
- Diagnosis and treatment should be relatively cost-effective.
- The screening should be an ongoing process.

For a screening test to be effective, early detection and treatment must lead to fewer deaths. An anaplastic carcinoma would carry such a poor prognosis that any screening test would make no difference to outcome. Similarly, earlier detection of tumours with a short latent stage is unlikely to help.

5.5   BCE

Based on randomised trial data from the 1990s, recommended excision margins for cutaneous primary melanomas are: 0.5 cm for *in situ* tumours; 1.0 cm for tumours with a Breslow thickness of 1 mm thick or less; and 2 cm for tumours thicker than 1 mm. These values, however, still remain contentious and more trials are in progress.

Randomised studies have shown no benefit of routine lymph node dissection when excising a melanoma. The use of sentinel node biopsy can make prophylactic local node dissection more rational. However, therapeutic nodal dissection does not improve survival by as much as 50%. Melanomas on the trunk and neck are associated with the male sex, those on the legs with the female sex.

5.6   BCEF

Hamartomas are not true tumours but represent overgrowth of one or more cell types that have normal constituents. However, they are arranged in irregular fashion (e.g. haemangioma, lymphangioma, lipoma and neurofibroma). Sarcoma is a malignant tumour arising in tissues of mesenchymal origin. Sarcomas of soft tissue and bone are rare and represent less than 1% of malignant neoplasms. A Krukenberg tumour is the name originally given to metastatic deposits on the ovaries secondary to a gastric tumour. Zollinger–Ellison syndrome is a gastrin-secreting pancreatic tumour associated with peptic ulceration; over 50% are malignant. A high fasting serum gastrin level is diagnostic. Barrett's oesophagus is a metaplastic change from squamous to columnar epithelium in the distal oesophagus. It is premalignant condition.

5.7   CD

Current opinion on breast carcinoma states that women with negative axillary lymph nodes will gain no additional survival benefit from a dissection. Axillary node dissection does, however, confer improved regional control. Breast conservation is the appropriate treatment for most women with stage I and II disease, so the mainstay of management of early breast cancer consists of a wide local excision of the primary tumour combined with an axillary nodal dissection (± radiotherapy depending on nodal status) and radiotherapy to the breast. Such management has similar survival and local control rates to mastectomy. Tamoxifen improves survival in both pre- and postmenopausal women for oestrogen-receptor-positive tumours. Adjuvant systemic therapy has reduced mortality by 30%.

5.8   Consent for surgical treatment
1. A   **Yes, surgery can proceed**
2. C   **Apply to make the child a ward of court**
3. A   **Yes, surgery can proceed**
4. B   **No, surgery cannot proceed**

1.   Surgery is needed for the preservation of life and can be performed despite the patient's inability to give consent. The patient's wife cannot give permission or stop her husband's operation. No adult can act as legal proxy for any other in the UK with regard to giving consent for surgical treatment.

↑ Parents

2.   The surgeon can either respect the patient's wishes and not subject the child to an operation or can make an application for the child to be made a ward of court and proceed with appropriate surgical treatment. In this case surgical treatment is essential and almost all surgeons would do the latter.

3.   The current Mental Health Act does not allow for the compulsory treatment of any medical condition other than a mental disorder. The orthopaedic surgeon may, however, proceed with surgery for the patient's fractured femur if he and the patient's psychiatrist agree that it is the best form of management for her. It is good clinical practice to also obtain a second consultant surgical opinion confirming the need for operative treatment and to involve the relatives in the decision-making process where possible. Every clinician should make detailed entries in the patient's records and sign and date them.

4.   No. Before the deterioration of this patient's condition he clearly refused to consent to operative treatment. Surgery cannot therefore be performed even when he is unable to express his refusal for such a seemingly essential intervention.

5.9   AC
The development of lymph node metastases dramatically reduces survival. When regional lymph nodes are involved the 5-year survival decreases to approximately 30%. Satellite lesions represent an aggressive tumour and microinvasion. Nodular melanomas are more aggressive than superficial spreading lesions. Other indicators of invasiveness include: vascular invasion; high mitotic rate; ulceration; and tumour-infiltrating lymphocytes.

5.10   ACD
Testicular tumours mostly spread to the para-aortic nodes, and not to the inguinal lymph nodes. Prostatic carcinoma characteristically produces metastases in the lumbar vertebrae as a result of the prostatic venous plexus drainage into the internal vertebral plexus. Prostatic tumours are adenocarcinomas with a variable degree of differentiation. This is reflected in their behaviour and the aggressiveness of their local and metastatic spread. Osteosarcoma preferentially spreads via blood to the lungs.

5.11   B

β-Naphthylamine exposure has been strongly linked with bladder tumours. The human bladder mucosa secretes the enzyme β-glucuronidase, which splits b-naphthylamine and releases a carcinogen. β-Naphthylamine is an aromatic amine and is a good example of remote carcinogenesis. The average latent period from exposure to disease development is 15 years. Other strong links with bladder carcinoma are from benzidine exposure and smoking.

5.12   Death and the law
1.   B   **Any medical practitioner**
2.   E   **Medical practitioner who attended during previous 14 days**
3.   A   **Coroner**
4.   C   **Registrar of births and deaths**

A doctor may issue a death certificate if he/she is a registered medical practitioner. In practice this usually means where the doctor attended within 14 days of the death. Only the coroner is entitled to hold an inquest on any case that is reported to him/her.

5.13   CD

In DCIS, the proliferating malignant epithelial cells are confined to the lactiferous ductal system and have not breached the basement membrane. Most women with DICS are asymptomatic and the disease is only picked up by mammography. FNAC is unable to tell us whether the basement membrane has been breached by malignant cells. A core biopsy is required.

DCIS accounts for less than 5% of symptomatic breast cancers and for 15–20% of breast cancers detected with screening mammography. Less than 1% of DCIS lesions are associated with regional metastases. Mastectomy for DCIS is associated with a cure rate exceeding 99%. Other treatments include lumpectomy with or without radiotherapy.

5.14   ADE

Tubular, medullary, colloid, papillary, cribriform and mucinous carcinomas are associated with a good prognosis. Around 30% of invasive breast cancers are from these histological groups. Axillary lymph node status is the single best prognostic indicator. Tumour size is also an important prognostic indicator, and correlates well with nodal involvement and the probability of distant metastases. The Nottingham Prognostic Index (NPI) takes into account the tumour size, the number of involved axillary nodes and histopathological grade according to the equation:

NPI score = (0.2 x maximum tumour dimension (cm)) + (Grade) + (lymph node stage).

Lymph node stage is defined as follows: no metastasis scores 0; tumour in 1–3 nodes scores 2; 4 or more nodes score 3. The NPI score is thus the culmination of the major independent prognostic factors in breast carcinoma. The 10-year survival rates for scores less than 3.4 is 90%, for scores between 3.4 and 5.4 is 70%, and for scores over 5.4 is 20%. Survival actually improves from ages 35 to 49 years but declines rapidly in the following decade. Overall, age extremes have a poorer prognosis. A deficiency in steroid receptors, such as oestrogen, is another poor prognosticator.

5.15   Cancer therapy options
1.   C   Systemic chemotherapy
2.   D   Surgical resection
3.   D   Surgical resection
4.   B   Hormonal manipulation
5.   A   Radiotherapy and steroids

Prolonged remission, or even cure, can be achieved using systemic chemotherapy for recurrent non-Hodgkin's lymphoma.

Isolated pulmonary metastasis from colorectal cancer (as occurs in 5% of patients) can be surgically removed with curative intent if the patient will tolerate a thoracotomy. It is only suitable if the primary tumour has been rigorously controlled and extrathoracic secondaries have been excluded.

Residual anal squamous-cell carcinoma post local radiotherapy is best treated by abdominoperineal resection with curative intent.

Metastatic prostatic carcinoma not involving bone is best treated by hormonal manipulation. If the bone is involved, radiotherapy is the treatment of choice, with or without internal fixation.

Multiple intracranial metastases are best treated with radiotherapy, whether over the whole brain or with stereotactic radiosurgery (gamma knife). Diffuse intracranial metastatic melanoma has an extremely poor prognosis. Short-term benefit may be achieved by radiotherapy with steroids; chemotherapy is of no benefit.

5.16   CDE

Prognostic indicators can be divided into pathological and biochemical. Pathological prognostic factors include lymph node status. It has been shown that the number of positive nodes correlates very well with prognosis. Indeed, axillary lymph node status is the single best prognostic indicator. Patients with more than five positive nodes have a 5-year survival rate of less than 20%. Tumour size is another important prognostic indicator, and correlates well with nodal involvement and the probability of distant metastases. Chemograde is also a good predictor of prognosis, as is vascular invasion and multicentricity. Tubular, medullary, colloid and papillary carcinomas are associated with a better prognosis. Inflammatory carcinoma *per se* is not a prognostic indicator. The biochemical prognostic factors include oestrogen-receptor status in the primary tumour. This is useful for predicting the response to endocrine therapy and for survival.

5.17   ABD

Absolute contraindications to conservative breast surgery include: two or more primary tumours in separate quadrants; first or second trimester pregnancy; previous radiotherapy to the region; persistent positive margins after surgery; and diffuse malignant microcalcifications. The only relative contraindication is a large tumour in a small breast. Axillary nodal involvement, a family history of breast carcinoma and subareolar tumours do not preclude conservative surgery. A tumour of greater than 4 cm is thought to be unsuitable for breast-conserving surgery. A tumour with proven metastases is not a contraindication to breast-conserving surgery as the treatment would primarily involve adjuvant chemotherapy having obtained the main tissue diagnosis.

5.18   ABDE

Staging of malignant lesions for individual patients allows only a statistical risk of outcome for that patient. Accurate tumour staging cannot be made on the basis of a histological specimen alone, and requires additional information on nodal and distant disease. Pathological staging may be altered by the response to chemotherapy or irradiation treatment, and is known as downstaging. Staging of tumours takes into account local tissue anatomy for individual primary tumour sites: e.g. invasion of tumours into the different layers of the wall of any viscus, and invasion into adjacent local structures.

5.19   AB
Bowen's disease is a skin disorder that may develop into squamous-cell carcinoma, histologically it is an intraepidermal carcinoma. It predominantly occurs on the legs. Keratoacanthoma is a benign self-involuting lesion, and molluscum contagiosum is an infective lesion. Basal-cell papillomas (seborrhoeic keratoses) are benign and have no malignant potential, as opposed to solar (actinic) keratoses, which do. A Spitz naevus is a variant of benign melanocytic lesions and can be mistaken histologically for malignant melanoma. It is most common in females under 30 years of age.

5.20   C
When melanocytes drop off the epidermis into the dermis they are known as naevus cells. If these cells clump at the dermis/epidermis junction, the lesion is known as a junctional naevus. If cells only clump in the dermis, the lesion is known as an intradermal naevus. If clumping occurs at both sites, the lesion is known as a compound naevus. None of the three varieties have a high malignant potential, though malignant change does occur. Halo naevi are confined to the dermis, and malignant transformation is very rare.

5.21   All false
Technically categorised as a stage 0 tumour, lobular carcinoma *in situ* (LCIS) mostly affects premenopausal women (aged 40–50 years) and is a marker of an increased risk for developing invasive breast cancer (risk is 15–25%). LCIS is typically multifocal, multicentric and affects both breasts. While it may be picked up on mammography, LCIS is normally found incidentally from a breast biopsy taken for another indication. The comedo variant is an architectural pattern that occurs in DCIS. Regular surveillance (regular clinical examination, self-examination, mammography) is the mainstay of management in patients found to have LCIS. Some women receive tamoxifen for up to 5 years, and those with great concern or a family history of breast cancer can undergo a prophylactic mastectomy.

5.22   Malignant melanoma
1.   **C   Lentigo maligna melanoma**
2.   **B   Acral lentiginous melanoma**
3.   **C   Lentigo maligna melanoma**
4.   **A   Superficial spreading melanoma**

Superficial spreading melanoma (65% of cases) is the commonest form of cutaneous malignant melanoma. Lentigo maligna is preceded by, or occurs within, a Hutchinson's melanotic freckle and is most commonly found on the face. Both of the above melanomas have a pronounced horizontal growth phase. Lentigo maligna melanoma and thin superficial spreading melanomas (<0.76 mm) have a good prognosis. Acral lentiginous melanomas have a predilection for sites of thick epidermis such as the sole of the foot, and have a poorer prognosis. Nodular melanomas have a pronounced vertical growth phase and hence a poor prognosis.

5.23   BD

Most malignant bladder tumours are transitional-cell carcinomas; 2–3% of bladder tumours are squamous-cell carcinomas. Adenocarcinomas are very rare. Colon and prostatic carcinomas are mostly adenocarcinoma in origin. Bronchial tumours are mostly squamous cell in origin (35%). Others include small-cell tumours (25%) and adenocarcinoma in 30%. 95% of cervical tumours are of the squamous-cell type; 5% are adenocarcinomas.

5.24   ABDE

Oncogenes are normal cell proteins that become abnormally activated in cancerous cells. They cause cells to proliferate through various mechanisms. Oncogenes and their corresponding oncoproteins are implicated when their encoded proteins become overexpressed, truncated, mutated or otherwise modified. The *erbB2* oncogene product, for example, is overexpressed in 20% of breast cancers. Oncogenes are also expressed during embryogenesis, regeneration and healing.

5.25   D

Surgical resection is the only chance of cure for patients with non-small-cell lung cancer. Suitability for resection includes: fitness for major surgery; ability to tolerate the loss of lung tissue; and the presence of sufficiently localised disease as to permit complete resection. Involvement of ipsilateral lymph nodes is not a contraindication to resection and in 85% of cases complete resection is still possible. Small (oat)-cell lung cancers are highly malignant and have usually disseminated at the time of presentation. Thus, chemotherapy is the treatment of choice for the majority of patients. Less than 5% of small-cell tumours are suitable for surgical management.

5.26   Histological tumour types

1. **C   Neoplastic polyp**
2. **A   Hamartoma**
3. **A   Hamartoma**
4. **B   Neuroendocrine tumour**
5. **B   Neuroendocrine tumour**
6. **D   Stromal tumour**
7. **B   Neuroendocrine tumour**

Hamartomas resemble tumours but they are not neoplastic. They result from a localised disorder of the relationships of normal tissues, leading to overproduction of one or more elements without the growth characteristics of tumours. Stromal-cell tumours arise from smooth muscle or Schwann cells. They have different grades of malignancy and spectrum of aggressiveness. They are relatively radioresistant and chemoresistant.

5.27   DEF

A tumour suppressor gene normally encodes products that inhibit growth and cell proliferation. It is a recessive gene as a mutation in one of the two copies of this gene will normally cause no harmful effect, as the remaining copy continues to code for a functional protein (Knudson hypothesis). Both copies must be affected before uncontrolled cellular growth and proliferation results.

Tumour suppressor genes were discovered as a result of studies in rare and inherited forms of cancer, particularly retinoblastoma. Retinoblastoma is the commonest malignant eye tumour of childhood. Most cases are diagnosed by the age of 3 years; 20–30% of cases affect both eyes. All of the bilateral cases and 15% of the unilateral cases are inherited as an autosomal dominant trait. The risk of retinoblastoma in the offspring of those with the genetic form of the disease is up to 50%.

TP53 is a tumour suppressor gene whose protein products cause cells to arrest in the G_1 phase of the cell cycle. Mutations of this gene are common in cancers, occurring in up to 60% of instances (e.g. Li–Fraumeni syndrome; breast, gastric, lung and thyroid cancer). Other examples of tumour suppressor genes include *APC, hMSH2, hMLH1* and the *BRCA1* and *BRCA2* genes.

In contrast to tumour suppressor genes, oncogenes are deemed dominant as only one copy of the two genes needs to be affected for carcinogenesis. The oncogene *erbB2* is implicated in breast, ovarian, gastric and bladder carcinoma. The transcription factor *c-myc* is involved in Burkitt's lymphoma, small-cell lung cancer, multiple myeloma, testicular and prostate cancer. *c-myc* plays a role in gene amplification. It is found in normal cells but functions with less restriction in tumour cells.

K-*ras* is an oncogene implicated in colorectal, pancreatic and lung carcinomas as well as leukaemia.

5.28   BDG
α-Fetoprotein is the fetal equivalent of plasma albumin and is produced by the fetal liver, yolk sac and intestine. It can be elevated in hepatocellular carcinoma (up to 90% of cases), testicular teratoma, pancreatic, biliary, gastric and bronchial cancers. Increased levels are also seen in hepatitis (viral). It is found in pregnancy, where high levels can be indicative of neural tube defects. A pure seminomatous germ-cell tumour does not produce α-fetoprotein.

5.29   BE
Malignant tumours have the potential to metastasise and therefore would include cholangiocarcinoma and adenocarcinoma. Adenocarcinoma tends to metastasise to the lymph nodes and liver. Cholangiocarcinoma spreads via lymphatics and the bloodstream.

Adenomas are benign tumours but can undergo genetic mutations and progress to neoplasia. However, only 5% of colonic adenomas will progress to adenocarcinoma and malignancy. Similarly, only a minority of gallbladder adenomas will become malignant. Breast fibroadenoma does not have malignant potential. Basal-cell carcinoma is the commonest skin malignant tumour and is typically slow growing and locally invasive. Metastases can occur, but are exceedingly rare.

5.30   All true
Squamous-cell carcinoma is the second most common cutaneous malignancy (the commonest is basal-cell carcinoma). It may arise in an area of Bowen's disease. Predisposing factors include exposure to sun, radiation, certain chemicals and albinism. Squamous-cell carcinoma is locally invasive and treatment involves excision with block dissection of draining nodes, if they are involved. Squamous-cell carcinomas also respond to radiotherapy and early lesions can be treated topically with 5-fluorouracil. Most cases follow actinic keratoses; those that do not, tend to be more aggressive.

5.31   Tumour markers
1.   **B   β-hCG**
2.   **A   α-Fetoprotein**
3.   **E   Acid phosphatase**
4.   **C   Carcinoembryonic antigen (CEA)**
5.   **D   Paraproteins**
Multiple myeloma is associated with the secretion of paraproteins, which may be seen on an electrophoretic strip. Light-chain protein (Bence-Jones) is secreted into the urine in myeloma.
A proportion of colorectal carcinomas secrete carcinoembryonic antigen (CEA). CEA has a limited role in the follow-up of patients with colorectal cancer. Interpretation and intervention of late rises in CEA remains controversial.
Hepatomas may secrete α-fetoprotein, and teratomas β-hCG. Though not diagnostic, they have some role in screening investigation of tumours. They are useful for follow-up of recurrence.
Acid phosphatase is now an uncommonly used marker of prostatic cancer, as it has a low specificity. Prostatic specific antigen (PSA) is a much better tumour marker in terms of sensitivity and specificity.

5.32   AC
The breast lies on the pectoralis major, serratus anterior and external oblique muscles. It is a modified apocrine sweat gland. The mammary gland is mainly supplied by the lateral thoracic artery, by branches that curl around the border of pectoralis major. In addition, there is a blood supply from the internal thoracic artery, intercostal and thoracoacromial arteries. The main lymphatic drainage is to the axillary and infraclavicular nodes. The gland contains approximately 15 main ducts that open separately on the summit of the nipple.

5.33   BCD

Renal carcinoma peaks around 65–75 years of age. Bilateral tumours occur in 3% of cases. In advanced cases, the tumour may extend into the ureter, renal vein and subsequently the IVC. The classic triad of haematuria, loin pain and mass only occurs in a small minority of patients diagnosed with renal carcinoma.

Histologically, most renal tumours are clear cell. Renal-cell carcinoma typically occurs in the cortex. Renal tumours are generally radioresistant and, thus far, relatively chemoresistant.

5.34   ACEF

Bronchial carcinoma is the most common malignant tumour in the western world, and now the third most common cause of death in the UK. It carries the highest mortality of all malignancies in the UK and the USA. Bronchial carcinoma is usually advanced at the time of presentation. Normally, once there is mediastinal lymph node involvement, a curative resection cannot be performed. The UK incidence of lung cancer is decreasing in men, but increasing in women and is likely to reflect the altered smoking habits of contemporary women. Due to paraneoplastic syndromes, ectopic ACTH may be produced, causing a fall in K^+, hyperglycaemia and an alkalosis. Similarly SIADH can result in hyponatraemia. SIADH is commoner in small-cell cancers and is therefore associated with irresectability. SCLC is the most radiosensitive of all lung cancers.

5.35   Chemotherapy regimens
1. **B   Colorectal carcinoma**
2. **D   Breast carcinoma**
3. **C   Testicular seminoma**

Several studies have now shown a limited survival benefit for Duke's C and Duke's B colorectal cancer using adjuvant treatment with combination 5-fluorouracil (5-FU) and folinic acid. Seminomas of the testis are sensitive to combination bleomycin, cisplatin and etoposide, and this has led to a marked improvement in survival rates in recent years. Adjuvant treatment for cancer of the breast using combination cyclophosphamide, methotrexate and 5-FU (CMF regimen) has been shown to prolong survival, especially in women who are node-positive and <70 years. Doxorubicin (adriamycin) has been shown to improve survival for breast cancer and is replacing CMF in some centres.

5.36   ADE

Approximately 50% of liver metastases originate from primaries in the gastrointestinal tract; mainly the colon and rectum, closely followed by stomach and pancreas. This can be attributed, in part, to the portal venous circulation. Outside the gastrointestinal tract, lung and breast carcinoma represent the most common sources. Unenhanced CT is not sensitive enough to detect smaller malignant deposits in the liver. Contrast CT or CT portography are superior methods. Liver resection for hepatic metastases in patients with breast cancer provides no improved survival benefit.

5.37   BCGH

Anal cancer is relatively rare. It is most commonly squamous or epidermoid in origin. Evidence suggests that it is more common in homosexuals and those with human papillomavirus (HPV) (types 6, 11, 16, 18, 31, 33) or HIV. Condyloma acuminata, or anal warts, are associated with anal cancer and are likely to reflect HPV infection. Anal cancer typically spreads to the perirectal and inguinal lymph nodes. In fact, inguinal lymphadenopathy may be the first sign of the tumour. Distant spread is rare, but can include the liver or lungs. First-line treatment is now chemoradiotherapy. Success is achieved in 70% of cases. The surgical option for the non-responder or recurrence is abdominoperineal resection.

5.38   CF

Radiotherapy is not the first-line treatment of oesophageal adenocarcinoma. Preoperative radiotherapy has conferred no advantage compared to surgery alone. In fact, adenocarcinomas are relatively resistant to radiotherapy. The primary treatment for gastric or rectal carcinoma is surgical resection. An adjuvant role for radiotherapy has been found by some studies of gastric cancer, particularly with regards to locoregional control. Radiotherapy is not, however, the primary mode of treatment of gastric cancer. Approximately 90% of oral and oropharyngeal tumours are squamous-cell carcinoma in origin, including those of the vocal folds. Early vocal fold tumours can be treated initially with radiotherapy. Advanced tumours may benefit from palliative radiotherapy. Cystosarcoma phylloides tumour is a mixed connective tissue and epithelial tumour of the breast. It is fast growing but only 15% are malignant. Treatment is local excision, but it may require chemo- or radiotherapy in metastatic cases. First-line treatment for anal cancer is now radiotherapy with or without chemotherapy.

5.39   ABE
Familial adenomatous polyposis is an autosomal dominant premalignant condition (accounting for 1% of all colorectal carcinomas). Multiple polyps are found throughout the colon and rectum by the early teens. If left untreated, the polyps will become malignant. Paget's disease of the nipple is nearly always associated with an intraductal carcinoma *in situ* and if left alone will progress to invasive cancer. Acanthosis nigricans is a skin condition that is associated with malignancy, but is itself not a premalignant condition. Patients typically develop pruritic hyperkeratotic plaques affecting flexor surfaces such as the axilla. The tumours associated with acanthosis nigricans are mostly intra-abdominal, classically gastric carcinoma. Histologically, a keratoacanthoma resembles a squamous-cell carcinoma. However, it is not premalignant. Typically, keratoacanthomas grow rapidly but do not infiltrate beyond the sweat glands. After several weeks of such growth a keratoacanthoma regresses.

5.40   ACE
Ascites is most commonly seen in ovarian and pancreatic tumours. Two-thirds of patients with ovarian carcinoma have ascites at some point during their disease. Malignant ascites is also a feature in other primary and secondary tumours of the abdominal cavity, including the terminal stages of metastatic liver disease. Malignant ascites is mainly due to tumour infiltration of the peritoneum causing increased production and reduced absorption of peritoneal fluid. Another mechanism is portal hypertension from liver metastases. A large ascites should be drained gradually or slowly to prevent massive volume and protein loss from the patient. Spironolactone or furosemide (frusemide) are sometimes used in the management of ascites. Denver and LeVeen shunts are still occasionally used in ascites to drain intraperitoneal fluid into the SVC. However, they are associated with complications including infection, shunt failure and DIC.

5.41   ABD
Prognosis of patients with colonic malignancy is related to the grade of tumour, spread (involvement of lymph nodes) and presence of clear tumour margins. Dukes staging is the most common, but Astler Collier and TNM grading systems are also used. Villous adenomas have the greatest malignant potential, followed by tubulovillous and tubular. Dukes B tumours have invaded through the muscularis propria. CEA is neither sensitive nor specific enough to be useful for the screening of colonic malignancy.

5.42   ACDEG

Smoking is an established risk factor in many tumours, particularly: colorectal, cervical, bronchogenic, pleural, oral, pharyngeal, laryngeal, oesophageal, and to a lesser extent bladder, kidney and pancreatic. Meat intake increases the risk of colonic tumours so vegetarians and vegans are relatively protected. Familial adenomatous polyposis is an autosomal dominant premalignant condition (accounting for 1% of all colorectal carcinomas). If untreated, the polyps will almost invariably become malignant. Ulcerative colitis increases the risk of colorectal tumours. The risk is directly proportional to the extent and duration of the disease. While diverticulosis and colorectal carcinoma can coexist, there is no evidence linking the two.

5.43   ABC   *not commonly*

Carcinoma of the caecum usually presents insidiously with a picture of iron deficiency anaemia. It is usually polypoid in nature. 25% of tumours cause obstructive symptoms and constipation may occur. Frank bleeding per rectum has a greater association with left-sided tumours. Caecal tumours typically have occult blood loss and are more common after 65 years of age.

5.44   CDEF

Papillary carcinoma accounts for 70% of thyroid tumours. It usually presents in children and young adults. Medullary carcinoma of the thyroid is associated with multiple endocrine neoplasia (MEN IIa and IIb). Following unilateral lobectomy or total thyroidectomy, papillary carcinomas are treated with thyroxine to suppress TSH levels, thereby reducing potential recurrence. Most thyroid tumour patients are euthyroid, and although hyperthyroidism can occur, it is relatively uncommon. The combination of adequate sampling with an experienced cytopathologist makes FNA a useful first-line modality for the detection of tumour cells. Surgical resection is the mainstay of therapy for papillary carcinoma of the thyroid. Radioactive iodine may be used as an adjuvant or to treat metastases. Since thyroglobulin is only synthesised by thyroid tissue, it has been proved to be a useful tumour marker. Tall and Hurthle cells are aggressive variants of papillary thyroid cancer. They have a greater potential for malignant behaviour.

5.45   BEF

The programme was initiated in 1986 after the Forrest Report and screens women between 50 and 64 at 3-yearly intervals. There been no major increase in benign biopsies, but there has been an increase in the proportion of early-stage disease detected.

5.46   B
Experience from both the USA and UK has shown that regular screening with Papanicolaou-stained (Pap) smears from the cervix can reduce mortality from cervical cancer. To date, studies on screening with regular chest radiographs or sputum cytology have shown no improved survival from lung cancer. Further trials are pending. There is no survival benefit for screening cancer of the ovary in the general population at present. However, there may be a strong case for screening a high-risk group with 'familial' ovarian cancer syndrome.

5.47   BCE
Malignant tumours are characterised by their invasiveness (an absolute criterion) and lack of ordered growth. They typically do not have a capsule. Malignant tumours contain cells with greater variation in size and shape, with increased cellular turnover and incomplete differentiation than benign tumours. Loss of cellular adhesion at the tumour primary site is a major step in metastasis formation. Oncogene activation can occur in both benign and malignant tumours. Tumours larger than 2 mm^3 will require angiogenesis to sustain them. Since larger tumours are, in general, more likely to metastasise, the presence of angiogenesis may indicate malignancy.

5.48   BCDEFG
Maxillary sinus carcinoma tends to affect African, Japanese and Arabic populations. It is much rarer in western Europe and the USA. 90% of cancers of the sinuses affect the maxillary and ethmoidal sinuses, with only 10% affecting the frontal and sphenoidal sinuses. Definite aetiological factors include hardwood dust and nickel. Other implicated factors include radiation, mustard gas production and materials used in boot-making. The clinical features include: nasal obstruction; epistaxis; toothache; loosening of teeth; destruction of bone, which may lead to proptosis and diplopia; invasion of nerves causing numbness of the facial palate; and invasion of the infratemporal fossa causing trismus. In 10% cases there is metastatic lymph node involvement.

5.49   AB C
Alkylating agents are perhaps the oldest class of anticancer drug and are still in frequent use. Alkylating agents form covalent bonds in cellular DNA, thereby resulting in their de-activation. Mitomycin C, for example, is used in the treatment of gastric and bladder cancer. It is both an antibiotic and an alkylating agent. Vinca alkaloids are a separate class of chemotherapeutic agent which prevent spindle formation.

C includes cyclophosphamide

5.50   CD

Neuroblastoma is a tumour of the sympathetic nervous system, and is usually highly malignant. It mostly affects children and infants. Since neuroblastic tumours are derived from neural crest cells, they can affect the adrenal medulla (and adjacent retroperitoneal tissue), sympathetic neurones and melanocytes. Males and females are affected equally. Around 75% of neuroblastomas have metastasised at presentation. The presence of c-*myc* in tumour cells is associated with increased aggressiveness.

5.51   ACD

Prostate cancer is mainly a disease of elderly men. Rectal examination and biopsy are the mainstay of diagnosis. Serum prostatic specific antigen (PSA) can assist in screening as well as in follow-up. Bone isotope studies, CT and MRI can be used in staging. Prostate cancer is relatively rare in the Far East, but is particularly common among North American Blacks. The tumour is predominantly an adenocarcinoma, affects the outer margins of the gland and is multicentric. Both lymphatic and haematogenous spread occur. Approximately 50% of cases have demonstrable metastases at the time of presentation. Organ-confined tumours can be treated with radical prostatectomy, radiotherapy or brachytherapy. Advanced or metastatic disease may respond to hormonal therapy. A PSA over 100 is highly suggestive of carcinoma, but not diagnostic. A PSA greater than 10 reflects increased odds of extracapsular disease. Bony secondaries in prostate cancer are more likely to be sclerotic.

5.52   CE

Audit is defined as 'the systematic, clinical analysis of the quality of medical care, including the procedures used for diagnosis and treatment, the use of resources, and the resulting outcome and quality of life for the patient'. There are three main elements to audit:
1. Structure: this refers to the available patient resources.
2. Process: this is what is done to the patient.
3. Outcome: is the result of clinical intervention.

Audit does not only concern doctors, but also other healthcare professionals. It can be consultant-led, but individual practices vary. Standards are ideally set by a multidisciplinary team. While audit aims to improve the quality of patient care, its prime interest is in whether standards have been met and not outcome analysis (which is better served by controlled trials).

5.53   ABE

CEA is a water-soluble glycoprotein. It is elevated in less than 5% of patients with Dukes grade A colorectal cancer, 25% of Dukes' B, 44% of Dukes C and approximately 65% of patients with distant metastases. It is not a useful diagnostic marker as it is increased in severe benign liver disease, inflammatory conditions (particularly of the gastrointestinal tract), trauma, infection, collagen diseases, renal impairment and smoking. It may assist in detecting tumour recurrence, especially in the liver following colorectal cancer resection. The half-life is 10 days.

5.54   ACE

Aromatic amines such as β-naphthylamine are associated with urinary tract (especially bladder) tumours in chemical workers who are particularly involved with dyes and pesticides. Painters, printers, mechanics and others working with petroleum derivatives and organic solvents (benzene exposure) are at an increased risk of developing leukaemia, lymphoma and multiple myeloma. Arsenic is used in pesticide manufacture and exposure also occurs in metal smelters. It is associated with skin and lung cancers as well as bladder tumours.

5.55   AD

Cancer registries obtain their data by identifying all death certificates that state 'cancer' as the cause of or contributing to death and then studying the notes of these patients. Postmortem findings contribute greatly to the accuracy of such data. Among other things, cancer registries can monitor the outcomes of ongoing treatment trials and compare current therapies and centres. In addition, they enable at-risk families to be identified for study and possibly screening. Whilst they are a source of valuable local data, they are of particular value in providing a large information source for the collection of national data, thereby enabling national features and trends to be identified and studied and regional variations to be highlighted.

5.56   ACD

Hamartomas are benign overgrowths of fully differentiated normal components of the tissues in which they arise. In a hamartoma the proportion and composition of these normal tissue components differs greatly from the normal tissue structure. The most common hamartomas are vascular and include birthmarks such as port-wine stains. The polyps of Peutz–Jeghers syndrome are gastrointestinal hamartomas, whilst the associated lesion at the vermilion border of the lips is due to increased pigmentation. Although not neoplastic, hamartomas are mass lesions and, unlike true neoplasms, they cannot grow autonomously. Hamartomas require surgery if they cause obstruction, intussusception or bleeding. Hamartomas can take over a decade to double in size.

5.57   A

Adenomas are benign tumours of ductal or glandular epithelial cells. Consistent with their benign nature they are typically encapsulated and not invasive, although they can be premalignant. Nuclear pleomorphism is characteristic of malignancy, although some colorectal adenomas can display cellular characteristics intermediate between normality and malignancy. Adenomas can contain dysplastic cells. Annular lesions which grow in hollow organs and can cause stricturing are typically malignant. Neoplasms of squamous, columnar or transitional epithelial cells are papillomas if benign, or carcinomas if malignant. However, it is thought that there are no truly benign transitional-cell papillomas.

5.58   BD

A Dukes B colorectal cancer has invaded through the bowel wall but has not involved lymph nodes (it is thus N_0). N_1-stage breast cancer indicates ipsilateral mobile axillary lymphadenopathy. Typically, the extent of locoregional nodal disease is a more important indicator of prognosis than tumour size, hence a T_2N_1 tumour will generally have a better prognosis than a T_1N_2 tumour. Evidence of regional node involvement is an indicator for radiotherapy or chemotherapy in many cancers.

5.59   ABE

Oncogenes are normal cellular genes with the potential to cause malignant transformation when structurally and functionally mutated or abnormally or inappropriately expressed. They tend to code for proteins (oncoproteins) involved in key cellular regulatory processes. They can cause malignancy not only when their gene product is altered by mutation, but when they are over- or underexpressed or expressed at an inappropriate stage of the cell cycle. Because of the key regulatory roles of their products, oncogenes tend to be fundamental to cellular activity and hence highly conserved throughout evolution. Their discovery and much research work hinged on the discovery of tumour viruses containing viral analogues of these genes, derived from cellular oncogenes, which act as vectors for their transmission and for malignant transformation of host cells. The H-*ras* oncogene in the Harvey rat sarcoma virus is found in a variety of common human cancers.

5.60   ABC

Metastasis is facilitated by the ability of neoplastic cells to secrete angiogenic and angioproliferative factors to promote the development of new blood vessels and hence their own blood supply (as they grow beyond 1–2 mm). Tumour growth and metastasis both require angiogenesis. To metastasise, cells must overcome their normal cohesion and be able to invade the tissue, a property facilitated by the secretion of the enzyme protease. Cancer cells must adhere to the basement membrane in order to pass through. Adhesion to the basement membrane requires the expression of integrins (cell-surface receptors for basement-membrane components) but not cadherins, which enhance cell-to-cell adhesion.

5.61   D

In the cell cycle, the growth and proliferation of normal cells is regulated, and changes in the regulatory mechanisms may result in neoplastic transformation. Immediately following cell division, cells enter the G_1 phase of high metabolic activity, but not DNA synthesis. DNA is synthesised in the next stage, the S stage. From there the cell enters the G_2 stage preparing for the M phase, or mitosis – which, as the DNA content of the cell is now double, results in the production of two diploid cells. All the stages, apart from G_1, have fairly fixed durations; hence the growth rate of a tissue depends on the length of time its cells spend in G_1.

5.62   BCDF

Combination chemotherapy is utilised to combat drug resistance. Combinations of drugs have at least as much toxicity, if not more than single agents. Many chemotherapy agents, such as doxorubicin and vinca alkaloids, are metabolised in the liver. Thus, toxicity would be increased in liver impairment. Highly emetogenic drugs require treatment with the serotonin antagonists ($5\text{-}HT_3$) such as granisetron. Bone marrow suppression may present as bleeding such as epistaxis. Hair loss due to chemotherapy is almost always reversible after the course treatment, even if the quality of regrowth may be altered. Creatinine clearance is a measure of renal function. Drugs excreted by the kidneys are therefore removed more rapidly when renal function is good.

5.63   ACDEF

The early complications of radiotherapy reflect the sensitivity of rapidly growing cells to radiation damage. They include desquamation lesions of the skin and gastrointestinal tract (inflammation, bleeding and ulceration), infertility and bone marrow suppression which can lead to bone marrow failure. Hypothyroidism is a late complication of exposure of the thyroid gland to radiation, and may also complicate radio-iodine treatment for thyroid malignancy. The production of secondary malignancies is now recognised as a late complication of radiotherapy and may develop from 3 years after therapy.

5.64   BEFG

Bromocriptine inhibits prolactin secretion and is used to suppress lactation in the treatment of galactorrhoea. Cimetidine is an H_2-antagonist used in dyspepsia. It interferes with cytochrome P450 in the liver and this leads to raised oestrogen levels sufficient to cause gynaecomastia. This is a dose-dependent side-effect. Similarly, liver disease can cause oestrogen/ androgen imbalance and gynaecomastia. Oral corticosteroids cause a redistribution of fat and Cushing's syndrome, but they do not lead to gynaecomastia. Pituitary tumours and hyperthyroidism may cause gynaecomastia. Around 10% of testicular tumours (usually teratomas) are associated with gynaecomastia.

5.65   B
Fibroadenomas are not true neoplasms as they do not develop from a single breast cell but from a single lobule. They occur most commonly in women in their twenties. Triple assessment should be performed; provided this is normal, it is acceptable to observe these lesions in older women not wishing excision. Carcinoma rarely develops in a fibroadenoma (incidence approximately 1 in 1000). When measuring over 5 cm they are known as 'giant fibroadenomas'. Phylloides tumours are fibroadenoma-like lesions, which are histologically benign but can behave in a malignant fashion.

5.66   BCE
Screen-detected lesions may be small, early tumours and often difficult to assess histologically. It is important that the best possible assessment is used. Frozen section may cause tissue distortion and make a precise diagnosis impossible, therefore formalin fixation and paraffin embedding prior to sectioning of the specimen must always be used in these cases. Surgical excision of these lesions can be guided either by insertion of a needle and positioning of a guide-wire or injection of a mixture of radio-opaque and coloured dyes into the lesion under mammographic control. Due to a degree of diffusion of the dye within breast tissue, the guide-wire technique is more accurate, although with an experienced operator results can be equally good with both methods. It is important to ensure excision by sending the specimen for radiographic confirmation that the abnormality is within the specimen before the operation is completed. It is essential to have a histological diagnosis on a radiologically suspicious lesion. This may be obtained by a stereotactic core biopsy.

5.67   ACE
The 5th edition of the condensed TNM criteria is set out below:

T_1	Tumour less than 2 cm in greatest dimension
T_2	Tumour more than 2 cm but less than 5 cm
T_3	Tumour greater than 5 cm
T_4	Tumour of any size with extension into chest wall or skin
N_0	No regional lymph node metastases
N_1	Metastasis to movable axillary node(s)
N_2	Metastasis to ipsilateral axillary node(s) fixed to each other or another structure
N_3	Metastasis to ipsilateral internal mammary lymph node(s)
M_0	No distant metastasis
M_1	Distant metastasis (including metastasis to the supraclavicular nodes)

Any of T_0, T_1, N_0 or N_1 tumours would classify as Manchester stage I. T_2N_{1b} tumours are stage II. T_3 or T_4 tumours are stage III. Finally, N_2, N_3 or M_1 tumours are stage IV.

5.68 AB

In terminal care, radiotherapy can be useful not only for managing bone pain but for reducing symptoms related to tumour bulk in surgically inaccessible or hazardous areas and reducing inoperable fungating lesions. Whilst steroids such as dexamethasone are useful in reducing problems due to peritumour oedema, especially where cerebral and spinal metastases are concerned, steroids are not useful for treating bone pain *per se*. Moreover, steroid usage may be complicated by osteoporosis, and even pathological fractures, exacerbating bone and joint pain. Steroid injections, often combined with local anaesthetic, may be useful when given into joints and specific pain trigger spots. Although recognition and treatment of a patient's depression may improve their tolerance of pain, antidepressants are not a specific treatment for bone pain. The antidepressant amitriptyline is useful in the treatment of neuralgia. Transcutaneous electrical nerve stimulation may help in the management of pain due to nerve compression or destruction.

5.69 ABF

A moral right is one that an individual can claim over other people, who must respect it regardless of their own wishes. Autonomy allows for an individual's right to self-determination, including their right to determine their medical future. It is necessary to attempt to ensure that a patient really understands the information that has been given to them before it can be considered that informed consent has been obtained. Even if a patient is detained for psychiatric treatment they may be capable of understanding and giving or withholding consent to a surgical procedure. Only if they are considered mentally incapable of this can the surgeon, together with the patient's psychiatric team, make a decision which they consider to be in the patient's best interests. Whilst the views of children should be considered and treated with respect, it is accepted that in many cases they may not be making a properly considered decision. It is for their parent(s) or guardian(s) to consent to or refuse treatment. Only when the surgeon considers that the parent(s) or guardian(s) may not be acting in the child's best interests may this be contested. A 16-year-old child is generally deemed capable of giving an informed consent and can sign a document form themselves.

5.70   BC

Drugs given in combination appear to give better results than drugs in isolation. One combination is cyclophosphamide, methotrexate and 5-fluorouracil (CMF). The drugs are most commonly given by intermittent injection, although there is increasing interest in continuous infusion via intra-arterial or intravenous pumps. Newer single agents such as doxorubicin are being introduced and in some centres replacing CMF. Chemotherapy is the treatment of choice for visceral metastases (especially liver and brain), and for inflammatory cancers. Clinical response is not merely confined to premenopausal women, though the gain in survival in postmenopausal women is modest.

5.71   AC

Oesophageal cancer has a very poor prognosis, with most patients being incurable at diagnosis. The overall 1-year survival rate is about 30%, and the overall 5-year survival rate is between 5 and 10%. Oesophageal cancer is associated with prominent lymphatic permeation, so producing microscopic metastases beyond the macroscopic limits of the tumour. Self-expanding, wire-mesh stents have been used to keep the oesophagus open and allow the passage of soft food. Stenting of upper-third tumours is poorly tolerated by patients and may also compromise the airway. Generally, only distal-third tumours are amenable to stenting. β-Naphthylamine increases the risk of developing bladder cancer.

5.72   BD

Radiotherapy has never been shown to improve overall survival from breast cancer, and in fact some trials have shown increased death rates from cardiovascular disease. However, postoperative radiotherapy clearly reduces local recurrence rates following conservative breast surgery. There is a high risk of severe arm lymphoedema following combined axillary clearance and radiotherapy. Radiotherapy should not therefore be applied to the axilla after a complete lymph node clearance, but may be given if the nodes have been sampled and are positive for tumour. A radiotherapy boost is often added to the internal mammary chain lymph nodes for medial tumours.

5.73   ACDE
Balanitis xerotica obliterans (BXO) is a dyskeratotic skin disorder affecting the prepuce, glans or urethral meatus. Similarly to condyloma, erythroplasia of Queyrat and Bowen's disease, BXO is considered precancerous. Paget's disease of the breast is associated with an underlying breast malignancy and is not premalignant. Both Peutz–Jeghers syndrome and familial adenomatous polyposis predispose to malignancies in the bowel. Severe metaplasia in a Barrett's oesophagus may also progress to oesophageal adenocarcinoma, the increased risk being approximately 20-fold.

5.74   ABEF
Testicular tumours account for less than 1% of all male tumours, but their incidence is rising and they are the commonest solid tumour in the 20–40-year age group. Most testicular tumours are germ-cell in origin, followed by seminomas, which are in turn more common than teratomas. Seminomas are more radiosensitive than teratomas. Untreated, teratomas have a greater metastatic potential and a worse prognosis than seminomas. However, the treatment for metastatic non-seminoma (e.g. teratoma) has been vastly improved since the 1980s. Chemotherapy now achieves cure rates of around 90%. In testicular malignancy, α-fetoprotein, β-hCG and LDH can be used as tumour markers.

5.75   ADE
Breast cancer is approximately 100 times rarer in men. Male breast cancer tends to present at a more advanced stage and affects older men (with greater comorbidity). Therefore, overall, men fare worse. There is an increased incidence in males with Klinefelter's syndrome. Despite the differing male hormonal physiology, the cancer can respond to tamoxifen; although the usual treatment is a radical mastectomy and radiotherapy, advanced disease may respond well to orchidectomy.

5.76   ADE
Results of screening programmes for cancer are limited by selection, length and lead-time bias. Selection bias arises from the tendency of people who enrol on screening programmes to be more health conscious and are therefore atypical of the general population. Length bias is the tendency for screening to detect a disproportionate number of cancers which are slow growing and have a better prognosis anyway. Lead-time bias occurs when screening advances the date at which diagnosis is made. This, therefore, lengthens the calculated survival time without necessarily altering the date of death.

5.77   CE

Finding results that are not statistically significant when the populations are actually different is known as type II error. The difference can be missed due to a combination of small sample size or high variability. Finding a statistically significant result when the populations are identical is called type I error. The Gaussian (normal) distribution plays an important role in statistical analysis. An unpaired *t*-test compares two groups on the assumption that the two populations are Gaussian. Paired   *t*-tests compare two paired groups. Parametric tests are used when data from population groups follow a Gaussian distribution. Non-parametric tests are used when data from the population group does not follow a Gaussian distribution.

5.78   BCD

The vast majority of colorectal carcinomas are thought to arise from pre-existing polyps. There is an increased incidence of colorectal carcinoma development following ureterosigmoidostomy, especially in the vicinity of the anastomosis. Chromosome 17 and 18 abnormalities are common and are thought to be involved in the progression of adenomatous polyps to carcinoma.

Dukes A tumours are confined to the muscularis propria, Dukes B tumours have traversed the bowel wall and Dukes C tumours have lymph node involvement. Longitudinal tumour spread is not a marked feature of colorectal carcinoma, and distal intramural spread more than 1 cm beyond the gross margins of the tumour is uncommon.

5.79   ABC

Other major contraindications to curative surgery in patients with non-small-cell lung cancer include vocal cord and phrenic nerve paralysis, tumour within 2 cm of the carina, cardiac tamponade, involvement of the main pulmonary artery, metastasis to the supraclavicular lymph nodes and severe pulmonary hypertension. A patient with an FEV_1 of >2.5 litres would be expected to tolerate a pneumonectomy.

5.80   CE

The mean of a set of values is the same as the average. The median is the middle value of the set of values. Standard deviation (SD) is a measure of the variability of a set of values: 68% of values lie within one SD on each side of the mean, and 95% within 2 SDs of the mean. Parametric tests are used for the assessment of data that follow a Gaussian (normal) distribution, and non-parametric tests for data not following a Gaussian distribution. The outcome of a rank or score has a limited range, and an arbitrary and artificial difference between scores. Such data cannot be Gaussian in distribution.

5.81   BD

Relative indications for mastectomy, rather than conservative breast excision, for breast cancer include multifocal disease, larger tumours (>4 cm), extensive DCIS, smaller breasts, salvage surgery and patient choice. Axillary lymph node involvement is not an indication in its own right. Absolute contraindications to conservative breast surgery include: two or more primary tumours in separate quadrants; first or second trimester pregnancy; previous radiotherapy to the region; persistent positive margins after surgery; and diffuse malignant microcalcifications.

5.82   ACDF

Potentially premalignant lesions of the oesophagus include: the Plummer–Vinson syndrome (oesophageal web); corrosive oesophagitis; achalasia; Barrett's oesophagus; and scleroderma involvement of the oesophagus. There is a 25-fold increased risk of developing oesophageal cancer in Barrett's. There is an increased risk of oesophageal cancer with achalasia and hiatus hernia.

5.83   B

Elective regional lymph node dissection (i.e. removal of clinically uninvolved nodes draining the area of the primary) has not been shown to increase the survival rate of patients with cutaneous malignant melanoma. Therapeutic regional lymph node excision (i.e. removal of clinically involved nodes), however, does improve survival in a proportion of patients, and is recommended in the absence of distant spread. Melanoma is a relatively chemoresistant and radioresistant tumour. Excision of solitary metastases, such as in the lung, is associated with improved long-term survival in only a minority of patients. The use of sentinel node biopsy can make prophylactic local node dissection more rational.

5.84   BCD

Testing for faecal occult blood has been shown to increase the detection of early colorectal tumours confined to the bowel wall and has resulted in a reduction in the number of deaths. The optimal period between repeat testing has yet to be established. Currently the most commonly used method of testing for faecal occult blood is Haemoccult. The Haemoccult FOBT relies on a peroxidase-type reaction, which turns a guaiac slide blue by oxidising it. However, Haemoccult can miss 25–50% of colonic cancers because of the phenomenon of intermittent bleeding. Around 1 in 10 patients with a positive faecal occult blood test have a colorectal tumour. A more likely cause for a positive test, however, is that they have a benign adenoma.

5.85   ABE

Carcinoid tumours can occur in the lungs and thymus, but are mostly found in the gastrointestinal tract (commonest site of all being the appendix). Carcinoid tumours of the colon and small bowel often behave in a malignant fashion, and often present with massive regional lymph node and hepatic metastases. The size of the primary tumour is a major prognostic factor.

The carcinoid syndrome is due to the release of serotonin (5-HT) and other hormonal peptides such as kallikrein into the systemic circulation. Therefore, malignant carcinoids of the gastrointestinal tract only produce carcinoid syndrome when metastases are present within the liver and the systemic circulation becomes involved. Small-bowel carcinoid tumours have the highest likelihood of spreading to the liver and causing carcinoid syndrome. 5-Hydroxyindoleacetic acid (5-HIAA) is a metabolite of 5-HT and is excreted in increased amounts in the urine. Therefore, a good biochemical test for carcinoid is a 24-hour urine assay for 5-HIAA.

5.86   ACD

Single-blinding refers to the patient not knowing which treatment he/she is receiving. Double-blinding is said to occur when both the patient and the investigator are unaware which treatment the patient is receiving. A trial participant can withdraw at any time. A control group is a group of patients observed after not receiving the index treatment. Historical controls are not as reliable as a group randomised to control.

5.87   ABD

Fibroadenomas of the breast arise from breast lobules rather than ducts. They contain both epithelial and stromal elements. There is a very slight increased risk of cancer development in patients with fibroadenomas (e.g. cystosarcoma phylloides tumours may arise in pre-existing fibroadenomas). Up to 40% of fibroadenomas spontaneously regress or resolve. They do not usually interfere with breast-feeding.

5.88   AC

Tissue from the centre of malignant lesions is often necrotic and will frequently provide insufficient information to establish a definitive diagnosis. Invasion may be multifocal and a single biopsy may not be representative of the whole of the lesion and therefore is insufficient to exclude a malignant process. Tissue should be taken from the junction of abnormal and normal tissue, as this gives the best chance of characterising the underlying histological abnormality. To prevent autolysis of tissue, specimens should be stored in formalin if there is going to be a delay in histological processing.

5.89   ABDF

Xeroderma pigmentosum is an autosomal recessive disorder in which there is increased susceptibility to sunlight-induced skin damage. There is a 1000-fold increased risk of developing cutaneous SCC. SCCs never regress to produce Bowen's disease. SCC seen in a long-standing venous ulcer is known as a Marjolin's ulcer. There is an increased incidence of cutaneous SCC in renal transplant recipients and other chronically immunocompromised patients. Less than 5% of cutaneous SCCs metastasise to lymph nodes. SCCs on the vulva and penis behave in a more aggressive fashion and thus have a worse prognosis.

5.90   Testicular tumours
1.   A   Teratoma
2.   B   Seminoma
3.   A   Teratoma
4.   A   Teratoma
5.   C   Choriocarcinoma

Teratomas produce α-FP in about 70% of cases, secrete β-hCG in about 60% of cases, and secrete either α-FP or β-hCG in about 90% of cases. Almost all choriocarcinomas secrete β-hCG, but they do not produce α-FP. Less than 10% of seminomas secrete β-hCG, and very rarely produce α-FP.

5.91   ACE
Bladder, cervical and laryngeal cancer are all smoking-related. No known association exists for the leukaemias and lymphomas.

5.92   AB
The blood supply to the breast is mainly from the lateral thoracic artery. The internal thoracic artery, perforating intercostal arteries and the pectoral branches of the thoracoacromial artery also contribute. Venous return simply follows the arteries mentioned above. The nipple is a reasonable reliable marker for the T4 dermatome. In the breast, 75% of the lymphatic drainage is via the axillary nodes. The retromammary space overlies the pectoralis major muscle.

5.93   AE
The clavipectoral fascia arises from the clavicle and encloses the pectoralis minor before fusing with the floor of the axilla. The thoracodorsal nerve supplies the latissimus dorsi. Damage to the long thoracic nerve (serratus anterior) causes a winged scapula. Level I nodes lie lateral to the pectoralis minor, level II behind and level III medial to the pectoralis minor. Division of the intercostobrachial nerve (T2) can lead to anaesthesia on the medial upper arm.

5.94   ABCD
Small lymphatic vessels from the breast cross the midline to the other breast, and also cross the diaphragm where they communicate with the whole breast and the lymphatics of the liver. The regional lymph nodes of the breast are found in the axilla and drain mainly the superior and lateral aspects, whilst those along the internal mammary artery may drain the inferior and medial parts. The subclavian lymph trunk emerges from the apical nodes of the axilla, and on the right drains into the subclavian vein or right jugular trunk. On the left it usually drains into the thoracic duct.

5.95   Thyroid cancer
1.   **D   Anaplastic carcinoma**
2.   **E   Lymphoma**
3.   **A   Papillary carcinoma**
4.   **C   Medullary-cell carcinoma**
5.   **B   Follicular carcinoma**

Papillary carcinoma of the thyroid is four times more common in women. It tends to affect younger people, is multicentric and metastasises early to lymph nodes. Follicular carcinoma of the thyroid, in contrast, tends to be solitary, encapsulated, invades the bloodstream and spreads to bone.

Medullary thyroid cancer is sporadic in 90% of cases. Familial cases may be associated with MEN II. Calcitonin is a good tumour marker for medullary thyroid cancer since it is known to be secreted from parafollicular C cells. Anaplastic carcinoma has one of the worst prognoses. It is a very aggressive tumour invading all local structures early.

5.96   ABE

The important feature is one of a changing lesion, which differentiates it from other pigmented lesion. Satellite lesions are a feature of melanoma, other features suggestive of a melanoma are:

A = asymmetry
B = irregular border
C= colour: variable; ulcerated when advanced (bleeds easily); may be
     depigmented
D = diameter >5 mm

The Glasgow 7-point checklist lists 3 major features:
1 – change in size
2 – change in shape
3 – change in colour
(one major feature indicates removal)

and 4 minor features:
4 – diameter of lesion >7 mm
5 – inflammation around lesion
6 – bleeding of lesion
7 – mild itching

5.97   B

Women have a better overall prognosis with melanoma compared to a controlled series of men. Breslow thickness is the best indicator of prognosis. Tumour thickness and ulceration are the two most dominant features of aggressive primary melanomas. Male sex, increased tumour thickness, the presence of ulceration, older age and mucosal involvement are also poor prognostic indicators. The prognosis also depends upon the lymph node involvement and growth pattern.

The 5-year survival rate is 90% for stage I, 50% for stage II, 30% for stage III and <1% for stage IV disease.

5.98   Hormone-secreting tumours

1. E   α-Fetoprotein
2. F   ACTH
3. A   Calcitonin
4. C   5-Hydroxytryptamine
5. B   Erythropoietin

α-Fetoprotein is secreted in high amounts by hepatocellular carcinomas (90% of cases) and teratomas.

Bronchial carcinomas may secrete a variety of hormones including ACTH, cortisol, ADH and parathormone.

Medullary thyroid carcinoma is known to secrete calcitonin (from parafollicular C cells), which can be used as a tumour marker.

Renal carcinoma may present with polycythaemia as part of a paraneoplastic syndrome. This is due to excess secretion of erythropoietin.

5.99   ACEFGH

Deaths reportable to the coroner include: dead on arrival; dead within 24 hours of emergency admission to hospital; deaths during or within 24 hours of an operation/anaesthetic/invasive procedure; deaths occurring as a result of an accident; unnatural, criminal or suspicious deaths, including those due to neglect, suicide or abuse; and deaths due to poisoning, drugs or acute or chronic alcohol abuse. Industrial or occupational diseases leading to death as well as deaths due to medical or surgical mishap should also be reported. Also reportable are: the death of a prisoner whilst in hospital; stillbirths; cases of hypothermia leading to death; deaths in public places, fires, police custody or prison; deaths where a property has been broken into; and deaths where the police are involved. Notifiable diseases have to be reported to the Consultant in Communicable Disease Control. At present, the reporting of AIDS to the CCDC is voluntary.

5.100   All true   ?B   incorrect

Patients require sufficient information before deciding to give their consent to a procedure, and therefore all the treatment options should be listed and explained. If a patient is not offered sufficient information as they reasonably need to make their decision (and in a form they can understand) then their consent may not be valid.

5.101   AC

Certain data is required for a surgical waiting list. The necessary information includes the diagnosis of the condition, the operation and the date of placement on the waiting list.

5.102   AC

Thrombophlebitis migrans is a condition producing recurrent thrombotic episodes in superficial veins, especially in the extremities. Many cases are idiopathic and show a diffuse inflammatory action. Thrombophlebitis migrans is a well-known feature of deep-seated carcinomas. The common sites of primary tumour associated with thrombophlebitis migrans are the pancreas, lungs, stomach and female genital tract.

PRACTICE PAPER 1 – MCQ ANSWERS

1 AB
Symptoms of aortic stenosis include syncope (at rest or on exertion) due to heart block (which may occasionally lead to sudden death), dyspnoea and palpitations.
Signs: BP tends to be low and the pulse is slow-rising. The murmur of aortic stenosis is an ejection systolic murmur that characteristically radiates into the neck.

2 A
A PCA pump can give a background infusion of analgesia to which boluses can be added and is under the control of the patient. A lock-out time is used to prevent overdose. Not all patients are suitable for PCA and therefore the choice of patient is important. Patients should be motivated and capable of understanding how to use the system. The pump should be treated as any other drug administered in hospital and therefore should be looked after by a qualified nurse or dedicated pain-control/anaesthetic team.

3 AB
Hereditary spherocytosis is an autosomal dominant condition in which there is a defect of the structural proteins of the red cell membrane. FAP is a rare disease which has an autosomal dominant inheritance pattern. The gene defect (APC gene) is on the long arm of chromosome 5. Cystic fibrosis shows a recessive pattern of inheritance. The gene defect is found on chromosome 7 and is carried by 1 in 20 white people. Trisomy 21 (or Down's syndrome) occurs when there is an extra chromosome 21, which can occur due to non-dysjunction or mosaicism. Haemophilia is a sex-linked, recessively inherited disorder of clotting factor VIII.

4 CD
Diazepam is a long-acting benzodiazepine with a half-life exceeding 24 hours. It is broken down into active metabolites, hence its long half-life. Its effects are reversed by flumazenil. Naloxone reverses the effects of opiates. An antegrade amnesia is produced by diazepam.

5   BC

Skin and ocular sarcoidosis are the commonest extrapulmonary presentations. Skin sarcoidosis is seen in 10% of cases and produces a chilblain-like lesion known as 'lupus pernio'. Bilateral symmetrical hilar lymphadenopathy is also seen in sarcoidosis. The other manifestations include anterior uveitis, hypercalcaemia, arthralgia and bone cysts. Hepatosplenomegaly is a rare manifestation of sarcoidosis and is rarely of any clinical significance. Cardiac involvement too is rare, occurring in 3% of cases. Ventricular dysrhythmias, conduction defects and cardiac myopathy with congestive cardiac failure are seen.

6   D

Sterilisation is defined as the complete destruction of all viable microorganisms including spores, viruses and microbacteria. In practice, this is defined in terms of the probability of a single viable microorganism surviving on one million items. Boiling in water only is a form of disinfection; it kills bacteria, some viruses and some spores but it does not sterilise. Sterilisation is achieved by steam, hot air, ethylene oxide, low-temperature steam–formaldehyde or gamma-irradiation.

7   ABE

There is a close relationship between potassium- and hydrogen-ion haemostasis in acidotic states. In acidosis, hydrogen ions will tend to be excreted in preference to potassium ions, whereas in alkalosis fewer hydrogen ions will be available for secretion and hence there will be an increase in potassium secretion. An exception to this is in renal tubular acidosis where there is a defect in hydrogen ion excretion. Mineralocorticoid deficiency present in Addison's disease may result in a raised serum potassium level. Plasma potassium levels rise progressively as blood is stored. However, elevated potassium is rarely a problem as prewarming of the blood increases red blood cell metabolism – the sodium pump becomes more active and potassium levels fall.

8   ABF

Pseudomembranous colitis (PMC) should be suspected in any patient on broad spectrum antibiotics who develops profuse watery, foul-smelling diarrhoea. PMC is due to overgrowth of the bacterium *Clostridium difficile* which responds to treatment with oral vancomycin or metronidazole. Antimotility agents are contraindicated as they may precipitate toxic megacolon.

9   AE

Bacteroides fragilis is a normal commensal of the gastrointestinal tract and is found at 10^{10}–10^{11} organisms per gram of faeces. It is a non-spore forming, Gram-negative anaerobe (strict). Vincent's angina is caused by *Borrelia vincenti* and *Fusiformis* spp. bacteria. Abdominal wound infections are usually caused by *Escherichia coli*, which in turn encourages the growth of *Bacteroides fragilis*.

10   ABCE

Brain abscesses are recognised complications of ear, sinus and dental infection. They are also associated with bronchiectasis and infective endocarditis. Cerebral tumour is a differential diagnosis of cerebral abscess. Postoperative infection causing abscess is a recognised complication of hypophysectomy, as is any skull fracture.

11   AE

The hemiazygos veins drain separately from their adjoining ends behind the oesophagus into the azygos vein. The azygos vein arches superiorly over the right bronchus. The vagus nerve lies just posterior to the right main bronchus, whereas the phrenic nerve is anterior.

12   ABCD

Atrophy is a decrease in the bulk of tissue or organ. It can occur physiologically and pathologically. Atrophy may occur at any time of life, including the gestational period. The ductus arteriosus and umbilical vessels remain as fibrous cords and are an example of atrophy in infancy. Localised atrophy occurs following ischaemia, pressure and denervation.

13   B

Pulmonary embolus is most commonly seen in the second week postoperatively, classically 10 days' postoperatively. Wound infections usually present after 3–5 days postoperatively but may occur later. A postoperative pyrexia may not always be due to an infection, but an atelectasis or a DVT. Pseudo-obstruction is a functional bowel disorder demonstrating identical signs and symptoms to mechanical large bowel obstruction.

14   DE

Split-skin grafts require several factors for optimal take, including a good vascular bed and absence of infection. The thickness of a split-skin graft can vary and does not affect its survival Split-skin grafts do not take on bone or tendon as they survive by imbibition for the first 24–48 hours and then by inosculation, which is the linking up of vessels between the graft and the wound bed. Pressure sores requiring surgical treatment are best managed by flap reconstruction as bulk is required. Split-skin grafts are most commonly harvested from the thigh or buttock; they can be stored for 2 weeks in the refrigerator and applied to wounds in patients on the ward.

15   BDE

Morphine and other opioids are commonly used for spinal analgesia. The advantage of an intrathecal opioid injection is that it relieves pain without the complication of a motor block, sympathetic block or even numbness. It is not suitable as analgesia following abdominal surgery. Patient-controlled analgesia using morphine is commonplace. It is necessary when using PCA to have a designated bolus dose and lock-out intervals. When assessing confusion in an elderly patient postoperatively, the drug prescription sheet must be carefully looked at as drugs are often the source of the problem. However, it is mandatory to carry out a full examination and investigate further.

16   AE

A characteristic sequence of events occurs in the first few days of wound healing. Neutrophils and monocytes are the first cells to appear. Neutrophils peak around days 1–3, monocytes marginally later around days 2–4. Macrophages act as phagocytes in wound healing. Macrophage infiltration is followed by the proliferation of fibroblasts (peak around day 6) which produce collagen. This is followed by an ingrowth of small capillary beds to form granulation tissue. Megaloblasts are erythroblasts with delayed nuclear maturation because of defective DNA synthesis (seen in megaloblastic anaemia). Megakaryocytes are found in the bone marrow and are precursors of platelets, but are not involved in wound healing.

17   BDE

The stress response to surgery involves a rise in the basal metabolic rate, protein catabolism and decreased gluconeogenesis with mobilisation of fatty acids, producing a negative nitrogen balance. Increased amounts of ACTH, ADH and aldosterone are secreted, reducing urinary sodium excretion and promoting water retention.

18   ABC

In response to hypovolaemia, baroreceptors in the carotid artery and aortic arch are stimulated. In addition, stretch receptors in the left atrium, pulmonary veins and juxtaglomerular apparatus are also stimulated. The resultant effect is a reduction in the flow of neural impulses from the baroreceptors to the brainstem, so causing an increased secretion of ADH. The release of ADH is stimulated by a decrease of 5–10% in the total circulating blood volume. In response to stress (i.e. hypovolaemia), there is an increased release of adrenaline, cortisol and growth hormone, all of which increase the blood glucose level. Due to the action of corticosteroids and mineralocorticoids on the distal renal tubule, hypokalaemia may occur.

19   BCDE

Deaths reportable to the coroner include: dead on arrival; dead within 24 hours of emergency admission to hospital; deaths during or within 24 hours of an operation/anaesthetic/invasive procedure; deaths occurring as a result of an accident; unnatural, criminal or suspicious deaths, including those due to neglect, suicide or abuse; deaths due to poisoning, drugs or acute or chronic alcohol abuse. Industrial or occupational diseases leading to death and deaths due to medical or surgical mishap should also be reported. Also reportable are: death of a prisoner whilst in hospital; stillbirths; cases of hypothermia leading to death; deaths in public places, fires, police custody or prison or deaths in a property that has been broken into, or when the police are involved. Notifiable diseases are those which the Consultant in Communicable Disease Control (CCDC) must be informed about. At present, the reporting of AIDS to the CCDC is voluntary.

20   ABCD

Low-molecular-weight heparins (LMWHs) act mainly through the inhibition of factor X. LMWHs have comparatively little antithrombin III activity. The activated partial thromboplastin time is not prolonged in LMWH treatment. However, when monitoring is required, anti-Xa assays are used. LMWH has a longer half-life and more predictable bioavailability than unfractionated heparin and therefore can be administered subcutaneously, once daily. It requires monitoring only if used long-term or if anticoagulation control is critical. It is at least as effective as (and may be superior to) unfractionated heparin in some patient groups in perioperative thromboprophylaxis. LMWH is safe and has revolutionised long-term anticoagulation in pregnancy.

21   BCD

Complications associated with massive blood transfusion include hyperkalaemia, hypothermia (blood is stored at 4 °C, fast-flow blood warmers may reduce the hypothermia and should be used routinely), disseminated intravascular coagulation, thrombocytopenia (dilutional – stored blood is low in functional platelets) and hypocalcaemia (due to citrate in stored blood).

22   BCD

The vagus nerve lies posterior to the lung root, whereas the phrenic nerve lies anterior. The azygos vein is formed from the union of the lumbar vein and the right subcostal vein; it enters the mediastinum through the aortic opening of the diaphragm under the shelter of the right crus. The azygos vein arches over the right bronchus at T4.

23   ABE

Wallace's Rule of 9s for adult burns states that the burn area for the head is 9%; for each arm 9%; for each leg 18%; and for the trunk 36%. Deep or full-thickness burns coagulate and destroy all areas of the skin, typically resulting in complete anaesthesia. Such burns do not blister and may have a mottled or waxy appearance. In addition to being a prognosticator, Wallace's Rule can be used to estimate how much fluid the patient would need. Burns involving more than 20% of the body surface area require IV fluids. Numerous fluid regimens, however, have been described. One, based on ATLS, advises 2–4 ml of Ringer's lactate/kg body weight per percentage (second and third degree) of the burn surface area in the first 24 hours. Fluid replacement can use a combination of crystalloid, albumin and colloid solutions. Regular clinical examination plus 4-hourly haemoglobin and haematocrit levels and hourly urinary output measurements would be valuable. Healthy skin is able to prevent the entry of microorganisms. Burns disrupt skin and tissue integrity so infection is one major complication. Common organisms include *Staphylococcus*, *Pseudomonas* and *Acinetobacter* spp. as well as *Streptococcus faecalis*.

24   E

The anterior compartment of the leg or extensor compartment contains the anterior tibial vessels and the deep peroneal nerve. In addition, the muscles tibialis anterior, extensor hallucis longus, extensor digitorum longus and peroneus tertius are found there. The muscles in this compartment are responsible for foot and ankle dorsiflexion. The tibial nerve gives off the medial plantar nerve which supplies the first dorsal cleft.

25   AC

Fat embolism is seen after closed and open femoral fractures, though it is more common in closed fractures. Fat emboli are believed to be released from most long-bone fractures, but fat embolism syndrome (in which the patient develops symptoms) is rare. It can present with petechial haemorrhages, confusion, hypoxia, restlessness and agitation.

26   CD

The purpose of the primary survey is to identify and immediately address life-threatening conditions. A chest film will demonstrate several such injuries (pneumothorax, haemothorax, widened mediastinum), whilst pelvic films can reveal fractures that can be accompanied by major haemorrhage. A lateral C-spine film demonstrating injury can be useful, though a negative one will not exclude C-spine injury. The new ATLS guidelines include only chest and pelvis films as mandatory in the primary survey. Routine C-spine X-rays have now been omitted and are only indicated if there is cervical spine tenderness or a palpable deformity. There is no indication for skull X-ray in the primary survey. A mini-neurological examination will provide the necessary information required for the initial management of the head-injured patient. The presence or absence of a skull fracture adds little useful information at this stage. Plain abdominal films likewise add little to the initial management of abdominal trauma or to the decision to proceed to early laparotomy. There is no indication for requesting extremity X-rays in the initial phase, they are often of poor quality and again provide little to the early management of the patient.

27   BCD

Characteristically a tension pneumothorax, cardiac tamponade or pericardial effusion would cause a low blood pressure with a high CVP. Massive pulmonary embolism may also give this picture. In septic shock, the blood pressure would be low, as would the CVP.

28   ABCD

The floor of the anterior cranial fossa roofs the orbits, ethmoidal sinuses and the nose. It contains the frontal lobes of the cerebral hemispheres and the olfactory and anterior ethmoidal nerves. A fracture of the anterior fossa would result in rhinorrhoea, anosmia and visual disturbance. Bilateral black eyes (periorbital ecchymosis, 'racoon eyes') are a sign of a basal skull fracture.

29   AD

The narrowest part of the GI tract that has to be negotiated is the pylorus. Observation would not be advisable in this case as the pin is open and therefore could potentially cause visceral perforation. MRI would be a contraindication as metallic objects are affected by the magnetic field. The pin may be removed by gastroscopy, an overtube or an oesophagoscope may be advanced over the pin and safely extracted. In the rare instances when the pin cannot be successfully removed by gastroscopy, a laparotomy may be required.

30   BE

Upper trunk brachial plexus injury is known as an Erb's palsy. It is due to root injury to C5, C6 and sometimes C7. The abductors (deltoid, supraspinatus) and external rotators (infraspinatus, teres minor) of the shoulder, supinators (biceps brachii) and elbow flexors (biceps brachii, brachialis) are paralysed. Weakness of finger and wrist extension is seen (extensor compartment muscles). Sensation will be lost over the lateral arm (C5–6 dermatomes). Lower root lesions lead to finger paralysis.

31   BCE

In addition to the separation of the fracture fragments, tissue interposition and poor blood supply, excessive movement will also cause non-union. Non-union can be either hypertrophic or atrophic. In hypertrophic non-union, excessive amounts of useless callus are formed. Very little callus is formed in atrophic non-union.

32   ACD

Flail chest occurs when a chest wall segment loses bony continuity with the rest of the thoracic cage, usually as a result of from trauma associated with multiple rib fractures. The 'flail' segment displays paradoxical movements with respiration. Disruption of the normal chest wall movement and underlying lung contusion may lead to respiratory failure. 50% of adults with a flail chest have an associated pulmonary contusion. Diagnosis may be difficult because of splinting of the chest wall. Treatment includes oxygen therapy with the establishment of adequate ventilation (around 35% of patients require artificial ventilation) and management of associated lung contusion by carefully controlling fluid infusions.

33   ABCDE

Major burns may lead to excessive fluid loss, thereby causing haemodynamic compromise. Myocardial suppression due to an associated myocardial depressant factor is also seen. Reduced RBC survival from increased capillary permeability and bone marrow suppression also occurs. An initial thrombocytopenia followed by a thrombocytosis is seen together with disseminated intravascular coagulation. Mast cells in burned skin release histamine. Immunoglobulin production is commonly decreased after a major burn, and this plays a role in increasing the risk of infection.

34   BCD

Tension pneumothorax produces acute severe respiratory compromise in association with profound hypotension, absence of breath sounds on the affected side, hyperresonance to percussion on the affected side, distended neck veins and tracheal deviation to the opposite side.

35   ACE

The diaphragm rises to the fourth intercostal space during full expiration, thus intra-abdominal viscera are at risk from penetrating lower chest wounds. Around 20% of lower chest stab wounds and 60% of lower chest gunshot wounds are associated with a significant intra-abdominal organ injury. Penetrating chest trauma requires chest drainage to deal with the associated pneumothorax and haemothorax. The mortality for pneumonectomy following trauma is over 50%, mostly attributable to right heart failure.

36   AB

Loss of fixation in two or more points is required to destabilise a ring structure mechanically. Acetabular fractures are usually evident on AP X-rays of the pelvis, though some posterior fracture-dislocations may not be obvious. They are best visualised on oblique X-ray films and spiral CT. Acetabular fractures are due to forceful impaction by the femoral head. Surgery can be delayed for a few days in closed acetabular fractures as this may reduce perioperative blood loss. Arthritis is common following acetabular fractures.

37   AE

The inspiratory capacity is the volume of maximum inspiration starting from the normal expiratory position. The total volume of both lungs is the total lung capacity. The vital capacity is the maximum volume of air that can be expelled from the lungs by forceful effort after a maximum inspiration. The maximum ventilation volume is the greatest volume of air that can be breathed in a given time (e.g. litres/min). The functional residual capacity includes residual volume which cannot be expelled into a spirometer.

38   AF

The manubriosternal joint is at the level of the lower border of the T4 vertebra. The structures which may be seen at this point are the thoracic duct, oesophagus, right vagus nerve, the left vagus, the left phrenic nerve and right phrenic nerve, the azygos vein, the superior vena cava, the trachea and arch of the aorta. The tracheal bifurcation occurs at level of T5; the left brachiocephalic vein is seen at a higher level.

39   ACD

The commonest cause of L5 root compression is a prolapsed intervertebral disc. Signs include weakness of the extensor hallucis longus, weakness of ankle dorsiflexion, wasting of the extensor digitorum brevis and reduced sensation in the L5 dermatome.

40   CD

The middle lobe of the right lung has two bronchopulmonary segments and is separated from the lower lobe by the oblique fissure. It is auscultated in the 5th intercostal space anteriorly (the lower lobe intervenes posteriorly). Both the right atrium and the dome of the diaphragm make large impressions on the lung surface.

41   ADE

Hypokalaemia is usually asymptomatic but severe hypokalaemia may cause muscle weakness, paraesthesia and reduced tendon reflexes. Hypokalaemia increases the risk of digoxin toxicity by increasing the binding of digoxin to cardiac cells. Hypokalaemia may also cause cardiac dysrhythmias and interstitial renal disease. The pathogenesis of the latter is incompletely understood. The ECG changes associated with hypokalaemia include flattened T waves and depression of the ST segment. Tall, peaked T waves are associated with hyperkalaemia.

42   BEFG

ARDS is a non-specific reaction to a wide variety of insults, either direct (e.g. smoke inhalation) or indirect (e.g. including trauma, sepsis, fat emboli and massive transfusion). Its pathophysiology is poorly understood but a reduction in surfactant levels and lowered lung compliance are observed. An increase in pulmonary capillary permeability and pulmonary vascular resistance are seen; the pulmonary capillary wedge occlusion pressure is characteristically low (<16 mmHg). ARDS presents with a refractory hypoxaemia and diffuse alveolar infiltrates on the CXR. Nitric oxide therapy can be used in an effort to reduce shunt (V/Q mismatch) in the lungs, though it has not been shown to significantly reduce mortality or morbidity.

43   All false

Features of atrial fibrillation include absent P waves and an irregular pulse. Atrial fibrillation does not produce any T wave changes directly; T-wave changes are associated with ischaemia which can result from fast AF. Carotid sinus massage will convert atrial flutter but not fibrillation. Intolerance of warm weather is a symptom of thyrotoxicosis, which is a cause of AF.

44   A

α-Adrenoreceptor (α-blockers) will cause postural hypotension, and thus decrease coronary artery perfusion. Thus, α-stimulation will cause increased coronary artery perfusion. All β-adrenoreceptor agonists dilate the coronary vessels.

45   DFG

1st heart sound represents atrioventricular (AV) valve closure.
2nd heart sound represents aortic and pulmonary valve closure.
In the cardiac cycle, the following waves/pressure changes are seen in the atria:
- 'a' wave is caused by atrial contraction (pressure rises by 4–6 mmHg).
- 'c' wave occurs when the ventricles begin to contract, caused by bulging of the AV valves backward toward the atria.
- 'v' wave occurs towards the end of ventricular contraction, and results from the slow build-up of blood in the atria while the AV valves are closed during ventricular contraction.

46   ADE

Disseminated intravascular coagulation (DIC) is a multisystem disorder characterised by simultaneous activation of the coagulation and fibrinolytic pathways. Common causes include sepsis, malignancy (especially adenocarcinoma), trauma and obstetric emergencies (e.g. placenta abruption, amniotic fluid embolism). Although DIC usually manifests as bleeding, some patients display thrombosis. Progressive consumption of all the coagulation factors and platelets leads to a characteristic laboratory profile of prolongation of the PT, APTT and TT and falling fibrinogen and platelets. Increased fibrinolysis is indicated by rising concentrations of fibrinogen degradation products or D-dimers. Although similar findings may be seen in hepatic insufficiency, DIC may be diagnosed by demonstrating deteriorating coagulation abnormalities in conjunction with a likely clinical cause. The mainstay of care is treatment of the underlying cause, replacement of the deficient factors with fresh-frozen plasma, cryoprecipitate and platelets.

47   BDE

The essential components of total parenteral nutrition are nitrogen, carbohydrate, fat, minerals (calcium, magnesium, iron, zinc, manganese, copper, fluoride, iodine, chloride) and vitamins.

48   ACE

The cisterna chyli runs between the aorta and the right crus of the diaphragm, passes through the aortic diaphragm opening and drains into the thoracic duct. The thoracic duct ascends anterior to the posterior intercostal vessels and has several valves. At the thoracic inlet, it lies to the left of the oesophagus and arches forward over the dome of the left pleura draining into the left brachiocephalic vein. The right bronchomediastinal trunk drains into the right subclavian vein.

49   ACE

The phrenic nerve arises from C3, 4, 5 deep to the scalenus anterior and medius, and runs on the scalenus anterior, over the anterior part of the dome of the pleura to enter the mediastinum posterior to the subclavian vein. Here the right phenic nerve spirals forward to lie on the SVC, right atrium and IVC, and traverses the diaphragm via the caval orifice. The vagus nerve gives off the recurrent laryngeal.

50   All true

Central venous-line insertion may cause trauma to adjacent tissues with consequent haemorrhage and pneumothorax. If it is left open then air may enter the blood causing venous air embolism. Systemic arterial air embolism may occur if the cannula is mistakenly placed in the carotid artery.

51   ACE

Pulmonary artery occlusion (or wedge) pressure can be directly measured by Swan–Ganz catheterisation. Cardiac index and left ventricular stroke work can also be derived from these measurements using the Fick principle. FiO_2 (concentration of inspired oxygen) and end tidal CO_2 (concentration of expired CO_2) cannot be measured by Swan–Ganz catheterisation.

52   BDE

Adjuvant chemotherapy has been shown to produce a modest survival advantage in Dukes C and some Dukes B colorectal cancers. Thus far, the best results have been with 5-FU administered alone or in combination with folinic acid (leucovorin). Other agents (e.g. vincristine and levamisole) have been tested in a few trials, with conflicting evidence for survival benefit. Irinotecan is used as second-line chemotherapy and in advanced cancers.

53   ABCF

Tumour markers are substances that are present in the body at a concentration proportional to the tumour burden. They are not always tumour-specific, for example, human chorionic gonadotrophin levels may be elevated in pregnancy, germ-cell tumours and gestational trophoblastic disease. Tumour markers are most commonly used to monitor therapeutic responses. However, they may also aid in diagnosis, have a role in the detection of relapse and provide prognostic information. For example, in the case of testicular germ-cell tumours, the level of tumour markers before treatment is an important predictor of outcome. CA-125 has not been detected in the normal ovary, but PSA is found in the normal prostate.

54   BDE

The absolute criterion for malignancy is invasiveness. Malignant tumours exhibit cells with greater variation in size and shape than benign tumours. There is increased cellular turnover and incomplete differentiation.

55   EF

Both volunteer- and population-based studies have found mammography to improve survival in breast cancer. Mammography is least useful in younger women because the breast tissue is relatively radio-opaque and abnormalities such as mass lesions and calcification are therefore more difficult to see. Ultrasound tends to be the first-line radiographic imaging technique for women <35 years. Studies in the under-50 age groups have shown smaller reductions in mortality with screening mammography. Women aged 50–64 years are currently invited for breast screening every 3 years. The service is available to older women on request. Mammography should be carried out in patients with an obvious carcinoma as it may reveal impalpable tumours in the same or the contralateral breast. The sensitivity of mammography is in the region of 90%. Ductal carcinoma *in situ* (DCIS) may cause microcalcifications that can be seen on mammography.

56   ADE

Non-cycling ('resting') cells are said to be in the G_0 phase of the cell cycle. RNA and protein synthesis occurs during the first growth phase, i.e. G_1. Duplication (replication) of cellular DNA occurs during the S phase which is followed by a second growth phase (G_2). This precedes mitosis (M). The duration of the cell cycle varies from 20 to 100 hours; 20–24 hours in rapidly growing cells. The rate of tumour growth decreases exponentially with time (Gompertzian pattern), therefore the growth fraction of small tumours is greater than that of larger ones. Cytotoxic drugs usually act on cycling cells and can be phase- or non-phase-specific.

57   All true   N ot A or D

Radiotherapy can result in nausea, fatigue and vomiting. Lymphoedema of the arm can occur following axillary clearance and is compounded by radiotherapy. Other side-effects include pulmonary fibrosis, telangiectasis, pneumonitis, oesophagitis, radiation myelitis and pericarditis.

58   BD

Needle-aspiration cytology is a tool for the detection of malignant cells. Cytology may reveal mitotic figures, increased nuclei and decreased cellular cohesion. It will give no information regarding staging. Gram-staining is used for bacterial infection investigation but is not used in needle-aspiration cytology. Needle-aspiration cytology is particularly effective in distinguishing between benign and malignant cells in breast, bone and soft tissue tumours.

59   ABCD

Informed consent must include explanation of the major risks of the procedure and the anaesthetic risks. The chance of short- and long-term success must be explained. There are now consent forms in circulation that outline all these points.

60   AC

Thrombophlebitis migrans is a condition causing recurrent thrombotic episodes in the superficial and deep veins, especially of the extremities. Many cases are idiopathic (or form a part of Buerger's disease) and show a diffuse inflammatory action. Thrombophlebitis migrans is also a well-known complication of a deep-seated cancer, the usual sites of primary tumour being the pancreas (tail and body), lungs, stomach and female genital tract.

61   ABCDE

Tamoxifen is a synthetic oestrogen that acts primarily by binding to oestrogen receptors. It is most widely used hormonal treatment for breast cancer. It has a half-life of around 7 days and it takes approximately 4 weeks to reach a steady state. Tamoxifen has a role in both breast cancer treatment and prophylaxis. As adjuvant treatment, it should be taken for a period of 5 years, as a longer period of ingestion would lead to an increased risk of endometrial carcinoma. Tamoxifen has been shown to decrease contralateral breast cancer by 47%. Other benefits include preservation of bone density (probably due to its partial agonist action on steroid receptors) and decrease in plasma cholesterol levels. The latter effect is thought to partly explain the reduced risk of cardiac disease. Side-effects include hot flushes and water retention. The standard daily dose is 20 mg. Tamoxifen increases the risk of both thrombophlebitis and embolic events, particularly when administered with cytotoxic agents. Tamoxifen is used in premenopausal women who are known to have oestrogen receptor positive tumours.

62   ABG

Malignant primary bone tumours are rare. Benign primary tumours such as osteomas are more common. The commonest bone tumour is a metastasis from a primary malignant tumour at another site. Ewing's sarcoma has an overall poor prognosis. Benign bone tumours tend to occur in adolescents and young adults. Primary malignant bone tumours are often very aggressive and tend to occur in adolescents and young adults. There is often a characteristic history of pain. Lesions can have ill-defined margins on X-ray (Codman's triangle, sunray spicules). Osteoporosis is the leading cause of pathological fractures.

63   CD

FOBT screening with Haemoccult is a guaiac-based test relying on a peroxidase-like reaction. Animal haemoglobin and certain vegetables containing the enzyme peroxidase may give rise to false positives. In a number of trials, early detection using FOBT has been shown to lead to a 15–30% reduction in the incidence of colorectal cancer-specific mortality in a number of trials, for example: Minnesota (33% reduction), Nottingham (15% reduction) and Funen (Denmark) (18% reduction). Approximately 10% of patients with a positive test will on investigation be shown to have a colorectal carcinoma.

64   ABE

Both t-tests and ANOVA (analysis of variance) are examples of parametric tests and can be used to assess Gaussian (normally) distributed data. The Wilcoxon and Mann–Whitney tests are non-parametric tests and are used for non-Gaussian data.

65   ABCD

Approximately 95% of gastric cancers are adenocarcinomas, and about 4% are lymphomas and 1% leiomyosarcomas. In most studies outside Japan, less than 5% of gastric cancers are limited to the mucosa and submucosa at the time of diagnosis, and regional lymph node involvement occurs in 60% of cases.

Predisposing factors include: blood group A, smoking, type B gastritis, pernicious anaemia, *Helicobacter pylori*; previous gastric surgery and work in the coal and other mining industries.

Anorexia and weight loss occur in over 95% of cases. Pyloric obstruction occurs mainly with distal lesions. Dysphagia occurs with proximal lesions. About half present with a palpable abdominal mass.

PRACTICE PAPER 1 – EMQ ANSWERS

Skin lesions

66 D S-100-positive on immunohistochemical staining
67 E Palisading basal cells at the periphery of tumour islands
68 B Keratin pearl formation
69 C Intraepidermal (*in situ*) squamous carcinoma
70 A Central keratin plug

Basal-cell carcinoma characteristically has palisading basal cells at the periphery of tumour islands.

Most cutaneous malignant melanomas stain S-100-positive using immunohistochemical techniques.

Squamous-cell carcinoma displays keratin pearl formation.

Bowen's disease is an *in situ* squamous-cell carcinoma. Lesions appear as reddened, scaly, slightly raised plaques. Invasion occurs only after many years, typically 15–20 years.

A keratoacanthoma is a self-limiting, benign cutaneous tumour. A small red swelling grows quickly into a pale dome-shaped mass with a central keratin plug. These lesions regress spontaneously.

Paget's disease of the breast represents intraepithelial spread from an underlying ductal carcinoma.

Local anaesthetic agents

71 B Amethocaine
72 A Bupivacaine
73 D Cocaine

Amethocaine is an ester that rapidly diffuses into the conjunctiva. Cocaine is also an ester but causes sympathetic stimulation, and so is reserved for situations where vasoconstriction is required (e.g. nasal procedures).

All the other local anaesthetics are amides. Bupivacaine binds to the myocardium and has caused a number of deaths when used in Bier's blocks. Thus, it is now contraindicated for use in Bier's blocks. Prilocaine binds poorly to the myocardium and so is the best agent for intravenous regional anaesthesia.

Operative management
74 A   Carry on with surgery regardless
75 A   Carry on with surgery regardless
76 C   Wait 4 weeks
Appendicitis in pregnancy may be difficult to diagnose due to upward displacement of the appendix and masking of guarding by the uterus. The later into the pregnancy, the greater is the mortality risk to the mother and fetus. A patient with acute appendicitis who is on the oral contraceptive pill should have an emergency operation. Neither pregnancy, nor taking the oral contraceptive pill is a contraindication to appendicectomy. The correct procedure for women on the oral contraceptive pill is to carry on with the surgery but take precautionary measures, such as thromboembolic deterrent stockings (TEDS), pneumatic calf compression and administration of heparin or low-molecular-weight heparins.

A patient requiring elective right inguinal hernia repair taking the oral contraceptive pill should have the surgery delayed, as the risk of potential complications (i.e. PE) would outweigh waiting for 1 month and then performing the surgery. During this 1-month delay, the patient should be advised to stop taking the oral contraceptive pill and to use other forms of contraception.

Mediastinal conditions
77 A   Aortic dissection
78 B   Carcinoma of the oesophagus
79 C   Mallory–Weiss tear
Aortic dissection produces tearing chest and back pain together with neurological deficits from spinal cord and cerebral ischaemia.

Oesophageal carcinoma is more common in elderly people and presents in advanced stages with progressive dysphagia.

Achalasia is the failure of the lower oesophageal sphincter to relax, with abnormal oesophageal peristalsis. It does not cause an anaemia unless there is malignant change.

A Mallory–Weiss tear produces a linear mucosal tear in the lower oesophagus close to the gastro-oesophageal junction, which results in haematemesis and later melaena.

Mediastinal masses

80 B Anterior mediastinum
81 D Posterior mediastinum
82 A Superior mediastinum
83 B Anterior mediastinum
84 C Middle mediastinum

The locations of mediastinal masses include:

Superior mediastinum: thyroid masses, lymph node enlargement, oesophageal tumours, aortic aneurysms, parathyroid lesions

Anterior mediastinum: thymic lesions, lymphoma, germ-cell tumours, pleuropericardial cysts, lymph node enlargement

Middle mediastinum: lymph node enlargement, bronchogenic cysts, enterogenic cysts

Posterior mediastinum: neural tumours, thoracic meningocele, oesophageal tumours, aortic aneurysms, paragangliomas

Tumour type

85 E Lymphoma
86 D Sarcoma
87 B Squamous-cell carcinoma
88 A Adenocarcinoma
89 A Adenocarcinoma

Epstein–Barr virus infection may lead to Burkitt's lymphoma, which usually first appears in the jaw, and which shows a 'starry sky' appearance of a few macrophages in a sea of lymphoblasts on histology. Epstein–Barr virus is also responsible for nasopharyngeal carcinoma.

Muscle tumours arise from connective tissue, rather than epithelium. They are therefore sarcomas and not carcinomas. Striated muscle malignant tumours are therefore rhabdomyosarcomas. Malignant tumours arising from smooth muscle are leiomyosarcomas.

The human papillomavirus types 16 and 18 are responsible for CIN, and ultimately carcinoma of the cervix or anus. 95% of these are squamous cell in origin, and 5% are adenocarcinomas.

Barrett's oesophagus arises as glandular dysplasia (from squamous to glandular epithelium), usually as a result of continued acid reflux.

Krukenberg tumours represent the transcoelomic spread of gastric carcinoma to the ovaries.

Death certificates
90   A   Report to the coroner
91   B   Issue a death certificate
Death should be referred to the coroner if:
The cause of death is unknown.
The deceased was not seen by the certifying doctor either after death or within 14 days before death.
The death may be due to an accident.
The death was unnatural, violent or suspicious.
The death may be due to self-neglect or neglect by others (as in scenario 90).
The death may be due to an abortion.
The death may be a suicide.
The death may be occupational/as a result of industrial disease.
The death occurred during/after detention in police custody or prison.
The death is during or within 24 hours of an operation/anaesthetic/invasive procedure
For scenario 91, it is common practice to telephone the coroner to get advice for death following an operation. However, according to the guidelines above, this is not strictly necessary.

Paraneoplastic syndromes
92   E   Thymoma
93   D   Renal carcinoma
94   A   Multiple myeloma
95   B   Pancreatic carcinoma
Myasthenia gravis is seen with some thymic tumours.
Polycythaemia may result from tumours of the kidney or cerebellum due to increased erythropoietin production.
Hypercalcaemia results from bone mobilisation from bony metastases and ectopic parathormone. It is most commonly seen in myeloma, breast and lung cancer.
Pancreatic carcinoma may lead to hyperglycaemia if enough β cells are destroyed – but this is rare.
Gout sometimes accompanies lymphoma.
Thrombophlebitis migrans is especially associated with lung and pancreatic cancer.

Mode of tumour spread
96 D Lymphatic spread
97 A Local invasion
98 D Lymphatic spread
99 B Blood-borne spread
100 C Transcoelomic spread
Seminomas of the testis and papillary thyroid carcinoma spread predominantly by the lymphatic route. Spread of testicular tumours follows their blood supply, and so drains into para-aortic lymph nodes. Remember that inguinal lymph nodes drain local skin, including the scrotum.
Cutaneous basal-cell carcinomas invade local structures and are hence termed 'rodent ulcers'. They rarely, if ever, spread to lymphatics or metastasise.
Follicular thyroid carcinomas spread predominantly by the bloodstream.
Ovarian carcinomas frequently spread transcoelomically.

Multiple endocrine neoplasia (MEN) syndromes
101 C MEN IIB
102 A MEN I
103 C MEN IIB
104 A MEN I
The multiple endocrine neoplasia syndromes are inherited in an autosomal dominant manner or they may occur as new mutations. MEN I consists of pituitary, pancreatic islet cell and parathyroid adenomas or hyperplasia. Patients with MEN IIA and IIB develop phaeochromocytomas and medullary thyroid carcinomas. In addition, those with MEN IIA develop parathyroid hyperplasia, but are phenotypically normal; however, those with MEN IIB tend to be Marfanoid and develop submucosal neuromas.

Arterial blood gas analysis/acid–base balance
105 A Metabolic acidosis
106 B Respiratory acidosis
107 C Metabolic alkalosis
The pH is low in scenario 105, representing a picture of acidosis. As the PCO_2 is reduced, this indicates that the cause is not respiratory. The bicarbonate is low, suggesting a metabolic acidosis.

In the second scenario, the pH is low, representing a picture of acidosis. The PCO_2 is raised, indicating a respiratory origin. The bicarbonate is normal so there has been no renal compensation. This picture may be seen in narcosis due to excess administration of opiates.

The pH in the last case is high, so representing an alkalosis. The bicarbonate level too is very high, so indicating a metabolic origin. The PCO_2 is slightly high due to respiratory compensation. An example of this is seen in gastric outflow obstruction.

Heart murmurs
108 B Continuous systolic murmur
109 E Split second heart sound
110 C Early diastolic murmur
A ventricular septal defect will produce a continuous systolic murmur – pansystolic murmur, whereas an atrial septal defect will produce a wide and fixed splitting of the second heart sound.

A patient with aortic regurgitation has an early diastolic murmur.

Pelvic fracture
111 B Rotationally unstable, vertically stable pelvic fracture
112 B Rotationally unstable, vertically stable pelvic fracture
113 C Rotationally unstable, vertically unstable pelvic fracture
114 A Rotationally and vertically stable
115 A Rotationally and vertically stable
Stable pelvic fractures include fractures not displacing the pelvic ring (such as avulsion fractures and isolated fractures of the iliac wing or pubic ramus) or minimally displaced fractures of the pelvic ring.

Rotationally unstable, vertically stable pelvic fractures include open-book fractures (pubic diastasis >2.5 cm) and lateral compression fractures.

Rotationally and vertically unstable pelvic fractures usually result from vertical shear injuries.

Chest injury
116 B   Pericardial injury
117 C   Pneumothorax
Scenario 115 is likely to be due to cardiac tamponade. Signs indicating this include a weak pulse, raised JVP, hypotension, tachycardia. The only other condition that may cause similar signs is a tension pneumothorax. However, he has a normal chest film which makes this unlikely.
The patient in Scenario 116 is likely to have a pneumothorax as he has absent breath sounds, dyspnoeic and is drowsy due to hypoxia.

Anatomy of the brachial plexus
118 D   Middle trunk
119 H   Anterior divisions
120 A   C7 root
121 E   C6 root
122 D   Middle trunk
123 H   Anterior divisions
124 A   C7 root
125 E   C6 root
The middle trunk is a direct continuation of the C7 root; there is no other contribution to the middle trunk.
Anterior divisions innervate the flexor compartment of the limbs.
The inferior cervical sympathetic ganglion sends postganglionic fibres to the C7 and C8 roots – other sympathetic contributions to the plexus are from the T1 ganglion to the T1 root, and the middle cervical ganglion to the C5 and C6 roots (the superior ganglion contributes grey rami to the upper 4 cervical nerves).
The long thoracic nerve arises from the C5, C6 and C7 roots.
The median nerve is formed from the medial and lateral heads of the medial and lateral cords, respectively. Only the upper trunk of the plexus possesses a branch, the suprascapular nerve.
The posterior cord is formed entirely by posterior divisions.
The medial cord is a continuation of the anterior division of the medial trunk; there is no other contribution to the medial cord.

PRACTICE PAPER 2 – MCQ ANSWERS

1   ABC
In the design of a new theatre suite, the operating theatres should be sited on the same level and adjacent to the intensive-care unit and surgical wards. A separate trauma theatre should be instituted as well as a septic theatre for infected cases. Ideally, a separate daytime emergency list should be instituted.

2   BCD
Suxamethonium is a very rapid-acting muscle relaxant and is ideal if crash intubation is required. Suxamethonium acts by mimicking acetylcholine at the neuromuscular junction but undergoes hydrolysis much more slowly than acetylcholine. Depolarisation is therefore prolonged, which results in neuromuscular blockade. Guanethidine is an adrenergic neuroblocker preventing the release of noradrenaline (norepinephrine) from the postganglionic adrenergic neurones. It is rarely used clinically, only for resistant hypertension. Pentazocine, like fentanyl, is an opioid analgesic. Bupivacaine is a long-acting amide local anaesthetic, commonly used for epidural and spinal anaesthesia. Local anaesthetics depress conduction in small unmyelinated fibres first and larger myelinated fibres last. It can also affect autonomic nerve fibres. Hexamethonium is an agent that causes a depolarising block on the postganglionic cell body. Although it was used for the control of blood pressure several years ago, it is now no longer in use.

3   AD
Hepatitis A is an RNA virus and hepatitis B a DNA virus. The incubation period of hepatitis A is between 2 and 3 weeks. Hepatitis A accounts for 20–40% of all cases of viral hepatitis. It affects children and young adults particularly. It rarely causes fulminant hepatitis and does not give rise to a carrier state.

4   ABE
Numerous organisms produce infection and abdominal pain in HIV-infected individuals. The well-documented organisms include: cryptosporidia; cytomegaloviruses; *Mycobacterium tuberculosis*; *Salmonella, Shigella* and *Campylobacter* spp.; *Neisseria gonorrhoea*; *Treponema pallidum*; *Mycobacterium avium-intracellulare*; *Listeria monocytogenes*; *Entamoeba histolytica*; *Giardia lamblia*; *Isospora belli*; *Candida albicans*; *Histoplasma* spp.; and herpes simplex virus. Kaposi's sarcoma is a vascular tumour.

351

5 ACD

Epidural blockade involves entering the epidural space with a needle, introducing a catheter and then infusing local anaesthetic. The dura may be inadvertently punctured by the needle or catheter, resulting in headache. The local anaesthetic prevents transmission in the sensory, motor and autonomic sympathetic nerve fibres. A sympathetic blockade would cause hypotension and bradycardia, a motor blockade would cause hypoventilation and urinary retention.

6 AE

A 50-year-old diabetic is at risk of cardiac disease and so U&E, FBC, CXR and ECG are all justified. The best assessment of diabetic control is glycosylated haemoglobin (Hb A_{1c}). His blood glucose may be controlled perioperatively by the Alberti regimen, which comprises a simultaneous infusion of 5% dextrose containing potassium chloride and intravenous insulin. The resulting blood sugar may be measured accurately by bedside tests, but the laboratory is required for measurement of the serum potassium concentration.

7 BC

Diathermy uses the heating effect of an electrical current. The smaller the area the current travels through, the higher the current density and the greater the heating effect. A high-frequency current is used as this causes fewer problems, e.g. unpleasant sensations, muscle contraction and ventricular fibrillation. However, high-frequency electricity can spark across gaps and a patient may receive an exit burn even though he is not touching an earth. Class 3 equipment is incapable of producing a burn. Although diathermy can be used in a patient with a pacemaker, the pad of a monopolar diathermy should be positioned well away from the pacemaker. Bipolar diathermy does not interfere with pacemakers and may be more suitable.

8 ACF

Strep. pyogenes is β-haemolytic and belongs to Lancefield group A. Staphylococci are found in clusters, streptococci are found in pairs or chains. *Streptococcus* spp. produces streptolysins O and S, hyaluronidase, streptokinase, leucocidin and an erythrogenic toxin that causes scarlet fever. It is associated with rheumatic fever, carditis and glomerulonephritis as immunological sequelae. It is sensitive to penicillins.

9   CDE

The predominant commensal bacteria of the skin is *Staphylococcus epidermidis*. Others include *Staphylococcus aureus*, micrococci, coryneforms and anaerobic cocci. The lower respiratory tract is usually sterile. The predominant bacterial flora of the oropharynx are *Streptococcus viridans*, coryneforms and *Neisseria* spp. Many anaerobic bacteria colonise the colon, especially *Bacteroides fragilis*. The other main groups of commensal skin bacteria include members of the genus *Clostridia*. Aerobic bacteria such as *Escherichia coli* and *Enterococcus* spp. are also present in large numbers. Lactobacilli are the predominant species in the vagina. Others include *Gardnerella vaginalis* and anaerobes.

10   BCD

From the results of prospective randomised controlled trials, antibiotic prophylaxis in surgery has been established to be of proven benefit. Infection is only prevented when antibiotics are given just prior to or at the time of surgery. With the exception of prolonged operations, single-dose prophylaxis is effective in most clinical situations. A further dose is given if the operation lasts longer than 4 hours. Full doses of the correct antibiotics should be given (ones with proven efficacy to prevent wound infection).

11   ADE

Phagocytosis is the process whereby cells – such as neutrophils and macrophages – ingest solid particles (involving adhesion of the target to the cell surface) facilitated by opsonisation. These cells fuse to form a phagosome, which further fuses with lysosomes leading to the formation of a phagolysosome. It is within these that intracellular killing of microorganisms occurs. The neutrophils produce microbicidal agents which act dependently or independently of oxygen. Oxygen-dependent mechanisms include hydrogen peroxide, peroxide anions and hydoxyl radicals. Oxygen-independent mechanisms involve lysozyme and lactoferrin. Elastase and collagenase are two enzymes released from lysosomes and cause damage to local tissues. They also activate factor XII and attract further leucocytes. They may classified as oxygen-dependent or oxygen-independent mechanisms. In the former, neutrophils produce hydrogen peroxide, peroxide anions, hydroxyl radicals and singlet oxygen. The latter mechanism involves lysozyme (muramidase), lactoferrin which chelates iron is required for bacterial growth, cationic protein formation and low pH inside phagocytic vacuoles. Release of lysosomal products from the cell damages local tissue by proteolysis by enzymes such as elastase and collagenase, activates coagulation factor XII, and attracts other leukocytes into the area. Some of the compounds released increase vascular permeability, while others are pyrogens, producing systemic fever by acting on the hypothalamus.

12   ACE

Morphine is the most effective analgesic for pain due to malignant disease. Morphine is more effective than pethidine as it has a relatively longer half-life, and is available in long-acting preparations. Opiate formulations such as fentanyl can be given as patches for transdermal drug delivery. It has been shown in many studies that psychological addiction to opiate does not occur, therefore morphine must not be withheld. An epidural is not appropriate for a patient in the terminal stages of life.

13   AE

Pyrexia in the first 24 hours after surgery is usually due to atelectasis (collapse of the small airways). Pneumonia occurs most frequently 5 days postoperatively. DVT is classically found at postoperative day 10. Wound infections classically occur at day 5 postoperatively. Urinary tract infections may occur at any stage postoperatively Thrombophlebitis is not a common complication of surgery but it may give rise to DVT. Urinary tract infections may occur at any stage postoperatively.

14   ABCE

There is an extremely high incidence of DVT after lower limb surgery and pelvic and lower limb fractures. They frequently occur following orthopaedic procedures such as hip and knee replacement. There are a number of risk factors for DVT, including increasing age; obesity; immobility; malignancy; trauma; pregnancy; past history of DVT/PE; oral contraceptive pill/hormone-replacement therapy; dehydration; and thrombophilia (factor V Leiden, protein C deficiency, protein S deficiency). DVT can be accurately diagnosed by duplex Doppler ultrasound, especially proximal to the popliteal vein. DVT may be prevented by the use of subcutaneous heparin, LMWH, thromboembolic deterrent stockings (TEDS) and pneumatic calf compression.

15   ABDE

α-Adrenoreceptor blockers are used for the treatment of hypertension and benign prostatic hypertrophy. Common side-effects include urinary frequency and incontinence. Haemorrhoidectomy can cause urinary retention as a result of pain. Bladder tumours can give rise to acute urine retention due to obstruction. Constipation, immobility, pain and stress can also cause urinary retention.

16 **ABCE**

Wound healing by secondary intention occurs when the wound edges are not brought together. This could be due to tissue loss or wound dehiscence caused by a wound infection. The surgeon may have chosen to allow the wound to heal by secondary intention, particularly in cases of dirty or contaminated wounds. The process of wound healing by secondary intention is much slower than primary intention, because the base of the wound has to fill with granulation tissue and epithelialisation needs to occur from the wound edges.

17 **AB**

At normal systemic blood pressure the renal vascular resistance adjusts the pressure in the renal arterioles so that renal blood flow remains fairly constant (autoregulation). In hypertensive patients there is a shift of autoregulation, so that they have a slightly reduced renal blood flow for a given blood pressure. Blood flow in the cortex is much higher than in the medulla. Autoregulation is impaired in shock, sepsis and low cardiac output states.

18 **BD**

Monofilament sutures generally cause less infection than braided sutures. Closure of the peritoneal layer is unnecessary. Closure of the abdomen may be performed using absorbable or non-absorbable suture material. The key element is to use a strong suture material such as nylon or PDS. Jenkins' rule is used to minimise abdominal wound dehiscence and states that 1-cm bites should be taken 1 cm apart and the suture should be four times the length of the wound.

19 **BDE**

Intravascular haemolysis may result from the mechanical destruction of red cells by prosthetic heart valves or arterial grafts, in arteriovenous malformations or after severe physical exercise. Immune-mediated intravascular haemolysis is only usually encountered in the potent antibody–antigen interactions seen following ABO-mismatched transfusion. Most autoimmune haemolytic anaemias produce red cell destruction in the reticuloendothelial system. Disseminated intravascular coagulation may cause microangiopathic haemolysis with red cell destruction in the microcirculation.

20   All false

Most haematologists now recommend that preoperative platelet transfusion should only be administered if the count is: $<100 \times 10^9/l$ for neurological and ophthalmic surgery; $<80 \times 10^9/l$ for most other surgical procedures, lumbar puncture or liver biopsy; and $<50 \times 10^9/l$ for minor procedures such as central venous catheterisation. These guidelines should be relaxed if there is an additional haemostatic defect or in the event of bleeding. Patients not requiring imminent surgery do not require platelet transfusion unless the count is $<10 \times 10^9/l$ as spontaneous bleeding is unlikely. Transfused platelets have a short half-life *in vivo*. They should be given as close to surgery as practicable, and given as often as indicated by the clinical state. Patients with immune thrombocytopenia will have a very poor response to transfused platelets, and therefore attempts to increase the platelet count before splenectomy should be performed with corticosteroids or intravenous immunoglobulin before resorting to platelet transfusion.

21   BCDE

Compartment syndrome is associated with closed fractures, particularly of the femur, elbow, forearm and proximal third of the tibia. It can also result from reperfusion of ischaemic tissue, tight casts and bandages, severe crush injuries or burns. It may present with one or more of pain, pallor, paraesthesia, paralysis and pulselessness. Paraesthesia (particularly loss of vibration sense and two-point discrimination) occurs relatively early. Pulses are palpable until very late in compartment syndrome when the osteofacial compartment pressure exceeds the arterial pressure. Compartment syndrome can lead to myoglobinuria, which can result in renal failure. Abdominal compartment syndrome can result in cardiopulmonary arrest, mainly due to reduced venous return to the heart from IVC compression.

22   ABCE

If oxygen delivery to the brain is reduced, agitation and coma can occur. Blood pressure may still be normal in compensated shock. Reduced renal perfusion and compensatory mechanisms to preserve vascular volume will reduce and urine output will fall. In a hypovolaemic state, peripheral vascular resistance is decreased to preserve flow to vital organs. The normal response to hypovolaemic shock is tachycardia; however, with progression, bradycardia and even cardiac arrest may occur.

23   BE
Central venous access should only be considered once peripheral access has been established. Peripheral access with two large-bore cannulas (14-gauge) in the antecubital fossae is recommended. Poseuille's law states that flow is proportional to the fourth power of the radius and inversely proportional to the length of the cannula. In ATLS, vascular access should follow Airway with cervical spine control and Breathing maintenance. Intraosseus infusions may be used in children under 6 years of age.

24   BCDE
Traumatic diaphragmatic rupture is easily missed unless a high index of suspicion is maintained. Evidence of irregularity or obliteration of the diaphragm, air-containing bowel or a nasogastric tube above the diaphragm should strongly suggest the diagnosis. More subtle associations include air-filled bowel, omentum and abdominal or retroperitoneal organs in the chest mimicking the appearance of a loculated pneumothorax, contralateral mediastinal shift, pleural effusion, lower rib fractures, pulmonary contusion and widening of the mediastinum or cardiac shadow caused by peritoneal contents herniating into the pericardial sac. The diagnosis is often delayed and, on occasion (particularly in small, right-sided lesions), may not be made for a considerable period after the injury.

25   All true
Children have a smaller mass, hence the force is transmitted over a relatively smaller area compared with adults. Children's bodies have less fat than adults, with their organs being located closer to the surface. Their skeletons are relatively uncalcified and hence more pliable, therefore the absence of fractures does not rule out underlying organ damage. Rib fractures, if present, are indicative of a large transference of energy, thus a high index of suspicion for the presence of an internal injury must be maintained. As there is a large surface area to mass ratio, hypothermia occurs quicker in children than in adults.

26   All true
Paediatric responses to hypovolaemia include:
Cardiovascular: a weak pulse, tachycardia (progressing to bradycardia), hypotension
CNS: lethargy, confusion, a dulled response to pain and coma
Renal: decreasing urine output, increased specific gravity
Peripheral: cool, pale, clammy, with reduced capillary refill.

27   CD

CXR is useful in about 50% of cases. Suspicious findings include an enlarged cardiac shadow, pneumopericardium and widening of the upper mediastinum. It is worth noting that the CXR has poor sensitivity and specificity for pericardial effusions. CT scanning of the heart is not usually performed because of long scanning times. Echocardiograms are the investigation of choice, being fast, reliable and non-invasive. ECGs can be helpful in about 30% of cases.

28   BDE

A compound fracture is one in which the soft tissue envelope of the limb has been breached so allowing the bone to communicate with the exterior. Within 6 hours of injury the wound may become colonised with bacteria. Internal fixation is not a contraindication for bone stabilisation. Internal fixation is thought to facilitate nursing care and allow access for potential plastic surgical flaps. Primary wound closure is rarely ever indicated.

29   ABE

In an 'open' or 'sucking' pneumothorax air passes preferentially through the chest wall with each respiratory effort along the path of least resistance, reducing alveolar ventilation and resulting in tissue hypoxia. Acute treatment is by creation of a flap-valve dressing occludes the defect during inspiration but allows expulsion of intrapleural air during exhalation. A chest drain can later be placed at a site away from the chest wall defect. Defects themselves usually require definitive surgical closure.

30   AE

A minimum of two large-gauge cannulas (14-gauge) in the antecubital fossae should be established during the early assessment of severely traumatised patients. ATLS recommends that initial fluid replacement should be with a balanced crystalloid solution such as Ringer's lactate. Normal saline can result in a hyperchloraemic metabolic acidosis owing to its high chloride content (the kidneys will excrete bicarbonate in exchange for its chloride). Acute haemorrhage results in movement of interstitial fluid into the intravascular space. Intracellular fluid will then fill this interstitial volume but this deficit must be corrected. Crystalloids are ideal fluids for initial resuscitation as they provide volume to fill this deficit. Hypovolaemic shock is treated with intravenous volume replacement. Vasopressive agents have no role in the initial stage.

31   ABDE

Signs of significant injury in penetrating neck trauma include a pulsatile or expanding haematoma, dysphonia, dysphagia and haemoptysis. Others include shock, external haemorrhage, reduced carotid pulsation, odynophagia, stridor, hoarseness, haemoptysis, haematemesis, subcutaneous emphysema, lateralised neurological deficit and aphasia.

32   ACDE

The common peroneal nerve supplies the lateral and anterior muscular compartments of the calf as well as the skin over the anterior aspects of the calf and foot. With foot drop, the patient trips on walking as the toes catch the ground. Cutaneous innervation of the sole of the foot is through the medial and lateral plantar branches of the tibial nerve. Inversion is weakened because of paralysis of the tibialis anterior muscle. Muscle wasting is a sign of lower motor neurone damage. The peroneus longus tendon is one of the supports of the lateral arch; when paralysed the arch is compromised.

33   ACE

At higher doses of adrenaline (epinephrine), α-mediated vasoconstriction reduces renal blood flow and can cause oliguria and precipitate acute renal failure. Noradrenaline (norepinephrine) is predominantly an α-agonist. Dopexamine is a potent splanchnic vasodilator, reducing afterload and improving blood flow to vital organs including the kidneys. Dobutamine reduces systemic vascular resistance, decreasing afterload and ventricular filling pressures, and is of use in cardiogenic shock and cardiac failure.

34   ABD

The thoracic sympathetic chain lies on the heads of the ribs, anterior to the posterior intercostal vessels, immediately under cover of the pleura, with the splanchnic nerves passing from the chain medially and anteriorly over the vertebral bodies. The thoracic sympathetic chain receives white rami from all intercostal nerves, and passes into the abdomen under the medial arcuate ligament of the diaphragm.

35   BDEFGH

Haemorrhage and septicaemia cause a low CVP and blood pressure. A high CVP is caused by any factor than impedes venous return to the heart or reduces the output from the right ventricle. This in turn leads to low cardiac output and thus low blood pressure.

36   BCD

The oxygen–haemoglobin dissociation curve is sigmoid-shaped, and a right shift is associated with a decreased affinity for oxygen. The curve shifts to the right with an increase in PCO_2, temperature, 2,3-DPG and an increase in hydrogen-ion concentration (decreased pH).

The curve shifts to the left with decreased PCO_2, temperature, 2,3-DPG and reduced hydrogen-ion concentration (increased pH).

37   AB

Cardiac surgery is performed with controlled hypotension together with hypothermia. The hypothermia is used to decrease cellular metabolism and reduce energy requirements of the tissues. However, surgery can be performed on a beating heart and at normothermic temperatures. Cardiac tamponade is a well-known complication of cardiac surgery; it usually presents in the early postoperative period with deteriorating cardiac function and cardiac arrest. Valvular surgery may be performed through a thoracotomy incision. Although bypass grafts can produce symptomatic relief of angina, vein grafts will occlude after a median time of 7–10 years.

38   ABC

Pulmonary artery occlusion pressure (PAOP) can be used to exclude oedema of cardiac origin. It may be useful in cardiogenic shock to allow more accurate fluid management. PAOP may be of use in abdominal aortic aneurysm surgery. The pulmonary artery wedge pressure is elevated in cardiogenic shock. Pulmonary artery wedge pressures are not routinely measured following a myocardial infarction.

39   ADE

The jugular venous pulsation has a double waveform. The 'a' wave corresponds to atrial contraction and ends synchronously with carotid artery pulse. The 'c' wave occurs when the ventricles begin to contract and is caused by bulging of the AV valves backward towards the atria. The 'v' wave is seen when the tricuspid valve is closed just prior to ventricular contraction – with and just after the carotid pulse. The 'v' wave represents the gradual build-up of blood in the atria while the AV valves are closed during ventricular contraction. The absence of 'a' waves is a feature of atrial fibrillation.

40   BDE

Hyperphosphataemia and hypocalcaemia may be seen in chronic renal failure. Stress ulceration is associated with ARF and may be prevented by sucralfate (cytoprotection and pepsin adsorption). Renal hypoperfusion is associated with avid sodium retention with minimal excretion into the urine (<20 mmol/l). Indications for renal biopsy include: unclear pathogenesis; suspicion of glomerular disease or interstitial nephritis; or prolonged (4–6 weeks) renal failure.

41   ACDE

The catabolic phase of the metabolic response to injury is accompanied by increased energy expenditure and a negative nitrogen balance. The size and duration of the response are directly related to the severity of the trauma or surgical insult.

42   C

The clinical diagnosis of ARDS is usually provided by a history of a catastrophic pulmonary event (e.g. aspiration or pulmonary sepsis), respiratory failure (exclusion of cardiogenic pulmonary oedema or chronic lung disease as the cause of respiratory failure) and diffuse pulmonary infiltrates on X-ray. Lung biopsy is not required. In ARDS, the lung is stiffer and therefore pulmonary compliance is reduced. The overall mortality is approximately 50%. Prognosis depends on the age of the patient, the presence of other organ complications and the severity of the lung injury.

43   ABE

The left coronary artery arises from the left posterior aortic sinus behind the pulmonary trunk. After a short course it divides into two main arteries: the circumflex and the left anterior descending (anterior interventricular artery). Typically, the left coronary artery supplies the left atrium, part of the right ventricle, most of the left ventricle, most of the interventricular septum and the sinoatrial node in 40% of cases.

44   ADE

The scalenus anterior inserts on the scalene tubercule. A groove is found on the 1st rib anterior to the scalene tubercule for the subclavian vein. The subclavian artery runs behind the scalenus anterior muscle. The 1st rib is related to the lower two roots of the brachial plexus C8 and T1. The cervicothoracic ganglion, otherwise known as the stellate ganglion, lies in front of the neck of the first rib.

45   A

The oesophagus is formed at the lower border of the cricoid cartilage. It is crossed anteriorly by the left main bronchus, lies behind the left atrium and passes through the muscular part of the diaphragm to the left of the central tendon through the muscular sling of the left crus. It is innervated, in part, by the recurrent laryngeal nerve, not the phrenic nerve.

46   DE

The clavipectoral fascia is pierced by the cephalic vein and lateral pectoral nerve, overlain by the C4 dermatome (acromial branches of the supraclavicular nerves), and the infraclavicular lymph nodes. The fascia splits to enclose the pectoralis minor and subclavius muscles, and continues beyond as the suspensory ligament of the axilla.

47   ACDE

The left brachiocephalic vein drains blood from: the cervical vertebrae via both vertebral veins; the thyroid gland by the inferior thyroid veins; the first left intercostal space via the left superior intercostal veins; and all anterior intercostal spaces by the anterior intercostal veins draining into the internal thoracic veins. The thoracic duct enters the vein at its commencement behind the left sternoclavicular joint. The bronchial veins drain into the azygos/hemiazygos systems.

48   ABDE

Factors predicting poor outcome in malignant melanoma include advanced stage at presentation, Breslow thickness, increasing age, male sex, presence of ulceration and anatomical location. In stage I and II disease, a positive sentinel node is a useful predictor of outcome. In stage III disease the number of positive regional (or in-transit) nodes is associated with a worse prognosis. In stage IV disease poor performance status, elevated serum LDH and the extent of metastases are predictive of poor outcome. The presence or absence of abnormal melanocytes adjacent to the tumour is not a reliable prognostic indicator.

49   ADE

A meningioma is a benign tumour of the meninges. A rhabdomyoma is a benign tumour of striated muscle (its malignant counterpart is termed a rhabdomyosarcoma). A chondrosarcoma is a malignant tumour of cartilage.

50   D

Metastasis is the spread of a tumour from one part of the body to another that is not directly interconnected. A variety of factors play a role: loss of cellular cohesion and cytoarchitecture, initiation of angiogenesis and adhesion molecules. Transluminal metastases are uncommon. Basal-cell carcinomas invade locally and metastases are rare. Osteosarcoma typically spreads via the bloodstream, most commonly to the lungs. It can also spread to other bones. The extensive venous plexus surrounding the prostate makes haematogenous spread likely. Lymphatic drainage nodes generally follow the path of arteries.

51   BCE

Fat necrosis is more common in obese and postmenopausal women. In at least half of cases there is no history of trauma. Benign calcification resembling carcinoma may be seen on mammography. Branching micro-calcification is a feature of malignancy.

52   ABEFG

Hypercalcaemia may be part of a paraneoplastic syndrome of numerous malignancies including carcinoma of the bronchus. Bone lysis occurs in multiple myeloma, giving rise to hypercalcaemia. Hypoparathyroidism reduces serum calcium, whereas hyperparathyroidism does the converse (as does hyperthyroidism). Renal failure can lead to secondary hyperparathyroidism, so raising serum calcium levels. Citrate used in the storage of blood binds ionised calcium and so reduces the serum level.

53   AD

In its classic form, osteosarcoma is a highly malignant tumour arising within the bone and spreads outwards to the periosteum and surrounding soft tissues. It is most common in the second decade of life. It may affect any bone, but most commonly involves the long bone metaphyses, especially around the knee and at the proximal end of the humerus. Frequently, the tumour extends beyond the cortex, elevating the periosteum, forming a 'Codman's triangle'. Formation of sunray spicules (tumour perpendicular to the bony margin) may also be present. Osteosarcoma may be a complication of osteogenesis imperfecta, Maffucci's syndrome (enchondromas, cutaneous haemangiomas and skin pigmentation) and multiple enchondroma. Osteochondroma is not known to lead to osteosarcoma.

54 BCDE

The commonest cause of nipple discharge is lactation. Microdochectomy is the treatment of choice for persistent troublesome discharge if only one duct is involved. Duct ectasia causes a thick green discharge. Bloodstaining occurs in intraductal papilloma. Clear serous fluid discharge may occur in fibroadenosis and in women on the contraceptive pill.

55 BDE

Postmenopausal hormone replacement therapy is thought to increase the risk of DVT, PE, MI, CVA, breast and endometrial carcinoma. HRT is thought to be protective against osteoporosis, colorectal and ovarian carcinoma. Unopposed oestrogen replacement therapy should not be given if a woman still retains her uterus, as the risk of endometrial cancer is high.

56 EG

Testicular tumour incidence peaks between the ages of 20 and 30 years for non-seminomas, and between 30 and 40 years for seminomas. Testicular tumours primarily metastasise to para-aortic nodes. Testicular tumours are more commonly seen in patients with maldescended testes (relative risk around 3.5). Where the maldescent is unilateral, both testes are at increased risk of malignancy. Testicular tumours should be removed via a transinguinal approach, as a trans-scrotal approach would cause tumour seeding. In view of the para-aortic nodal spread of testicular tumours, CT of the abdomen and thorax is advocated. The tumour markers used to monitor progression of the disease include α-fetoprotein and β-hCG (particularly in non-seminomas) and LDH (particularly in seminomas).

57 ABDE

Squamous-cell carcinomas are the second most common cutaneous malignancy. They are otherwise known as epidermoid carcinomas or epitheliomas. Sun damage is a major risk factor, resulting in carcinoma *in situ*, followed by an invasive carcinoma.

A Merkel-cell carcinoma (otherwise known as trabecular carcinoma) is a rare but highly aggressive tumour derived from the Merkel-cell population, which are primitive neuroendocrine (APUD) cells in the skin. These tumours occur mostly in elderly people. They tend to occur on sun-exposed sites, particularly the head, neck and limbs. The prognosis is poor, with local recurrence developing in 40% of cases and nodal metastases in up to 65%. Approximately half the patients are dead within 2 years.

A dermatofibroma is a red or brown small papule or nodule containing fibroblastic tissue, usually found on the legs and with no known aetiology or malignant potential.

Bowen's disease is a skin disorder that may develop into squamous-cell carcinoma; histologically it is an intraepidermal carcinoma. It predominantly occurs on the legs. Bowen's disease of the glans of the penis is called erythroplasia of Queyrat.

A solar (actinic) keratosis is a potentially precancerous condition, frequently seen on the head and face, typically in sun-exposed older people. Treatment can be by excision, cryotherapy or the use of 5-FU cream.

58   ABE

Bronchial carcinoma is the most common malignant tumour in the western world, and now the third most common cause of death in the UK, behind heart disease and pneumonia. It carries the highest mortality of all malignancies in the UK and the USA. In the UK approximately 35,000 people die each year from bronchial carcinoma, with a male to female ratio of 3.5:1.

Bronchial carcinoma may be divided into small-cell (SCLC) and non-small-cell lung carcinoma (NSCLC). NSCLCs include squamous, large-cell, adenocarcinoma and alveolar cell carcinoma. In the preoperative assessment, radionuclide, CT scanning and mediastinoscopy will assess the spread of tumour.

Absence of any mediastinal spread favours curative resection. At present, mediastinal lymphadenopathy precludes resection, although hilar lymphadenopathy does not. Surgery is the only treatment of value for NSCLC. Only 20% of all cases are suitable for resection. If the patient can tolerate the procedure then NSCLC tumours are resected, providing they are no more advanced than stage IIB (i.e. $T_2N_1M_0$ or $T_3N_0M_0$). Some surgeons may opt to operate on more advanced cases but only if complete resection is deemed probable. A lung tumour causing a malignant pleural effusion is classified as T_4, and is thus considered inoperable.

Following surgery for NSCLC, radiotherapy and chemotherapy are often used to prevent relapse. SCLC tends to present at an advanced stage and is usually irresectable. It is therefore usually treated with chemotherapy and radiotherapy.

Around 80% of lung cancer cases in the UK have been attributed to smoking. Smoking carries a greater relative risk for small- and squamous-cell lung cancers (not adenocarcinoma).

59   CE
Although typically consultant-led, clinical audit in surgical practice can be led by any interested appointed party (e.g. medical or nursing staff, or administrator) with access to the required data. Unlike a trial where one patient may receive a different treatment to another, audit does not typically require patient consent. Audit offers the ability to alter clinical practice if findings suggest improvements can be made (completing the audit cycle). Detailed clinical information is not always required if only a particular aspect of outcome or care is being assessed.

60   BDE
FAP is an autosomal dominant disorder. Affected individuals (normally early teens) have multiple large-bowel polyps with a virtually inevitable tendency to malignant transformation over the next 20 years. There is an associated long-arm deletion at q21–q22 of chromosome 5. About a third of cases are sporadic, arising as new mutations without a positive family history.

61   DE
The p value is a probability with a value ranging from zero to one. The threshold p value for significance is traditionally set at 0.05. If two means are compared, the null hypothesis is that the two populations have the same means. A p value of 0.001 is more significant than a p value of 0.01. The smaller the p value, the more significant the result: in other words, the more likely that the differences found did not occur solely due to chance.

62   ABD
Curling's ulcers are associated with burns patients and are thought to be due to increased stress following injury. ARDS is a well-recognised, but uncommon, complication of burns. The clinical indicators of inhalation injury include facial burns, singeing of the eyebrows, carbon deposits and inflammation in the oropharynx, history of impaired mentation or history of explosion. Full-thickness burns characteristically have a waxy-white or leathery appearance. Partial-thickness burns have a red/mottled appearance and a blistered and broken epidermis which is very painful and tender.

63   CD

The total volume of cerebrospinal fluid (CSF) is approximately 150 ml. The rate of CSF production is about 550 ml per day. The composition of CSF is essentially the same as that of brain extracellular fluid. The pH of CSF is 7.33, whereas that of plasma is 7.4 due to the higher PCO_2 in CSF than in plasma. The protein, glucose, lactic acid, cholesterol, potassium and calcium concentrations of CSF are all lower than in plasma. However, CSF does contain more glucose than nasal mucus, thus a positive glucose dipstix test of clear nasal discharge indicates a CSF leak. The lumbar CSF pressure is normally 7–18 cmH$_2$O.

64   ABDE

Complications of TPN can be divided into those at the time of central line insertion, metabolic/electrolyte disturbances and fatty liver. Others include hyperlipidaemia or hypertriglyceridaemia. The calorific delivery of TPN is insufficient to produce obesity, particularly in the highly catabolic states requiring its use, e.g. sepsis.

65   BD

Studies have shown a reduction in mortality and local recurrence with preoperative radiotherapy. Cancer of the rectum can be treated by an anterior resection or abdominoperineal resection if low. A distal clearance margin of 2 cm is adequate. The precise indications and time course for preoperative radiotherapy are unknown and are a subject for further trials and investigation. One popular course of management is for patients to undergo a course of radiotherapy for middle or lower third tumours, or fixed tumours. Mobile or upper third rectal tumours need no preoperative radiotherapy. Total mesorectal excision or total anatomical dissection, which serves to remove the fascial envelope containing the lymphatic tissue surrounding the rectum, has been shown to reduce local recurrence. Total mesorectal excision should be used for middle and lower third rectal cancers.

PRACTICE PAPER 2 – EMQ ANSWERS

Microorganisms
66 B *Streptococcus pneumoniae*
67 G **None of the above**
68 C *Clostridium difficile*

Ludwig's angina is bilateral infection of the submandibular, sublingual and submental spaces – usually arising from dental sepsis. Streptococcal infection spreads in deep cervical and pharyngeal fascial planes. It may cause airway obstruction.

Vincent's angina is due to the symbiotic action of fusiform bacteria and the spirochaete *Borrelia vincentii*. It is a pharyngeal infection with ulcerative gingivitis.

Following broad-spectrum antibiotic therapy, infection with *Clostridium difficile* may lead to pseudomembranous colitis

Hepatitis B
69 C **Positive HBeAg in serum**
70 A **Raised titre of anti-HBs antibody**
71 A **Raised titre of anti-HBs antibody**
72 D **HBsAg**

The hepatitis B virus consists of an outer surface coat (HBsAg), and an inner core particle (HbcAg and HbeAg). Inside the core particle is the HBV DNA, and DNA polymerase. The whole virus is called the Dane particle. In acute infection, HBsAg is found in the blood and usually disappears after 3 months, at which point anti-HBsAg appears indicating immunity. HBeAg will also be seen early, and also disappears by 3 months, after which anti-HbeAg antibodies will be seen. In the 10% of patients who do not recover from the acute hepatitis infection, there is progression to chronic infection and the HBeAg and HBsAg will continue to be seen in the blood. This indicates continuing infection with the virus. If anti-HBe antibodies are present, the patient has seroconverted and his/her infectivity is lower. HBeAg represents replication of the virus and high infectivity. HBsAg represents a carrier status, if present for more than 6 months from onset of infection.

Sterilisation techniques
73 B   Hot air
74 C   2% glutaraldehyde

Sterilisation by steam is only effective if trapped air is removed. Air-tight containers are best sterilised by dry heat. This method can also be used to sterilise non-aqueous liquids. Delicate fibre-optic instruments are easily immersed in glutaraldehyde. Note that **most** bacteria are killed in less that 10 minutes (disinfection), but that at least 3 hours of exposure is needed to kill **all** microbes (sterilisation).

Anatomy of the heart
75 I   Sulcus terminalis
76 A   Right coronary artery
77 J   Left atrial appendage
78 B   Coronary sinus

The sinoatrial node lies over the sulcus terminalis of the right atrium.
The right coronary artery originates from the anterior aortic sinus; the left from the left posterior sinus.
Both atrial appendages overlie their respective coronary arteries.
The coronary sinus drains into the right atrium just above the septal cusp of the tricuspid valve.

Skin conditions
79 E   Necrotising fasciitis
80 C   Pyogenic granuloma

Necrotising fasciitis is a condition which is caused either by streptococcal infection or, more commonly, by mixed aerobic and anaerobic bacteria. It may occur in leg ulcers in patients with vascular insufficiency (and usually diabetes), as well as the perineum and scrotum (Fournier's gangrene). The patient is pyrexial and ill and the affected part becomes anaesthetic and gangrenous. The treatment is debridement of all necrotic tissue and antibiotics (penicillin-based).

A pyogenic granuloma is a haemangioma, which commonly occurs on the lips and fingers. This should not be confused with pyoderma gangrenosum, which is an ulcerated nodule or pustule with a tender, blue necrotic edge associated with inflammatory bowel disease, myeloproliferative disorders and inflammatory arthritides.

Surface/radiological anatomy of thorax
81 I   3rd intercostal space
82 H   1st right costal cartilage
83 E   Manubriosternal joint
84 B   Left sternoclavicular joint
The hilum of each lung lies behind the 3rd and 4th costal cartilages and intervening 3rd intercostal space, on each side.

The commencement of the superior vena cava (confluence of the left and right brachiocephalic veins) lies behind the lower border of the right 1st costal cartilage.

The lower border of the arch of the aorta bisects the transthoracic plane, the surface marking of which is the sternal angle.

The thoracic duct drains into the left brachiocephalic vein at its commencement (confluence of the left subclavian and left internal jugular veins) – all these structures lie behind the left sternoclavicular joint.

Statistics
85 B   Paired *t*-test
86 A   Wilcoxon test
87 B   Paired *t*-test
88 D   Chi-squared test
For normally distributed data, a Student *t*-test may be used.

For non-parametric (non-Gaussian) data, the Mann–Whitney or Wilcoxon tests are used. The Mann–Whitney test is used to compare two unpaired groups. The Wilcoxon test is used to compare paired group data.

The chi-squared test is used to compare one group to a hypothetical value, or 2 unpaired groups, or 3 or more unmatched groups.

Acid–base balance/status
89 A   Pulmonary embolus
90 B   Acute renal failure
91 C   Pyloric stenosis
Pulmonary embolus (small or medium sized) usually produces a lowered PCO_2 due to increased respiratory rate.
A flail chest occurs when a segment of the chest wall has no bony continuity with the rest of the thoracic cage. This usually results from trauma associated with multiple rib fractures. Underlying lung injury and restricted chest wall movement will contribute to the patient's hypoxia.
Vomiting due to pyloric stenosis causes volume depletion and loss of H^+. The obstruction between the stomach and the duodenum also results in a decreased loss of HCO_3^-. A resultant metabolic alkalosis may occur if duodenal secretion continues and renal excretion of HCO_3^- is insufficient to correct for the plasma rise in HCO_3^-.

Drug classification
92 B   Alkylating agents
93 C   Corticosteroids
94 A   Antimetabolites
95 D   T-lymphocyte suppressor
96 A   Antimetabolites
Cyclophosphamide is activated by hepatic microsomal enzymes to produce several alkylating metabolites which cause crosslinking between DNA strands, thus preventing division of immunocompetent cells.
Azathioprine is a cytotoxic immunosuppressant that is metabolised to 6-mercaptopurine, within the liver. 6-Mercaptopurine is a purine antagonist reducing DNA and RNA synthesis in dividing cells.
Ciclosporin acts at an intracellular level to block the proliferation of cytotoxic T lymphocytes. The actions of corticosteroids include: reduction of macrophage activity and motility; reduction of circulating T-cell populations; and stabilisation of lysosomal and cellular membranes.

Cardiac physiology
97 B   HR, 50; SV, 140; PP, 50
98 F   HR, 200; SV, 35; PP, 50
99 C   HR, 100; SV, 70; PP, 70
Marathon runners have a high stroke volume and a resultant bradycardia. The resting cardiac output is approximately 6 litres/min.
Uncontrolled hyperthyroidism leads to a tachycardia and the most common arrhythmia is atrial fibrillation. It has no effect on the pulse pressure (PP). The cardiac output in these cases may be elevated.

Shock
100 A Fat embolism
101 B Thromboembolism
102 D Hypovolaemic shock
Fat embolism occurs in patients with multiple closed fractures, but has been reported in those with other skeletal trauma and burns. Fat embolism causes a pyrexia, tachycardia, shortness of breath, confusion and petechial haemorrhages, especially on the chest and conjunctivas.
Postoperative day 7 is the characteristic time for a thromboembolism.
Scenario 102 describes a leaking abdominal aortic aneurysm (AAA). Management involves immediate transfer to the operating theatre for laparotomy and emergency grafting of his AAA.

Dyspnoea
103 A Left tension pneumothorax
104 D Pulmonary embolus
105 C Left haemothorax
The patient in Scenario 103 has signs of a tension pneumothorax. No tracheal deviation is seen in cardiac tamponade.
In Scenario 104, the characteristic ECG changes seen in pulmonary embolus are: S_1, Q_3, T_3.
Dullness to percussion is indicative of fluid in the pleural space, hence the most appropriate answer for Scenario 105 is a haemothorax.

Peripheral nerve anatomy
106 C Axillary
107 I Thoracodorsal
108 G Suprascapular
109 D Radial
110 A Long thoracic
The axillary nerve passes just below the capsule of the shoulder joint and is damaged here in about 5% of shoulder dislocations. The nerve gives off the upper lateral cutaneous nerve of the arm, and also motor branches to the deltoid and teres minor muscles. The multipennate fibres of the deltoid muscle contract isometrically when carrying weights in the hand. The strap/unipennate anterior and posterior slips of the muscle are used for flexion and extension and, when contracting together, take over from the supraspinatus muscle to abduct the arm beyond the first 15°.
The thoracodorsal nerve is most vulnerable to damage during axillary surgery, when the arm is laterally rotated and abducted, because it bows into the axilla from the posterior wall. Paralysis of the latissimus dorsi

muscle is detected clinically if the patient is unable to fold the arm behind her back and reach up to the opposite scapula. The intercostobrachial (sensory) nerve is also vulnerable and occasionally has to be sacrificed.

The suprascapular nerve, which is motor to the supraspinatus and infraspinatus muscles, may be damaged by sudden tightening of a car seat-belt (upper trunk injuries of the brachial plexus and clavicular fractures may also occur). Paralysis of both muscles weakens the rotator cuff, destabilising the shoulder joint. In addition, the supraspinatus abducts the arm from 0° to 15°, and the infraspinatus is a powerful lateral rotator of the humerus. Since the teres minor muscle is unaffected (axillary nerve), some lateral rotation is preserved after suprascapular nerve damage.

Mid-shaft fractures of the humerus can damage the radial nerve in the spiral groove. The branches to the triceps are given off before the nerve enters the groove and so the muscle remains functional. All other extensors are paralysed, resulting in wrist drop. Although the cutaneous branches no longer conduct, compensatory overlap by adjacent nerves restricts the paraesthesia/anaesthesia to the dorsal skin over the first interosseous muscle. The brachioradialis reflex is mediated by the radial nerve and is thus lost. The triceps reflex remains intact for reasons explained above.

The long thoracic nerve usually escapes damage during axillary surgery because it is bound to the serratus anterior muscle by overlying fascia on the medial wall, posterior to the mid-axillary line. When the nerve is injured, however, part or all of the serratus anterior muscle is paralysed, resulting in a 'winged scapula'. There is loss of protraction and weakness of rotation of the scapula (the later movement is, however, preserved by the action of the intact trapezius muscle – spinal accessory nerve).

5-year survival rates of tumours
111 G **>95%**
112 F **90–95%**
113 B **5–10%**
114 A **<5%**
115 C **25%**
116 E **70–75%**

The overall 5-year survival rates of patients with carcinoid tumours depend on the site of the primary. Those of the vermiform appendix have an approximate 98% 5-year survival, those of the rectum an 85% survival and those of the small bowel have the lowest survival rate.

The 5-year survival rates associated with Dukes A, B, and C rectal cancers has improved from the easily memorised '90%, 60%, and 30%, respectively, to 92% (A), 71% (B), 40% (C1) and 26% (C2).

Oesophageal and pancreatic cancers have a grave prognosis, and surgical cure is uncommon.

Metastatic prostatic cancer can frequently be temporarily controlled by hormonal manipulation.

Nosocomial infection
117 D   Escherichia coli
118 E   Staphylococcus aureus (MRSA)
119 C   Pseudomonas aeruginosa
120 B   Legionella pneumophilia

An outbreak of *E. coli* is rare in hospital, but it necessitates closure of the ward to prevent spread of the infection. There are various forms of *E. coli*, but the one that most commonly causes problems is the enteropathogenic form.

Staph. aureus is coagulase-positive and is the most common organism grown from infected wounds. Up to 5% of the population are carriers of *Staph. aureus* in the nares.

The most common organism grown from urine cultures is *E. coli*, both in hospital and in the community. However, in hospital, especially with instrumentation and catheters, *P. aeruginosa* is the most common organism. Nosocomial UTI may also be caused by *Proteus* and *Klebsiella* spp.

L. pneumophilia occurs in individuals staying in hotels or hospitals where the cooling systems or shower facilities have been contaminated with the organism. In 50% of cases GI symptoms occur, the patient is tachypnoeic and has a dry cough which later becomes productive.

Haemorrhagic shock
121 D   Blood loss of 0.75 litres
122 C   Blood loss of 2.5 litres
123 B   Blood loss of 1.7 litres
124 C   Blood loss of 2.5 litres
125 E   Blood loss of 1 litre

The effects of blood loss can be monitored in terms of physiology, i.e. pulse rate/blood pressure/pulse pressure/respiratory rate/urine output/CNS or mental status. Shock is graded I to IV depending on the amount of blood loss, and each grade is associated with certain physiological changes. Class I shock occurs when up to 15% of the blood volume is lost (up to 750 ml in a 70-kg adult); class II between 15 and 30% (750–1500 ml); class III between 30 and 40% (1500–2000 ml), class IV >40% (2000 ml). The percentages are best remembered as the scoring system in a tennis match.

INDEX

Locators are in the form chapter number.question/answer number. Thus 3.34 refers to chapter 3 question 34 and P1.36 to practice paper 1 question 36.

Index

Index

Index

Index

PASTEST COURSES

PASTEST: the key to exam success, the key to your future.
PasTest is dedicated to helping doctors to pass their professional examinations. We have 25 years of specialist experience in medical education and over 3000 doctors attend our revision courses each year.

Experienced lecturers:
Many of our lecturers are also examiners and teach in a lively and interesting way in order to:
✔ reflect current trends in exams
✔ give plenty of mock exam practice
✔ provide essential advice on exam technique

Outstanding accelerated learning:
Our up-to-date and relevant course material includes MCQs, colour slides, X-rays, ECGs, EEGs, clinical cases, data interpretations, mock exams, vivas and extensive course notes which provide:
✔ hundreds of high quality questions with detailed answers and explanations
✔ succinct notes, diagrams and charts

Personal attention:
Active participation is encouraged on these courses, so in order to give personal tuition and to answer individual questions our course numbers are limited.
Book early to avoid disappointment.

Choice of courses:
PasTest has developed a wide range of high quality interactive courses in different cities around the UK to suit your individual needs.

What other candidates have said about our courses:
'Absolutely brilliant – I would not have passed without it! Thank you.'
Dr Charitha Rajapakse, London.
'Excellent, enjoyable, extremely hard work but worth every penny.'
Dr Helen Binns, Oxford.

For further details contact:
**PasTest Ltd, Egerton Court, Parkgate Estate
Knutsford, Cheshire WA16 8DX, UK.**

**Telephone: 01565 752000   Fax: 01565 650264
e-mail: courses@pastest.co.uk   web site: www.pastest.co.uk**

PASTEST REVISION BOOKS FOR MRCS

Look out for this book's sister title:

MRCS System Modules: The Complete Test
C L H Chan   1 901198 19 7
This book offers you:
- *5 chapters of MCQs and EMQs based on the System syllabus:*
  Locomotor; Vascular; Head, Neck, Endocrine and Paediatric;
  Abdomen; and Urinary System and Renal Transplantation
- *2 practice papers to challenge candidates knowledge*
- *includes answers and expanded teaching notes*

Also Available from PasTest for MRCS revision:

MRCS System Modules Essential Revision Notes
C Parchment Smith   1 901198 41 3
MRCS System Modules Practice Papers
C L H Chan   1 901198 46 4

MRCS Core Modules Essential Revision Notes: Second Edition
S Andrews   1 901198 71 5
MRCS Core Modules: Practice Papers
C L H Chan   1 901198 45 6

Viva Practice for MRCS
C L H Chan   1 901198 54 5
Surgical Short Cases for the MRCS Clinical Examination
C Parchment Smith   1 901198 44 8

To order any of the above titles, please contact PasTest on:

01565 752000

PasTest Ltd, FREEPOST, Knutsford, Cheshire, WA16 7BR
Fax: 01565 650264; E-mail: books@pastest.co.uk
Or order online at www.pastest.co.uk